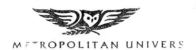

Intervention Planning
for Children with
Communication Disorders

Intervention Planning for Children with Communication Disorders

A Guide for Clinical Practicum and Professional Practice

Harriet B. Klein, Ph.D.
New York University

Nelson Moses, Ph.D.
Long Island University, Brooklyn Campus

Prentice Hall
Englewood Cliffs, New Jersey 07632

Library of Congress Cataloging-in-Publication Data

Klein, Harriet B.
   Intervention planning for children with communication disorders :
a guide for clinical practicum and professional practice / Harriet
B. Klein, Nelson Moses.
     p. cm.
   Includes bibliographical references and index.
   ISBN 0-13-138421-X
   1. Language disorders in children—Treatment. 2. Speech disorders
in children—Treatment. I. Moses, Nelson. II. Title.
   [DNLM: 1. Language Disorders—in infancy & childhood. 2. Language
Disorders—rehabilitation. 3. Speech Disorders—in infancy &
childhood. 4. Speech Disorders—rehabilitation. WL 340 K635i
1994]
RJ496.L35K54 1994
618.92'855—dc20   93-25685
DNLM/DLC   CIP
for Library of Congress

Acquisitions editor: Charlyce Jones-Owen
Editorial assistant: Nicole Signoretti
Editorial/production supervision and
   interior design: Bill Stavru
Cover design: Carol Ceraldi
Production coordinator: Mary Ann Gloriande
Page layout: Joh Lisa

© 1994 by Prentice-Hall, Inc.
A Paramount Communications Company
Englewood Cliffs, New Jersey 07632

Printed in the United States of America
10 9 8 7 6 5 4 3 2 1

ISBN 0-13-138421-X

Prentice-Hall International (UK) Limited, *London*
Prentice-Hall of Australia Pty. Limited, *Sydney*
Prentice-Hall Canada Inc., *Toronto*
Prentice-Hall Hispanoamericana, S.A., *Mexico*
Prentice-Hall of India Private Limited, *New Delhi*
Prentice-Hall of Japan, Inc., *Tokyo*
Simon & Schuster Asia Pte. Ltd., *Singapore*
Editora Prentice-Hall do Brasil, Ltda., *Rio de Janeiro*

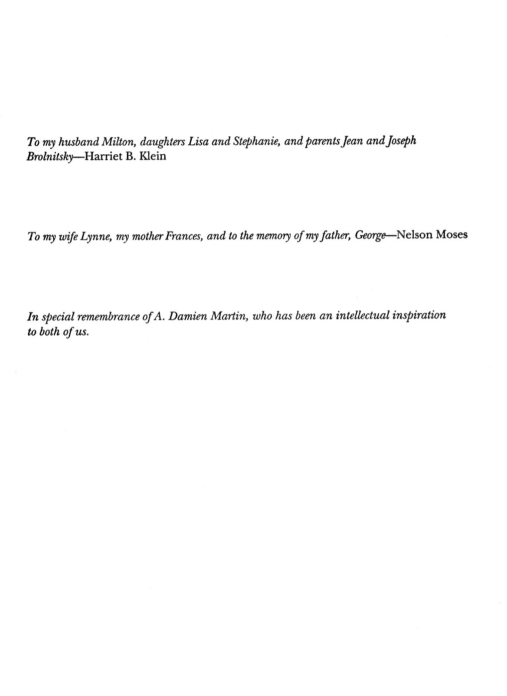

To my husband Milton, daughters Lisa and Stephanie, and parents Jean and Joseph Brolnitsky—Harriet B. Klein

To my wife Lynne, my mother Frances, and to the memory of my father, George—Nelson Moses

In special remembrance of A. Damien Martin, who has been an intellectual inspiration to both of us.

Contents

3

BASELINE DATA AND INTERVENTION PLANNING   67

4

PHASE 1 OF THE INTERVENTION PROCESS   94

5

PHASE 2 OF INTERVENTION:
THE IDENTIFICATION OF SHORT-TERM GOALS
AND DELINEATION OF PROCEDURAL CONTEXTS   129

6
PHASE 3: PLANNING SESSION GOALS AND PROCEDURES   176

7
COLLABORATION WITH ALLIED PROFESSIONALS AND FAMILIES   247

8
CLINICAL SUPERVISION FOR INTERVENTION PLANNING

Preface

In writing this book we were motivated primarily by a question frequently asked by our practicum students in speech-language pathology—"What should I do first?" Attempting to answer this question made us aware of its complexity. We realized that students needed to conceptualize an overall intervention plan before addressing the client's first session. We also realized that the conceptualization of this plan involved engaging students in a problem-solving, decision-making process that transcended any specific speech-language disorder. This intervention process may be described as "top down," moving from the development of long-term goals and procedures to specific session goals.

Clinical decision making involves the management of complex information. The current thinking is that speech and language disorders in children typically involve an interaction among semantic, syntactic, phonologic, and pragmatic components. In addition, impaired speech and language performance may rest on the relationship between linguistic and nonlinguistic behavioral systems (such as cognitive, sensorimotor, and psychosocial). Thus, it became clear to us that there was a need in the field of speech-language pathology for a book that deals with problem solving and decision making in intervention planning.

We believe that our book fulfills this need. It stresses the importance of understanding general principles underlying the formulation of an intervention plan. It includes information on how to make management decisions at three major points in the intervention process, regardless of speech-language disorder type and severity. This book addresses semantic, syntactic, and pragmatic components of language and behavioral systems interacting with language as factors maintaining speech and language performance. It is clinically and practically oriented, containing numerous examples of the application of these principles to specific speech-language disorder types and levels of severity.

Chapter One begins with an overview of what is involved in the intervention process. The three phases of intervention are introduced: Phase 1, developing long-term goals and a general procedural approach; Phase 2, identifying short-term goals and delineating procedural contexts; and Phase 3, developing session goals and procedures. Issues that must be addressed at each phase of the process are specified. These include clinician accountability, the clinician's conceptual framework, baseline data, factors maintaining communication disorders, and language-learning theories. Chapter Two provides a history of efforts to describe intervention, decision making, and problem solving in speech-language pathology. Chapter Three presents baseline data on four children who will be followed throughout the book. These children represent four different disorder types: language, phonology, fluency, and voice. Chapters Four, Five, and Six each deal with one of the three phases of the intervention process. These chapters are organized so that they deal with the kinds of decisions that need to be made regarding goal setting and procedure planning, and then they present case-study data from the four children with communication disorders.

Chapter Seven provides information on collaboration with allied professionals and families in intervention planning. This is in line with the present movement toward a collaborative model of service delivery in the field of speech-language pathology.

Chapter Eight provides a framework for practicum supervision aimed at helping students develop the complex skills involved in intervention planning. Attention to teaching clinical problem solving addresses the movement toward examining quality education at the university level.

The book is intended to be used as a primary text in upper-level undergraduate and graduate clinical practicum courses (i.e., clinical methods and materials, practicum seminars, and student teaching courses). It provides important and fundamental information for approaching the clinical situation for the first time; it may also be used as a guide throughout the clinician's professional career. The content of this book presumes some basic coursework in speech and language acquisition, communication disorders, and diagnostics.

Acknowledgments

We would like to thank the many people who have contributed to the writing of this book. We begin by acknowledging those who have inspired our work—our clients and students. Working with children who have communication disorders during the past two decades has laid the foundation for our model of intervention planning. Our students' questions and anxieties about clinical interactions were a major impetus for translating our experiences into a coherent model of intervention planning. For this we thank the students from New York University and Long Island University. We thank our students also for their questions, comments, and suggestions about earlier drafts and their patience with the many changes we made on the way to completion. Special thanks go to those students who contributed research time and editorial assistance—Goduwah Abdullah, Emma Cortese, Allison Garvin-Cullen, Livia Hoffman, Rosalie Schoeller, Heidi Volosov, Michele Waksbaum, and Aileen Zeits.

We also thank our colleagues who have contributed much time and expertise. We are especially grateful to Moya Andrews, who provided data on voice and was always available for consultation and editorial comments; Stephen A. Cavallo, who provided the foundation for the sensorimotor section of Chapter One; and David Shapiro, whose thoughts about fluency disorders and supervision are an integral part of this book. Other colleagues have given us immeasurable support by reading and commenting on earlier drafts of the manuscript. Special thanks to Elaine Altman, Anne Karpel-Freilich, and Cecile Spector. We also thank Brenda Lyons for her untiring efforts in the preparation of the displays that appear throughout the book. In addition, we appreciate the careful critiques of the reviewers for Prentice Hall: Peter LaPine, Michigan State University; Judith Harrington, University of Northern Iowa; and John Bernthal, University of Nebraska–Lincoln.

We are deeply grateful to our spouses and families for tolerating the diversion of so much time and energy spent in the creation of this book. Lastly, we would like to thank each other for a stimulating and enjoyable collaboration, and for the laughter along with serious writing efforts. Our collaboration represents an equal partnership, with the order of names merely alphabetical.

1

Introduction to the Intervention Process

THE INTERVENTION PROCESS AND WHY IT SEEMS SO COMPLEX

As speech-language pathologists, we have found that approaching a new client can be overwhelming, anxiety provoking, threatening, and sometimes even immobilizing. These feelings may relate to our awareness of the complexity of speech-language intervention planning. What makes intervention planning so complex? We must make important decisions—decisions about *what* to modify in a client's speech-language behavior and *how* to facilitate this modification. Although we have made decisions all our lives, making decisions in new areas, especially when they affect other people's lives, may be particularly disconcerting. Two primary factors contribute to the complexity of intervention planning: (a) the unpredictability inherent in clinical interactions and (b) the many interacting variables that can affect communication performance.

Unpredictability

The unpredictability inherent in clinical interactions is often the first factor that clinicians associate with intervention planning. Interactions among people are always somewhat unpredictable and potentially problematic—especially interactions among clinicians and their clients. We can never be absolutely certain how well a treatment plan will work. We can never know for sure whether a child will want to play with a particular toy, whether a child will follow instructions, or whether the child's parents will be pleased with our work. We must be prepared for "on-the-spot" decision making and problem solving. Intervention planning may be seen as an effort to anticipate factors that need to be addressed in session in order to minimize clinical problems and manage those that do arise.

Interacting Variables

A full awareness of the complexity of intervention planning may emerge as we try to anticipate factors that need to be addressed given a particular client. In this process, we begin to appreciate the complex nature of speech-language behavior. Speech-language behavior involves an interaction among semantics, syntax, phonology, and pragmatics. Each of these linguistic components affects the others during every communicative event. Consequently, any of these components may be implicated in any type of speech-language dysfunction. Furthermore, speech-language behavior is affected by the context in which an individual communicates as well as behavioral systems other than speech and language that the individual engages when communicating—that is, thinking processes (cognition), sensory and motor systems, and emotions. Thus, these variables, too, may be contributing to speech-language disorders. Figure 1–1 is a graphic illustration of the construct that speech-language performance is the product of a number of interactive linguistic factors influenced by nonlinguistic behavioral systems.

What Should I Do First?

Often our reaction to this complexity is to ask, "What should I do first?"—and then, not too much later, "What should I do next?" There must be a program guide somewhere that offers fail-safe therapeutic recipes!

FIGURE 1–1.   Interactions among linguistic and nonlinguistic behavioral systems.

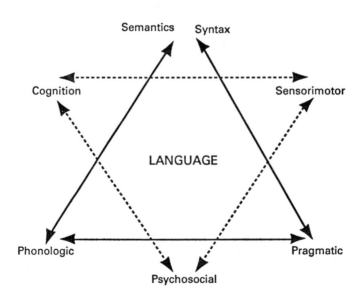

There is not. From our point of view, one can only arrive at answers to such questions at the *end* of a decision-making process in which consideration is given to all the variables that interact to maintain a speech-language disorder and to affect changes in communication performance. It is our intention to detail this process—which we term "intervention planning"—and its underlying principles. We believe this description will provide useful guidelines for the clinician making decisions about intervention goals and procedures.

DEFINING INTERVENTION GOALS AND PROCEDURES

The essence of intervention planning is the determination of intervention goals and the development of procedures. An intervention goal is a potential achievement by an individual with a speech-language dysfunction directed toward the improvement of speech-language performance. An intervention procedure represents the clinician's plan of action in which interactions and contexts are designed to facilitate the achievement of desired linguistic goals.

Intervention Goals

The definition of an intervention goal emphasizes, first, that a goal is a potential achievement by an individual with a speech-language dysfunction. This implies that goal setting follows a thorough assessment of speech-language functioning in which a problem is identified and evaluated. This also makes explicit that a goal represents the *client's* achievement, not the clinician's actions in therapy.

The definition of an intervention goal further indicates that the achievement of a goal will improve speech-language performance. That is to say, the clinician must be able to specify how achievement of the goal will advance the child in the direction of improved communication. Sometimes improved communication is achieved by modifying speech-language behaviors directly. In other instances, achieving the goal involves eliminating, modifying or compensating for factors contributing to the speech-language dysfunction. Eliminating or modifying indicates that the behavior or physical structure is remediable and that the emphasis in therapy is on facilitating better function (e.g., producing an /s/ without linguadental articulation). Compensating signifies that the problematic behavior or physical structure is not remediable and that the emphasis in therapy is on stimulating a different behavior or physical structure to assume its function (e.g., using the tongue blade rather than the tongue tip, or producing a medial /t/as [tʰ] if a flap is unattainable).

Intervention Procedures

The definition of an intervention procedure indicates, first, that it is a clinician's plan of action. This makes explicit that a procedure represents the clinician's actions, not the client's.

The definition also indicates that intervention procedures represent plans about how best to facilitate the achievement of goals. These plans include the clinician's consideration of (a) factors maintaining the disorder, which need to be eliminated, modified, or compensated for, and (b) contexts (i.e., conditions) presumed to be optimum for learning, including how the clinician will encourage the child to express the target behavior, what materials will be available for the client, and how the clinician will respond to the client's behavior.

In Box 1–1 we highlight the essential characteristics of intervention goals and procedures. These characteristics typify intervention goals and procedures in general. In intervention planning, however, we write different types of goals and procedures—traditionally, long-term, short-term, and session. It is our view that developing these different types of goals and procedures involves three phases of decision making. Next we will provide a brief introduction to these three phases of intervention planning and to the goals and procedures that are the products of decisions made at each phase.

The Three Phases of Intervention Planning

The first phase of intervention planning involves setting long-term goals, which are the ultimate expectations for change in the client. The first phase also involves envisioning a procedural approach. A procedural approach represents an initial set of hypotheses about (a) maintaining factors that will need to be addressed in creating optimal contexts for language learning and (b) principles derived from language-learning theories that will guide clinical interactions.

BOX 1–1. ESSENTIAL CHARACTERISTICS OF SPEECH-LANGUAGE INTERVENTION GOALS AND PROCEDURES

Intervention goals are:
1. Clients' expected actions
2. Directed toward the accomplishment of efficient speech-language performance
3. Directed toward the modification of or compensation for factors contributing to a speech-language dysfunction

Intervention procedures are:
1. Clinician's plans about how to best facilitate the achievement of goals
2. Plans about optimum therapy contexts and interactions
3. Clinician's actions during a therapy session

The second phase involves the prioritization of short-term goals and the delineation of a procedural context. Short-term goals are intermediate speech-language achievements expected of a child on the path toward reaching the long-term goal. The duration for achieving a short-term goal is generally regulated by the clinical facility (frequently, this duration is a semester). The procedural context represents an initial plan about types of materials and interactions that would best facilitate language learning. These materials and interactions should be consistent with the principles of language learning and maintaining factors identified during the first planning phase.

The third phase addresses session goals and procedures. This includes the determination of those steps (behavioral objectives) necessary to achieve each short-term goal and the specific materials and interactions for a particular session. The third phase also entails the modification of session goals and procedures during and after an actual therapy session. Box 1–2 summarizes the three phases of intervention planning. We will examine each phase in depth in Chapters 4, 5, and 6.

Additional Considerations Regarding Goals and Procedures

The basic feature of an intervention goal is that it represents the *client's* achievement in therapy. The basic feature of an intervention procedure is that it is a statement about the *clinician's* actions. These essential aspects of the definitions presented here may cause some confusion for clinicians because of the different perspectives from which therapy goals and procedures may be

---

BOX 1–2.   THREE PHASES OF INTERVENTION PLANNING

Phase I involves decisions about:
- The client's ultimate linguistic achievements (long-term goals)
- The maintaining factors to be modified or compensated for in order to facilitate speech-language development
- The principles from learning theories that will guide clinical interactions

Phase II involves decisions about:
- The prioritization of short-term goals expected to lead to the achievement of long-term goals
- The types of materials and interactions that will facilitate the achievement of short-term goals

Phase III involves decisions about:
- The steps within a series of behavioral objectives leading to the accomplishment of short-term goals
- The specific session materials and interactions

viewed. Confusion can emanate from (a) the tendency of some clinicians to refer to their own actions as intervention goals rather than procedures, (b) the possibility that clinicians may be working on two types of goals during intervention planning (goals for the client and professional performance goals for themselves), and (c) the possibility that some clinicians may associate the term *procedure* with certain client actions in therapy.

Distinguishing Intervention Goals from Procedures.   It is notable that clinicians frequently refer to their own actions as goals for the client. This is seen in the following attempt at a goal statement: "To *teach* Mary to identify the difference between a rough and smooth voice production." *Teaching* is the *clinician's* job. The goal for the *child* is "to identify rough and smooth voice qualities." Consequently, the goal statement should refer only to those behaviors expected of the child. The procedure statement will refer to the clinician's teaching behavior. It is important that clinicians make this distinction so that the *client's* performance may be targeted and evaluated appropriately during the session.

Distinguishing Intervention Goals from Professional Goals.   Confusion about the use of the term *goal* in intervention planning may also stem from objectives of supervision. Clinicians, with their supervisors, may wish to set professional goals for themselves—such as "to write an effective intervention plan" or "to develop professional expertise as a speech-language clinician." (Anderson, 1988; Dowling, 1992). Although these are important objectives from the standpoint of supervision, it is necessary to recognize at the outset that our primary frame of reference in this book is the derivation of intervention goals and procedures for *children with communication disorders*. We devote Chapter 8 to supervision and to the derivation of professional goals and procedures for clinicians relevant to the achievement of expertise in intervention planning.

Distinguishing Procedures from Goals.   Although we indicated that intervention procedures represent the clinician's actions in therapy, some clinicians may associate the term *procedure* with certain client actions in therapy. For example, suppose that in the voice case cited above the clinician had planned a game involving two identical puppets with different voices. The child would refer to the puppet with the rough voice as "ruffy" and the puppet with the smooth voice as "smoothy." One might wish to state that the child's talking to the puppets represents a procedure, since playing with puppets does not seem to be as critical for achieving long-term objectives as distinguishing between two vocal qualities. Discriminating vocal qualities may appear to be the true objective (i.e., goal) of the therapy session. Descriptions of both aspects of the child's behavior belong in the goal statement, however, because each description conveys specific information relevant to remediation of the presenting problem. Thus, the goal statement reads: "Mary will state 'I hear ruffy' in response to a puppet talking with a harsh voice and 'I hear smoothy' in response to a puppet speaking with an efficient voice." In such goal statements, the first part targets the child's speech-language production; the second part relates to the conditions under which the production is expected to occur (e.g., it is presumed to be easier and more motivating for the child to identify vocal qualities in a play context than in a direct instructional interaction with an adult). We will elaborate on these aspects of goal setting in the chapters that follow.

CATEGORIES OF KNOWLEDGE THAT GUIDE INTERVENTION PLANNING

Three categories of knowledge are basic to intervention planning. These are the clinician's knowledge of (a) the components of speech and language, (b) nonlinguistic and linguistic factors that maintain communication disorders, and (c) principles of learning theories that specify processes that underlie the learning of new behaviors. The clinician's knowledge of these areas will guide the derivation of goals and procedures. Knowledge of behaviors that constitute speech and language is the basis for determining speech-language structures targeted for change. Knowledge of factors affecting speech-language performance will guide the clinician in both goal and procedure planning. Knowledge of principles from learning theories is used primarily in the creation of intervention procedures. In the remainder of this chapter we will present some foundational information in the three areas of knowledge that the clinician may find useful in intervention planning.

The Nature of Speech and Language: Interacting Components

Regardless of a child's presenting communication problem, one body of knowledge that will guide intervention planning concerns the behaviors that constitute speech and language. It is our view that Lahey's (1988) definition of language as *a code for representing ideas about the world through a conventional system of arbitrary signals for communication* best details those behaviors and how they interact. Thus, we have adopted Lahey's definition as the most useful way to think about speech and language for intervention planning (see also the original statement of this definition in Bloom & Lahey, 1978.)

Content, Form, and Use. Lahey's definition refers to three *interacting* components of language: ideas, or *content;* a conventional system of arbitrary signals, or *form;* and communication, or *use.* Language content is "what individuals talk about or understand in messages" (Lahey, 1988, p. 1). This component is frequently termed *semantics* (e.g., Newhoff & Leonard, 1983). Language form refers to sounds, how they combine to form words, and how words combine to create more complex units (Bloom & Lahey, 1978). Language form includes phonology, morphology, syntax, and the suprasegmental features of prosody. Language use "has to do with the reasons why individuals speak...the ways in which individuals construct conversations, and in doing so use different forms of messages" (Lahey, 1988, pp. 1–2). This area is typically referred to as *pragmatics* (Lund & Duchan, 1988). Since language comprises three interacting components, formulating a management plan necessitates a consideration of (a) the component(s) of language which require(s) modification and (b) the potential effects of the interacting components.

We would like to emphasize that Lahey's definition of language is applicable to intervention planning across disorder categories. The definition subsumes the range of speech-language behaviors that may be targeted in intervention goals. Although it may not be immediately obvious, voice and fluency may be viewed as aspects of language form. Their function is to support the realization of phonology, morphology, and syntax. Furthermore, the definition underscores the interaction among all components of speech and language in communication disorders. We will examine the implications of these interactions as we illustrate intervention planning across disorder categories throughout this book. Figure 1–2 highlights knowledge about components of language that guides intervention planning.

FIGURE 1–2.   Knowledge that guides intervention planning: Components of language.

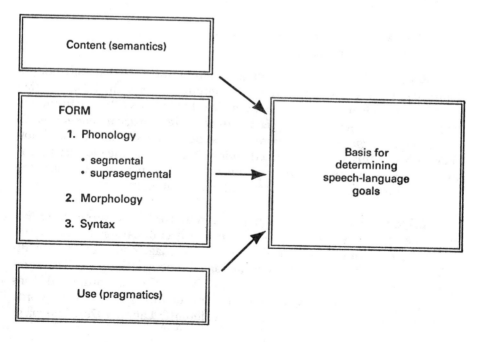

Maintaining Factors

In thinking about changing speech and language behavior we must also be knowledgeable of the behavioral systems that affect our client's communication performance. We identify four such systems: cognitive, sensorimotor, psychosocial, and the linguistic system, itself. Impaired functioning of any of the systems can contribute to the maintenance of any speech-language disorder. Thus, we anticipate that changes in each system will facilitate desired changes in speech-language behavior. Each system should be evaluated in the course of goal setting and procedural planning.

The specification of factors maintaining a speech-language disorder will provide information useful for both goal setting and procedural planning at each phase of the intervention process. The way in which information about maintaining factors is used in goal setting or procedural planning will change across phases. We will present an overview of the maintaining factors next. In subsequent chapters, we will show how knowledge of these factors contributes to goal setting and procedural planning at each phase of the intervention process.

Cognition. When we encounter a child with a communication disorder who is not exhibiting an expected cognitive achievement, it raises the possibility that the cognitive domain is maintaining the disorder. Cognition involves reasoning, problem-solving skills, mental representation, and awareness (e.g., Case, 1985; Fischer, 1980; Karmiloff-Smith, 1986a; Piaget, 1971). The major emphasis in the literature is on the relationship between cognition and semantics and syntax; less attention is given to potential relationships between cognition and other aspects of communication, such as voice and fluency. It will be necessary, however, to address cognitive factors in planning for all types of communication disorders.

An overview of proposed cognition–speech-language relations. It is generally agreed that cognition supports speech and language, although the nature of this relationship is controversial (Rice, 1983; Rice & Kemper, 1984; Lahey, 1990). Rice and Kemper (1984) have summarized the various hypotheses regarding the relationship between cognition and language. These have focused on how cognitive skills that are products of specific stages of cognitive development, such as the ability to find displaced objects at the end of the sensorimotor stage, relate to speech-language attainments, such as the use of single words (e.g., Gopnik, 1984; Tomasello & Farrar, 1984). These hypotheses have ranged from the position that cognitive structures are a basis for speech-language functioning to the position that certain language structures (especially syntactic structures) are independent of precursory or parallel cognitive structures. (Much of the literature involved in this controversy centered on attempts to correlate the onset of early words and word combinations with Piaget's Sensorimotor Stages 5 and 6; e.g., Gopnik, 1984; Tomasello & Farrar, 1984.)

Although there is much lack of agreement about the relationship between cognition and language, we pursue it as an important potential maintaining factor. The disagreements that have been cited concern "how much of early speech-language acquisition is accounted for by cognition" (Rice & Kemper, 1984, p.13) and how best to measure the relationship between these two domains (Lahey, 1990). The existence of a relationship between language and cognition is not at issue.

The existence of this relationship is based on general acceptance of two related notions: (a) cognitive skills (such as searching, comparing, reflecting, conserving) contribute to the representation of ideas about the world (Piaget, 1954; Piaget & Garcia, 1991) and (b) the representation of ideas about the world is an essential function of language (e.g., Bloom & Lahey, 1978; Lahey, 1988). There is a third idea that can have an impact upon intervention planning as well—that thinking about speech and language itself (i.e., "metalinguistic" reasoning) contributes to the development of speech and language (Karmiloff-Smith, 1979, 1986a).

Researchers have specified those cognitive skills that contribute to the development of ideas about the world and thus influence the evolution of language content. For example, Lahey describes how searching for objects, causing objects to disappear, and acting on different objects contribute to the emergence of the earliest content categories (i.e., existence, nonexistence, recurrence, action, locative action). Some researchers have related later cognitive achievements, such as classifying, ordering, and conserving, to later emerging language content, such as causal, temporal, comparative (Forman & Hill, 1984; Miller, 1984; Moses, Klein, & Altman, 1990). Still others view thinking about speech and language itself (i.e., metalinguistic knowledge) as central to the learning of subtle aspects of language content, form, and use (e.g., Karmiloff-Smith, 1979, 1986a; Osherson & Lasnik, 1990).

Because of our focus on the identification of maintaining factors for intervention planning, our concern is with those cognitive skills that can influence the development of speech and language. Based on the available literature, we identify a number of cognitive skills that deserve attention in intervention planning. Box 1–3 describes these cognitive activities and their likely effects on speech and language.

Implications for intervention planning. The information in Box 1-3 is organized with reference to stages of language development from the prelinguistic period through the production of complex sentences. Each period of linguistic development is associated with salient cognitive skills. We also suggest the way in which these skills are reflected in the acquisition of specific aspects of speech and language.

Knowledge of the cognitive skills presumed to be related to speech-language attainments is essential information for planning the goals and procedures of intervention. During the evaluation process we gather information about a child's cognitive functioning to determine whether cognition is

BOX 1–3.   COGNITIVE ACHIEVEMENTS RELATED TO LINGUISTIC PERFORMANCE

Stage of Linguistic Performance	*Associated Cognitive Skills*	*Effect of Cognitive Skill on Speech and Language*
Prelinguistic[a]	Circular reactions (the child notices his or her own behavior and repeats it)	Relates to reduplicative and variegated babbling
	Imitation of caregiver's production of sounds and gestures already generated by the child	Facilitates caregiver-child communication
		Supports the development of intentional sound production and gestures, turn taking, and other preconversational devices
	Intentional means-end behavior (intentionally setting a goal, such as getting daddy to repeat a favorite behavior, and using a familiar action, such as smiling to achieve a goal)	Relates to intentional communicative functions: instrumental, regulatory, interactional, personal, heuristic
Single words through the beginning of syntax (two- to three-word combinations)[b]	Object constancy (knowing that objects exist, even when displaced)	Provides a foundation for naming objects, commenting on their absence or recurrence
		Involves reflecting on objects, actions, and relationships
	Creation of new means not already in the child's repertoire to achieve goals and solve problems (e.g., using a chair to retrieve a box of cereal from the top of the refrigerator)	Provides a framework and reasons for talking about objects, actions, and locations

(continued)

BOX 1–3 *(continued)*

	Single scheme and combinatorial pretend play (combining and separating objects and representing objects and their functions with toys)	Exercises skills that may be used in representing objects and actions with words
	Imitation of novel gestural and vocal movements not already in the child's repertoire	Promotes the representation of movement patterns
		Provides a basis for articulating phonologic units
Two- to three-word combinations through complex utterances[c]	Multischeme pretend play and script play (planning pretend activities involving a series of actions and pretending at familiar activities, such as going to a restaurant)	Relates to talking about more complex ideas and producing narratives
	Early part-whole relations, classifications, and seriations requiring the manipulation of objects (involves distinguishing parts from the whole, grouping and regrouping objects according to attributes, and ordering objects according to a specific dimension [e.g., size])	Provides a foundation for talking about attributes, quantity, possession, and feeling
		May support linguistic comparatives and causal utterances that focus on observable causes
	Later, complex part-whole relations, classifications, and seriations in which various possible combinations of wholes and parts can be envisioned without the presence of concrete objects	Facilitates the use of language for planning and problem solving.
		May support complex causal utterances
	Awareness of speech and language as comprising units that may be manipulated (i.e., sounds, syllables)	Supports the ability to talk about sounds, voice quality, rate, language use, word and sentence meaning, and syntax (metalinguistic knowledge)

(continued)

BOX 1–3 *(continued)*

Sources:

a. Bates, Benigni, Bretherton, Camaioni, Volterra, 1979; Greenfield & Smith 1976; Olswang & Carpenter, 1982a; Piaget, 1954; Uzgiris & Hunt, 1978.

b. Gopnik, 1984; Gopnik & Meltzoff, 1987; McCune-Nicolich, 1981; Olswang & Carpenter, 1982b; Piaget, 1962; Sinclair, 1970; Tomasello & Farrar, 1984; Werner & Kaplan, 1964; Westby, 1980.

c. Gallagher & Reid, 1984; Johnson, 1985; Kamhi, Lee, & Nelson, 1985; Kamii, 1985; Karmiloff-Smith, 1979, 1986a; Klein, Lederer, & Cortese, 1991; McCune-Nicolich, 1981; Moses, Klein, & Altman, 1990; Nelson, 1986; Nesdale, Herriman, & Tunmer, 1984; Piaget & Inhelder, 1969; Wansart, 1990.

---

proceeding normally. Early goals and procedures will be influenced by knowledge of a cognitive impairment. Goals may be directed to establishing the cognitive skills associated with a particular linguistic attainment. For example, a goal for a child who has not begun to produce single words might involve the retrieval of hidden objects. As noted in Box 1–3, knowing that objects exist even when displaced provides a foundation for naming objects. On the procedural side, knowing that object constancy needs to be attained gives us direction in selecting materials and games during a treatment session. Another example comes from the last linguistic period in Box 1–3. At this point in linguistic development the corresponding cognitive attainment is a child's ability to manipulate aspects of speech and language as though they were objects. This cognitive skill manifests itself, for example, in the metalinguistic ability to play with or talk about sounds, syllables, and words (e.g., Kamhi, Lee, & Nelson, 1985; Klein, Lederer, & Cortese, 1991; Magnusson, 1991) or to change vocal registers (Bloom & Lahey, 1978). This relationship between cognition and language may be applied to children with voice, fluency, or articulation disorders. Children with such problems may need to describe aspects of their voice quality, dysfluencies, or articulatory movements as part of the treatment process. How knowledge of relationships between cognition and language guides intervention planning is exemplified throughout the book.

Alternate views of cognition. The cognitive skills cited in Box 1–3 reflect a developmental orientation to cognition and the cognition-language interaction. It has been popular in the field of speech-language pathology to focus on cognitive structures and processes that are thought to be involved in the processing of information, such as attention, sequencing, short-term memory (retrieval, recall, strategy, organization), and long-term memory (retrieval, recall). We view these structures and processes as interactive with and dependent on the developmental cognitive and linguistic achievements summarized in Box 1–3. Thus, we give these factors secondary consideration in intervention planning. We will develop this idea in the section on information processing in Chapter 2 and in subsequent chapters.

Sensorimotor. How a child receives information from the environment, moves, and senses his or her own movement constitutes a second behavioral system—the sensorimotor system—that can maintain a speech-language disorder. As such, the clinician's knowledge of the contribution of the sensorimotor system to speech-language functioning is central to competent intervention planning.

Due to our emphasis on intervention planning for children with communication disorders, we are concerned with *four areas of sensory processing, movement, and perception:* (a) sensorimotor functioning of the peripheral speech mechanism, which is central to speech-sound production (i.e., articulation); (b) speech-related perception; (c) maintenance and movement of the body through space (this aspect of sensorimotor functioning supports learning through play and the activity of the peripheral speech mechanism); and (d) the processing of feedback (the interaction between the processing of sensory information and motor control).

Peripheral speech mechanism. In assessing the possible contribution of the peripheral speech mechanism to normal speech-language production, it is useful for the clinician to be aware of developmental achievements in the structure and function of this mechanism and their corresponding impact on speech and language production. These sensorimotor achievements are considered when planning intervention for communication disorders involving articulation, voice, and fluency. If we observe a structural anomaly or suspect a deviation in sensorimotor functioning, our intervention planning will be directed toward modifying or compensating for the condition. With intervention planning in mind, we will next highlight the characteristics of the peripheral speech mechanism and their relation to speech-language production from infancy to puberty. This presentation will be organized according to Ingram's (1976) stages of phonological development.

1. An overview of development. The prelinguistic period spans the time from birth to twelve months. Many changes take place in the child's oral-motor, laryngeal, and respiratory structures during this period of time. In the newborn, the tongue sits completely within the oral cavity. The velum and larynx are closely approximated, separating the oral cavity from the airway (which permits infants to swallow and breathe at the same time). Due to the high vertical position of the larynx in the neck, the size of the newborn's pharyngeal cavity is very small (Crelin, 1973; Laitman & Crelin, 1976). Consequently, infants—unlike adults—sound nasal (Kent & Murray, 1982). Figure 1–3 illustrates differences between the adult and infant vocal tracts.

Structural changes during the first year of life include the separation of the larynx and nasopharynx and growth of the mandible down and forward. In addition, the larynx begins a gradual descent to its mature position (Crelin,

Adult

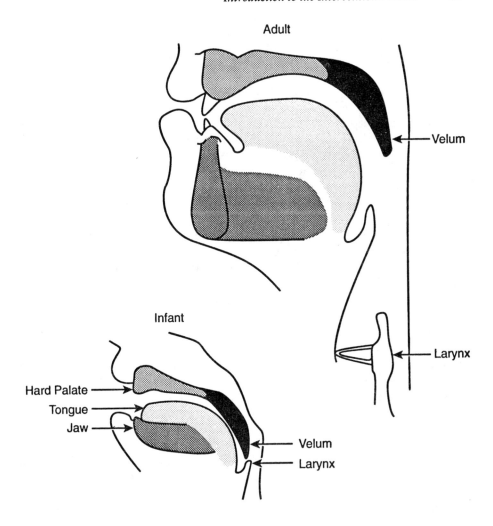

Infant

Hard Palate

Tongue

Jaw

Velum

Larynx

Velum

Larynx

FIGURE 1–3.   Anatomical differences between vocal tracts of adults and infants. Modified from Kent, R.D., and Murray, A.D. (1982). *JASA, 72,* 353–365.

1976; Kahane, 1983; Laitman & Crelin, 1976). There are also neuromuscular changes, which are reflected in increased tongue and lip mobility and greater control of breathing and vocalization (Netsell, 1980; Netsell & Daniel, 1979). These improvements in muscle function in turn contribute to the emergence of vowel- and consonant-like sounds, beginnings of CV segments and babbling sequences, and changes in resonation (e.g., decrease in nasality) and intonation patterns (e.g., Oller, 1980; Stark, 1980).

The period of the simple morpheme describes changes that occur from approximately one to three years of age. During this period, the larynx begins a descent to its mature physiologic position. The descent of the larynx (and resulting disengagement of the velum and epiglottis) creates a larger pharyngeal cavity and reduces infantile nasal resonance. Structurally, there is also a lowering of the tongue to form the anterior wall of the upper pharynx (Crelin, 1976; Kahane, 1983; Laitman & Crelin, 1976). During this period of time, there is further refinement and coordination of articulatory, laryngeal, and respiratory movements (although some variability in coordination is still evident, e.g., Netsell, 1980). These structural and neuromuscular changes are associated with an increase in the variety of consonant-vowel combinations and the beginning of the elimination of many phonological processes. There are greater distinctions between voiced and unvoiced plosives as a consequence of changes in voice onset time distribution from shorter to longer durations.

The next two periods comprise the completion of the phonetic inventory (four to seven years), and morphophonemic development (eight to twelve years). During these time periods the tongue and larynx complete their descent and the vocal tract assumes an adult contour (Hirano, Kurita, & Nakashima, 1981; Kahane, 1983; Laitman & Crelin, 1976). Motor control continues to increase in precision (Kent, 1980, 1992). Remaining phonological processes are eliminated and morphophonemic patterns and stress contrasts in noun-verb pairs are acquired. (e.g., Ingram, 1976). Box 1–4 presents a developmental schedule of sensorimotor achievements related to linguistic performance.

2. Implications for intervention planning. The information contained in Box 1–4 is presented as a resource for goal setting and procedure planning across speech-language disorders. Knowledge of the structural integrity of a child's peripheral speech mechanism and awareness of developmental relations between structure and function in speech production are essential in making decisions about how to treat children with communication disorders. This knowledge may be used in the formulation of goals and procedures directed toward modifying sensorimotor functions associated with a desired linguistic attainment.

Consider, for example, a five-year-old child with a harsh voice and a number of unsuppressed phonological processes—these include stopping, final consonant deletion, liquid simplification, and cluster reduction. The child appears to manifest a larynx that is not appropriately descended and some restriction in the range and differentiation of oral motor actions that might normally be expected of a five-year-old (exhibits problems imitating speech sounds, problems with oral motor activity, and drools when engaged in fine motor activity). Additionally, there appears to be tension in the chest and neck area. The speech-language pathologist, in collaboration with an occupational or physical therapist, may wish to target the differentiation and refinement of oral-motor movements (through a program involving positioning and movement activities). This would be an effort to alleviate problems that may be maintaining impairments in voice and articulation.

BOX 1-4   SENSORIMOTOR ACHIEVEMENTS RELATED TO LINGUISTIC PERFORMANCE

Stage of Linguistic Performance	Associated Anatomic and Physiologic Achievement	Prespeech-Speech Behaviors
Prelinguistic[a] Birth–1 month	Larynx and nasopharynx closely approximated. Respiration primarily nasal. Tongue (at rest) entirely within the oral cavity	Cry-discomfort and vegetative vocalizations predominate. Vocalizations nasalized, vowel-like, of short duration
2–4 months	Increased tongue and lip mobility (3–5 mos.). Considerable development of nerve myelinization (3–6 mos.). Ventilatory system achieves upright posture. Oral tidal respiration develops (3–5 mos.). Greater independence of mandible from tongue	Decrease in crying after 12 weeks. Vowel-like sounds predominate but consonant-like sounds (Cs) emerge (n, b, d, g, t, k, w, l, j). Beginning CV segments (/gu/). Glottal Cs appear (e.g., h, ?)
4–6 months	Separation of larynx and nasopharynx and improved velar functioning. Development of the ability to breathe orally. Increased duration of exhalation. Increased control of laryngeal and articulatory mechanisms	Expansion of phonetic repertoire. Increased number of C segments. Greater variety of V segments. Increased CV syllable production. Increased variation in intonation. Emergence of voiced-voiceless and nasal–non-nasal contrasts (6 mos.)
6–10 months	Breathing patterns more adult-like (7 mos.). Considerable growth of mandible down and forward. Significant lowering of the larynx. Upper airway assumes more mature dimensions. Integration of many infantile reflexes into CNS	Reduplicative babbling with CV, CVC constructions. Consistent variation of intonational patterns. Early nonreduplicative CV syllables. Duration of exhalation increases from 2 to 4 syllables per breath
10–12 months	Completion of myelinization of major neural pathways. Stabilization of musculoskeletal functions. Walking may begin	Increase in variety of CV, CVC combinations. Approximation of single word utterances

(continued)

BOX 1–4 *(continued)*

Simple morpheme: single words through simple sentences[b]

1–3 years	Refinement of articulatory movements	Speech movements slower and more variable than adults'
	Gradual descent of tongue to form the anterior wall of the upper pharynx	Many phonological processes are eliminated (unstressed syllable deletion, final consonant deletion, consonant assimilation, reduplication, velar fronting, diminutization, prevocalic voicing)
	Continued descent of larynx	
	Variability in timing of laryngeal and supralaryngeal adjustments during speech acts (affecting fundamental frequency, vocal tract posturing, and timing of laryngeal and supralaryngeal articulatory adjustments)	Voice onset time distribution begins to change from shorter to longer durations
		Continued variability in fundamental frequency

Completion of phonetic inventory[c]

4–7 years	Tongue completes descent	Most complex articulatory gestures acquired and combination of complex gestures mastered
	Increased precision of motor control	
	Descent of the larynx completed	Remaining phonological processes eliminated (cluster reduction, epenthesis, gliding, vocalization, stopping, depalatalization, final devoicing)
		Continued improvement in producing longer words and sentences

Morphophonemic development

8–12 years	Vocal tract approximates an adult contour	Acquisition of morphophonemic patterns (vowel alterations),
	Mature structures achieved after puberty	Production of stress contrasts (e.g., noun-verb pairs)

Sources:

a. Kahane, 1983; Kent, 1976; Kent, 1992; Kent & Bauer, 1985; Kent & Murray, 1982; Laitman & Crelin, 1976; Locke, 1983; Oller, 1980; Proctor, 1989; Stark, 1978, 1980; Stoel-Gammon & Dunn, 1985.

b. Bernthal & Bankson, 1988; Grunwell, 1981; Kahane, 1983; Kent, 1976, 1992; Ingram, 1974; Klein, 1981a, 1981b; Stoel-Gammon & Dunn, 1985.

c. Klein, Lederer, & Cortese, 1991; Nesdale, Herriman, & Tunmer, 1984.

Based on a diagnosis that a sensorimotor deficit is irremediable, a clinician may decide to help a child compensate for the damage rather than modify the damaged structure. An example would be the goal of producing the phoneme /t/ by positioning the tongue on the teeth (as opposed to the alveolar ridge) in the case of a child with a macroglossia (enlarged tongue). We will utilize information from Box 1–4 in developing management plans for specific children in Chapters 4, 5, and 6.

Speech-related perception. The prior section on sensorimotor development has focused solely on speech-sound *production*. We attempted to associate changes in anatomic and physiologic achievements with changes in prespeech and speech production skills. We believe that such information about sensorimotor achievements will be helpful in intervention planning by highlighting potential physiological impairments maintaining a speech-language disorder.

Developing parallel to and interacting with the production of sounds is the *perception* of sounds (Vihman, 1988) and other stimuli relevant to communication—for example, vocal qualities and facial expressions (Benner, 1992; Stern, 1985). Perception involves the ability to distinguish among stimuli. Speech-language clinicians typically address perceptual abilities in children with communication disorders. Children are taught to attend to, compare, and distinguish among stimuli such as facial features, vocal qualities, and speech sounds. Thus, the clinician's awareness of perception as a potential factor maintaining a communication disorder will be useful. For intervention planning, it is helpful to consider the child's perceptual abilities prior to the onset of language and during the language-acquisition period.

1. Prelinguistic development. We now know that infants within the first months of life can perceive contrasts among a variety of specific stimuli relevant to speech and language. They have been shown to discriminate stimuli along the lines of familiar versus nonfamiliar voices (Friedlander, 1970); facial features, especially eyes (Stern, 1985); prosody (Kaplan, 1970); and consonant-like stimuli (see Eimas, 1985, and Werker & Pegg, 1992, for reviews of pertinent research). We infer this from their reactions to novel stimuli—for example, facial excitement, diffuse tension or relaxation, and other, less-observable reactions, such as heart-rate and sucking changes (Eimas, 1985).

Researchers using specially designed research paradigms have shown that infants perceptually differentiate sounds contrasting in voice onset time (e.g., p, b), place of articulation (e.g., labial, dental, velar), and manner of articulation (e.g., stops versus nasals or glides). It should be noted, however, that the infant's ability to make distinctions does not extend to all possible contrasts. For example, Eilers (1980) showed that perception for speech sounds such as fricatives develops later. These findings regarding early perceptual behavior suggest that perceptual capacities are innate and may underlie linguistic comprehension and expression (Eimas, 1985; Ingram, 1989a).

This information on perception highlights the child's ability to respond differentially to contrasting stimuli even before the onset of language. Thus, in our work with infants and children—especially those with severe developmental disabilities—we will target responses to a variety of contrasting stimuli. Goals aimed at increasing the range of stimuli to which a child might respond can be developed on the basis of the child's demonstrated perceptual abilities. For example, a child with Down's Syndrome has demonstrated a response to sounds such as a toy train's "choo choo." The clinician noticing this perceptual ability might set a goal for the child to direct its gaze to the clinician's face when the clinician mimics the sound of the train.

2. *Linguistic development.* The infants' perceptual distinctions described above did not involve the processing of language. For example, the infants were not required to differentiate sounds with reference to differences in meaning. After the onset of language, children perceive contrasts among stimuli that have linguistic significance. Information about perception after the onset of language that has most influenced speech-language pathology has come from research on phoneme perception. This research has focused on the recognition of speech-sound contrasts and the relation of this ability to speech-sound production.

Over the past two decades, a number of studies were directed toward the identification of a developmental hierarchy in the acquisition of phoneme contrast *in words* (for reviews of this material see Ingram, 1989a; Vihman, 1988). In general, these studies of early linguistic speech perception have indicated that, although children between one and three can differentiate a variety of speech-sound contrasts, no universal hierarchy can be established.

Vihman (1988) summarized a number of studies undertaken by her and others that attempted to explore the relationship between perception and production. These studies examined the relationship between the presumed ease of perception of phoneme contrasts and the ability to produce these same phonemes. The researchers were interested in finding out whether production errors were necessarily related to errors in perception. Although in some cases they were (e.g., /Θ/ versus /f/), it is interesting that some production errors showed no evident relation to perception. That is, children were able to perceive sound contrasts that they could not produce (e.g., /k/ versus /kʰ/). It may be that some errors are based more on motor than perceptual skills.

Unfortunately, the research to date on speech-sound perception gives us no clear-cut direction for intervention planning. There is no apparent hierarchy that we can use as a guide for targeting the acquisition of speech-sound distinctions. For this reason, the decision to target perceptual distinctions among speech sounds must be based on an evaluation of a child's pattern of speech-sound error productions (Locke, 1980). Additionally, we cannot assume that by targeting speech-sound discrimination we will automatically be correcting a misarticulation. We must also consider the production component.

Stability and locomotion. With reference to the sensorimotor domain, our focus thus far has been speech perception, the function of the peripheral speech mechanism, and the effect of its maturation on the development of speech. We must not, however, lose sight of the impact that the child's overall motor development has on speech-language functioning. Specifically, the child's ability to stabilize and move the body in space supports the development of language content and adequate functioning of the peripheral speech mechanism (Bobath & Bobath, 1981; Connor, Williamson, & Siepp, 1978; Fiorentino, 1972; Mysak, 1980). Thus the child's stability and locomotor skills should receive attention in intervention planning.

Stability and locomotion involve tonicity and the differentiation, coordination, and integration of sensorimotor actions shaped by the primitive motor reflexes (Fiorentino, 1972). The earliest movement patterns observed in the infant are influenced by primitive reflexes that can be elicited during the first six months of life. Reflexes are suppressed and intentional motor skills develop as the child learns how to roll over, side lie, prone prop, crawl, sit, stand, and walk. The development of such competencies also takes place as the child manipulates the environment from supine, prone-prop, sitting, and standing positions. These sensorimotor abilities allow the child to learn about the world through manipulating, exploring, and playing with objects and people. These competencies also support adequate functioning of the peripheral speech mechanism.

For example, the extension of the body achieved as the child rolls, prone props, crawls, and sits may contribute to the elongation of the neck and the descent of the larynx and tongue (Connor, Williamson, & Siepp, 1978). These achievements, in turn, are reflected in changes in resonation patterns from those associated with "cooing" to those associated with "babbling." The child's ability to achieve and sustain antigravity positions of sitting, standing, and walking translate into the ability to sustain adequate subglottal pressure for continuous speech and more differentiated and coordinated speech movements (Davis, 1987). These achievements support phonologic and syntactic competence, as the child is able to generate speech movements whenever motivated to speak—regardless of posture or ongoing activities. Generally, we work with the physical or occupational therapist in evaluating and planning intervention goals and procedures related to stability and locomotor issues. We discuss collaboration throughout the book, especially in Chapter 7.

Feedback. There is another sensorimotor issue that merits attention in intervention planning: the interaction between the processing of sensory information and motor control. Every motor act has a feedback component (Mysak, 1980; Kent & Lybolt, 1982). This feedback component involves the sensing of movement. The sensing of movement involves proprioception (feeling where the body is in space and sensing pressure on the joints), vestibular activity (detecting and maintaining balance and uprightness), and tactile sensation (perceiving and tolerating deep and light touch). Children need to be able to sense their movements (i.e., receive and process feedback information) in order to learn how to control them (Bobath & Bobath, 1981; Mysak, 1980,). They also use feedback to represent objects that they interact with during play and other sensorimotor activities (Piaget,

1971). It is precisely this interaction between the motor act and its feedback component that underlies the acquisition, maintenance, and generalization of speech-language behaviors. Consequently, this interaction has important implications for goal setting and procedural planning.

Children with a range of communication disorders involving voice, articulation, and content-form interactions may present feedback processing problems. The speech-language pathologist, in collaboration with a sensorimotor specialist, may wish to target improved integration of sensory information and adopt facilitating procedures. The issue of feedback and its relation to intervention planning is developed throughout the book.

Psychosocial. Psychosocial factors that may have an impact upon the child's interpersonal relations represent a third domain of behavior that may contribute to a speech-language disorder. Psychosocial factors that affect speech-language functioning include (a) the child's ability to engage in and benefit from social interactions; (b) the child's typical affect and strategies for adapting to environmental demands, including reactions to communicative successes and failures; (c) the caregivers' efforts to facilitate communication development and their reactions to the child's communicative attempts; and (d) the characteristic composition of the child's environment (caregivers, peers, siblings, disciplinary measures, culture, socioeconomic background, affect, languages spoken). (For comprehensive overviews of the development of psychosocial skills, see discussions by Owens, 1992, and McLean & Snyder-McLean, 1978, on the social and communicative basis of early language and Bloom & Lahey, 1978, on the development of language use.)

The development of psychosocial abilities has been described in a number of recent books and articles from two major perspectives: (a) the child's developing ability to contribute to and benefit from potentially nurturing interactions with caregivers and (b) the caregivers' contribution to this interaction ("motherese"). It appears clear from these writings that both the normally developing child and the caretaker contribute to interpersonal interactions from birth (e.g., Murray & Trevarthen, 1986).

The child's contribution. Within the first weeks of life infants are attuned to a mother's face, eyes, smiles, vocalizations—aspects of a caregiver's communication. Moreover, infants signal this sensitivity to the caregiver by gazing, smiling, and vocalizing (Murray & Trevarthen, 1986). By eight to ten months, children can initiate routines such as "peek-a-boo" (Bruner, 1983; Ratner & Bruner, 1978) and other intentional communication acts (Halliday, 1975; Sugarman, 1978). These early psychosocial achievements are precursory to children's learning of conventions for engaging in and making conversation—conventions that include, for example, eye contact, turn taking, topic initiating and extending, and joint referencing (see Lahey, 1988). As children develop, their interpersonal skills become more complex. They learn to play cooperatively (sharing, taking turns, and planning together). They learn to take another's point of view (as in role playing and being sensitive to the expectations of others). Such psychosocial achievements have been associated with the development and progress of general language functions, such as requesting, regulating, and commenting (e.g., Dore, 1974; Halliday, 1975; Tough, 1977). Psychosocial achievements have also been associated with the development of discourse skills. These include conventions for requesting action (Garvey, 1975), issuing directives (Ervin-Tripp, 1977), asking questions (James & Seebach, 1982; Schwabe, Olswang, & Kriegsmann, 1986), answering questions (Parnell, Patterson, & Harding, 1984), and producing appropriate pronouns (Schiff-Myers, 1983).

The caregiver's contribution. Caregivers play a complementary role in the child's psychosocial development. They must provide an environment which is conducive to the acquisition of psychosocial skills associated with language learning. The establishment of contexts supportive of conversational interchange is one major contribution of caregivers. Mothers initially use verbal and nonverbal devices to get and maintain the child's attention (i.e., to highlight objects and actions). As the child matures, the mother provides salient opportunities for the child to produce vocal and gestural responses and ultimately language (e.g., omitting words in well-known game and song routines). The mother's supportive techniques have been referred to as "scaffolding" (Ninio & Bruner, 1978; Ratner & Bruner, 1978).

The mother's language and conversational style has also been viewed as an important factor in language development. In the past two decades, there has been much research into the nature and effect of caregivers' input. DeVilliers and DeVilliers (1978) reviewed a large number of studies describing the language typically used to address normally developing children. These studies supported a description of generally simplified and redundant phonology, syntax, and vocabulary. This language register, reserved for young children, has become known as "motherese."

Later studies on "motherese" were expanded to include the effects of particular linguistic structures and interaction styles on the child's developing language. It is generally agreed that maternal speech supports the child's development of syntax by engaging the child in linguistic interaction and providing illustrations of the structures the child needs to acquire (e.g., Hoff-Ginsberg, 1990). However, correlational studies with normally developing children have presented conflicting results regarding the *most efficient* language input for the developing child. Conflicting results have produced conflicting conclusions. Some researchers feel that the mother's speech style (with specific reference to particular syntactic structures) directly affects the child's syntactic development (e.g., Furrow, Nelson, & Benedict, 1979). In contrast, other investigators have argued that the effect of the mother's speech on the child's language acquisition is in a large part interactive with predispositions of the learner (Newport, Gleitman, & Gleitman, 1977; Gleitman, Newport, & Gleitman, 1984; Pinker, 1990; Yoder & Kaiser, 1989). (Differences in findings among many of these studies have been summarized by Scarborough & Wyckoff, 1986; and Yoder & Kaiser, 1989.)

Given these disparate findings, as well as ideas about the child's innate propensity to learn language, some researchers believe that individual differences in "motherese" may be unimportant as long as some degree of adequacy is achieved (Scarborough & Wyckoff, 1986). In other words, it appears that conversation with an interested adult is more crucial than any particular technique or structure.

The contribution of the context. We have already alluded to a finding that appears throughout the literature on children's and caretakers' contributions to psychosocial development: Context plays an important role in the development of psychosocial competencies. We need to say a few preliminary words at this point about the term *context,* since it is so central to intervention planning.

The term *context* signifies the conditions that surround a behavior. Context may refer to the materials or people that the child is interacting with when communicating. For example, dolls, doll houses, cups, and saucers constitute typical contextual materials about which young children often communicate. Context may also refer to the linguistic behavior of the child or others. For instance, a mother modeling the word "man" while reading a book represents a linguistic context in which a child may learn how to say "man."

We are all aware of how changes in environmental conditions can have an impact upon how we communicate. For instance, as adults we know that it is often easier to say something in the presence of a small group of friends than to say the same thing in front of a large group of people at a conference presentation. Speaking in the presence of that large group may affect our fluency, voice, or syntax—even our ability to formulate the ideas we wish to express. Having the concrete object about which we are communicating in front of us, as opposed to trying to remember it, often facilitates the communication. Context clearly affects all aspects of communication performance.

Since communication performance is so context sensitive, it makes sense that the clinician will, in developing intervention plans, engineer contexts that facilitate speech-language performance. Considerations of context will affect both goals and procedures. We will be exploring the ways that we address context in intervention planning throughout this book.

For children, play is a context that often facilitates communication. Play, when it includes others, sets the stage for the expansion of language functions and the development of conversational skills. Characteristics of conversations are evident in the earliest playful interactions between infant and caregiver (i.e., reciprocal gaze, turn taking, anticipation). In the context of play, children learn to cooperate with and accommodate to others (Forman & Hill, 1984), assume reciprocal roles and envision events from another's perspective (Inhelder & Piaget, 1969; Ratner & Bruner, 1978; Sutton-Smith, 1979). These developing psychosocial skills reportedly correlate with the development of certain pragmatic achievements, such as taking the listener's knowledge into account when presenting new information, observing rules of conversation (e.g., initiating, responding to, maintaining, and extending topics), and using alternative forms of reference (e.g., deixis). In appropriate cases, the clinician may target such psychosocial competencies as intervention goals and design intervention contexts to facilitate such behavior. (For comprehensive discussions of pragmatic achievements see Owens, 1992; Rees, 1978.) Features of psychosocial development and their relationship to the development of speech and language are highlighted in Box 1–5. Correspondences between stages of language development, the child's psychosocial attainments, the effect of these attainments on language learning, and the role of the caregiver are also described. This information is meant to serve as a guide for identifying delayed psychosocial achievements or inappropriate parental behaviors as possible factors maintaining a communication problem.

Application to intervention planning. As with the other behavioral systems related to speech-language acquisition, we gather information about a child's psychosocial functioning during the assessment process. A child's level of psychosocial achievement and the parents' presumed contribution to this achievement will be important data for intervention planning. These data will be useful for designing the context in which a target linguistic achievement is expected (i.e., the goal context). These data will also be essential for the development of intervention procedures that may involve family or peers.

In the area of goal planning, information about psychosocial behavior is useful in establishing the psychosocial achievements associated with a particular speech-language achievement. For example, a goal for a child who has not begun to produce single words might involve *imitating* a caregiver's model of form-content interactions. As noted in Box 1–5, utilizing a caregiver's model may be supportive of the child's productions of single words. On the procedural side, knowing that a caregiver's models of form-content interactions are important would suggest that modeling be incorporated as an action of the clinician or caregiver. Another example comes from the last linguistic period in Box 1–5. At this point in linguistic development, the corresponding psychosocial attainment is a child's ability to take another's perspective. This psychosocial skill manifests itself in the pragmatic language skills that require differentiating self and listener's perspectives. This skill may be reflected in appropriate deictic reference, such as pronoun use (i.e., differentiating *I, me,* and *you;* Schiff-Myers, 1983). It is also a skill that may underlie the ability to comment on voice and fluency patterns associated with a variety of feelings, roles, and listeners (Andrews, 1986). Knowing that later language development involves the psycholinguistic attainment of taking another's perspective will guide the clinician in goal and procedure planning. For example, a goal for differentiating smooth from rough vocal quality might involve reflecting on a puppet with a very hoarse voice. On the procedural side, the clinician will encourage the child to talk about how the hoarse voice sounds and feels. How

BOX 1-5. PSYCHOSOCIAL ACHIEVEMENTS RELATED TO LINGUISTIC PERFORMANCE

Stage of Linguistic Performance	Child's Psychosocial Achievement	Effect on Speech-Language	Caretaker Contributions
Prelinguistic[a]	Can engage in reciprocal behaviors with caregivers: joint attention, co-occurring and alternating sound play, physical interactions involving touch, cuddling, cradling	Introduces the sense of being able to regulate others through joint attention, the use of language, and conversational turn taking	Orients child's attention (gaze) to self and objects
			Engages with child in play routines (e.g., "peek-a-boo")
			Responds to child's efforts at sound play by varying intonation, imitating child's vocalizations, and smiling
			Initiates sound play by producing sounds within child's repertoire and novel sounds with exaggerated intonation and facial expressions
	Can notice caregiver's responsiveness to his or her communication attempts	Reinforces the regulatory uses of intentional communication	Touches and cradles child
Single-words to beginning syntax[b]	Can imitate caregiver's modeling of form-content interactions that code a child's play and other nonlinguistic behaviors	May provide a support for the child's single-word and early multiword utterances	Models form-content interactions corresponding to activities child observes or participates in

(continued)

BOX 1-5 *(continued)*

Can respond to expansions of his or her utterances by caregiver		Expands child's attempts at form-content interactions
Can establish and maintain neutral affect during cognitive-linguistic activity	May enable the child to receive and process information	Engages with child in play routines that reenact familiar experiences
Can engage in cooperative play (play with others referencing and sharing toys and initiating, sharing, and shifting play topic)	May support the development of conversational skills, including turn-taking patterns, topic initiation, and topic shift	Mediates child's problem-solving activities by offering strategies and directions
Later language development[c] Can take another's perspective (as seen in role taking and other activities during play)	May support the development of pragmatic language skills that require differentiating self and listener's perspective, such as pronoun reference, deixis, ellipsis, differentiating voice qualities and fluency patterns	Mediates child's problem-solving activities by offering strategies and directions
Can perform more complex cooperative play skills: planning, imagination, and formal rule setting	May support the development of more complex conversational skills, including the ability to converse about events with some distance in space and time	Helps child reflect on past experiences and future possibilities
Can utilize caregiver directives to mediate problem-solving activity	May support the development of the problem-solving functions of language	

(continued)

27

BOX 1–5 *(continued)*

Can utilize caregiver mediation of experiences consistent with the sociocultural milieu	May provide a cultural framework for learning dialectal variations in content-form-use interactions
Can be comforted and gain security from parental-family stability	May support all aspects of language learning

Sources:

a. Bloom, 1988; Ginsberg & Kilbourne, 1988; Murray & Trevarthen, 1986; Platt & Coggins, 1990; Stern, Jaffe, Beebe, & Bennett, 1975.

b. Bloom, Beckwith, Capatides, & Hafitz, 1988; Bloom & Capatides, 1987; Bruner, 1975; Furrow & Nelson, 1986; Gleitman, Newport, & Gleitman, 1989; Hoff-Ginsberg, 1990; Ratner & Bruner, 1978; Rondal, 1980; Scarborough & Wyckoff, 1986; Scherer & Olswang, 1989; Tomasello, Conti-Ramsden, & Ewert, 1990; Yoder & Kaiser, 1989.

c. Emslie & Stevenson, 1981; Forman & Hill, 1984; Lund & Duchan, 1988; Musslewhite, 1986; Schiff-Myers, 1983; Taylor, 1986; Tough, 1977; Vygotsky, 1987; Wertsch, 1979, 1984; Westby, 1980; Wozniak, 1972.

knowledge of relationships between psychosocial development and language guides intervention planning is exemplified throughout the book.

Additional considerations. Note that Box 1–5 does not delineate correspondences between specific parental input (e.g., length, type, complexity of syntax) and children's output; rather, more general parental behaviors are listed (e.g., modeling, expansion, and clarification). This is because it is not yet clear if any specific types of structures are most facilitative for language learning (see the discussion on the caregiver's contribution above).

It should be noted, further, that the information in Box 1–5 is based on research with normally achieving children and their caregivers. In a review of the literature on caregiver-child interactions, Lahey (1988) was unable to find clear-cut trends in comparing caregiver input to normally achieving children with caregiver input to youngsters with language disorders. Her comparisons were based on complexity of input, number of questions and directives posed, use of expansions and corrections, and utterances about the attentional focus of the child. She attributed her findings primarily to methodological issues, such as differences in criteria for matching subjects (Chronological Age–CA versus Mean Length of Utterance–MLU) and inadequacies in using MLU as a criterion for comparing subjects. In addition, Lahey pointed out that it is impossible to determine from the studies what factors were guiding parents in their responses to children: the linguistic performance of the child or the child's general lack of responsivity. Lahey concluded that, despite inconclusive findings, "certain interactional patterns can interfere with the language learning of some language disordered children. Input that includes aberrant speech or language behaviors, lack of clarity in communicating, topics that are not the child's focus of attention, or lack of responsiveness to the child's attempts to communicate is certainly not designed to enhance language learning" (p. 356).

We did not include information about such psychosocial variables as motivation, dependency, or task orientation in Box 1–5, although research with school-age language-learning disabled children suggests that problems in these areas may play a role in language functioning (Shriberg & Kwiatkowski, 1982a). There is some disagreement as to whether motivation and task orientation are independent personality characteristics. Some researchers see the strength of these factors as related to other variables, such as the child's interests, prior experiences, cognitive functioning, task demands, and the novelty of a problem (e.g., Reid & Hresko, 1981; Reid, 1988). We agree. Thus, in intervention planning the clinician must assess and manipulate the above variables as factors potentially maintaining, for example, the client's motivational level or task orientation. We develop this idea further in subsequent chapters.

In summary, we have presented an overview of three nonlinguistic behavioral systems; impairments in these systems could contribute to the maintenance of a speech-language problem. Knowledge of functional status of these systems, therefore, provides a basis for (a) determining which behaviors to modify so that speech-language development may be facilitated and (b) designing client-clinician interactions and contexts to facilitate goal achievement. Figure 1–4 highlights the knowledge about nonlinguistic maintaining factors that guides intervention planning.

The Language System as a Source of Language Dysfunction.   We have thus far cited three nonlinguistic behavioral systems as possible maintaining factors that may represent the source of a language dysfunction. There is a fourth behavioral system that can maintain a language dysfunction—the language system, itself. The language system can be viewed as a mechanism for abstracting, organizing, and generating linguistic data (Chomsky, 1982a; Pinker, 1984; van Riemsdijk & Williams, 1986). Syntax and phonology, in particular, display unique organizational properties apparent in no other behavioral system (Piatelli-Palmarini, 1980). If that aspect of the neurological system responsible for processing linguistic information is impaired, a child will have difficulty learning language. This position has been argued historically by neuropsychologists (e.g., Lenneberg & Lenneberg, 1975). This viewpoint is also basic to the identification of a population of children who have been categorized as exhibiting specific language impairments (see Leonard, 1979, 1989, and Lahey, 1988, for reviews of the characteristics of this population).

FIGURE 1–4.   Knowledge that guides intervention planning: Nonlinguistic maintaining factors.

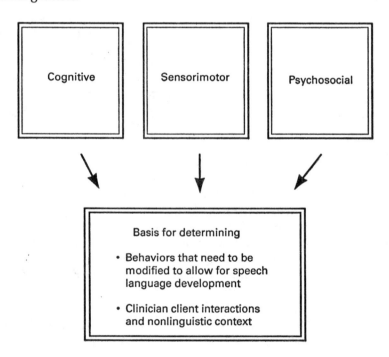

Though we may not give it any thought, we are actually addressing the language-learning system with each goal and procedure we plan. Intervention goals in general are designed to change (improve) existing speech-language behaviors. Thus, by implementing such goals we are attempting to affect the language system directly. We do this in addition to focusing on nonlinguistic behavioral systems that may be having a negative impact upon speech and language. This effort to affect the language-learning system directly brings us to another area of knowledge central to intervention planning: learning theories.

Learning Theory

Theories about how children learn language play an important role in decision making at each stage of the intervention process—especially in making decisions about procedures. It is our experience that when we raise the issue of theory in college classrooms or at workshops on speech-language intervention clinicians can be quickly turned off. They are sometimes explicit about what turns them off: "We want to know what to do, not some abstract ideas about processes that we can't observe and that nobody agrees on, anyway." Unfortunately, no cookbook exists that contains an exhaustive list of therapeutic procedures. No list presented in this text would be exhaustive, either. What we need for intervention planning is a way—given any clinical context—of creating appropriate procedures. Theories about language learning serve this function.

Theories about language learning are sources of *principles*. A principle is a general rule derived from a theory that indicates, though not always directly, (a) a behavioral event that can be explained and, perhaps, modified; (b) how to go about modifying that event (i.e., procedures); and (c) the reason that the procedures inferred from the theory ought to work (i.e., rationales). Principles derived from learning theories offer premises about what can be learned and the nature of interactions that facilitate learning. Consequently, such principles are handy tools. They aid the clinician in creating procedures.

For example, two principles that can be derived from operant learning theory are (a) observable behaviors that can be stimulated in a child can be learned and (b) events that follow a behavior can strengthen or weaken the behavior. Referencing these principles in teaching a child to articulate /k/ would lead the clinician to devise a way to provoke the child to produce a /k/ and to create an event following the child's production of the /k/ that would provoke the child to produce it again (for instance, presenting the child with an M & M). If the child succeeded in producing and replicating the /k/ sound, the clinician could refer to the principle to explain this success: the M & M following the child's production of a /k/ sound reinforced that behavior. Thus, unlike lists of procedures, principles derived from learning theory—in concert with the clinician's creativity—are inexhaustible sources of procedures.

There is some truth to the clinician's comment, above, that the learning theories from which principles are derived are "abstract ideas about processes that we can't observe and that nobody agrees on, anyway." It is true that learning theories often reference theoretical events as opposed to observable, "factual" data. Theories, in fact, are *belief systems* about learning. It is also true that there are many different learning theories—i.e., belief systems about language learning—and that they sometimes appear to conflict with one another. Several recent clinically oriented texts and articles summarize these theories (Carrow-Woolfolk, 1988; Cornett & Chabon, 1988; Hegde, 1985; Nelson, 1993; Perkins, 1982; van Kleeck & Richardson, 1986). We discuss language-learning theories at greater length in Chapter 2.

Efforts undertaken to make learning theories accessible to clinicians, although quite helpful, may in some ways contribute to confusion surrounding learning theory. For example, different authors sometimes use different terms to reference the same theory; e.g., learning theories based on Vygotsky's work are termed *social learning theory* by van Kleeck and Richardson (1986), and *cognitive organization theory* by Carrow-Woolfolk (1988). Others summarize theories that explain *what* needs to be learned and theories that focus on *how* learning takes place (Perkins, 1982; van Kleeck & Richardson, 1986) without explicitly distinguishing the different purposes of these different kinds of theories.

It is our view that theory does not need to be as intimidating and confusing as it is at present. To reiterate, we view learning theories as sources of principles that are tools for clinical decision making. There are steps that can be taken to abstract principles from learning theories and to make these principles accessible for clinical decision making.

Initially, we ask two questions of each learning theory in order to abstract information about two important issues. First, what does the theory tell us about what can be learned—that is, about the nature of the information to be learned? Second, what does the theory say about how learning takes place— that is, about the action of the learner, the action of the teacher (if there is one), and the conditions preceding and following the action of the learner? With reference to these areas of information, we believe that learning theories can be grouped into a manageable set of four categories: operant, constructivist-cognitive, social-cognitive, and motor learning.

Operant Theories.   Operant theories focus exclusively on observable behaviors—not internal processes, feelings, schemes, or concepts. Operant theories also concentrate on the *environment* as the locus of control for learning and behavior. The idea is that a behavior (or class of behaviors) can be shaped by stimulating the behavior and then following it with a consequence (or class of consequences) that will increase the probability that the behavior will be expressed again. It is essentially the immediate and historic consequences of a behavior that are seen as underlying the learning and maintenance of that behavior (Chiesa, 1992).

Cognitive Learning Theories. The next two categories—constructivist- and social-cognitive learning theories—differentiate a number of learning theories that are typically grouped together under the common heading *cognitive learning theories.* The tendency to group these theories together reflects a common focus. Unlike operant theories, which concentrate exclusively on observable behavior and on how environmental consequences of behavior control learning, each category of cognitive learning theory focuses on *internal aspects of behavior and the child's regulation of learning.* Cognitive learning theories, as they have been applied to explain speech-language acquisition, focus on developmental aspects of language. *Developmental* signifies that these competencies are acquired in a particular order and that certain competencies have to be acquired before others can emerge. Examples of developmental aspects of language include Bloom and Lahey's content categories, syntactic structures, and the functions of intentional communication. (The concept of *developmental* is examined in greater depth in Chapter 2, on the history of intervention planning, and Chapters 4 and 5, which deal with the long- and short-term planning phases.) Although the two categories of cognitive learning theories reviewed next both focus on internal aspects of behavior, their explanations of *how* these behaviors are acquired differ in significant ways.

Constructivist-cognitive learning theories. Constructivist theories (e.g., Case, 1985; Fischer & Pipp, 1984; Karmiloff-Smith, 1979; Piaget, 1985; Pinker, 1991) hold that some aspects of speech and language—especially the developmental aspects—are not learned directly from others. They are, instead, modified as children interact with the environment in creative ways—especially in the context of problem solving. Speech-language behavior is affected, too, by children's use of feedback from their own actions in the process of problem solving.

By reflecting on feedback during problem-solving children can become aware of objects and attributes (Piaget, 1977). This activity supports the development of language content. Furthermore, by reflecting on their own speech and language behavior, children can become aware of these behaviors. Awareness of speech and language behaviors, such as sound production, voice, and syntax, has been termed *metalinguistic knowledge* (e.g., Karmiloff-Smith, 1979; Pinker, 1984). The acquisition of such knowledge through problem solving may contribute to the development of phonology (e.g., Klein, Lederer, & Cortese, 1991), morphology and syntax (Karmiloff-Smith, 1979, 1986b; Pinker, 1984, 1990), voice (Andrews & Summers, 1993), and fluency (Shapiro, personal communication, September 11, 1992). In essence, the child's own creative (i.e., constructive) activities are seen as central to speech and language development.

Social-cognitive learning theories. Social cognitive theories—like constructivist theories—try to explain how children acquire internal components of speech and language. These theories often focus on information-processing skills, such as the ability to discriminate stimuli. Discrimination is often trained in intervention for articulation, voice, fluency, and language problems. Social-cognitive theories are especially interested in explaining how children acquire internal control over learning and problem solving (termed *learning how to learn*; e.g., Reid, 1988; van Kleeck & Richardson, 1986; Wertsch, 1979). Social-cognitive theories also focus on the learning of conversational skills and knowledge about communication (commonly termed *pragmatic skills*). Unlike constructivist-cognitive theories, social-cognitive theories generally propose that *adults* mediate children's development. Characteristics of speech and language are acquired as children internalize verbal directions, imitate problem-solving procedures, or attend to relations and distinctions (e.g., among sounds, words, and objects) that are highlighted or modeled by their caretakers. Recently, social-cognitive theories have emerged that indicate that children can learn speech and language skills from their peers in cooperative play and problem-solving activities (Nelson, 1993).

Motor-Learning Theories.   Motor-learning theories (e.g., Kent & Lybolt, 1982; Prinz & Saunders, 1984) represent a third learning-theory category. Motor-learning theories are concerned with the learning of sensorimotor schemes—which are patterns of behavior, not conscious ideas or cognitive processes. Learning mechanisms cited in these theories include the exercise of motor patterns, self-correction in response to problematic feedback, and the differentiation, integration, and coordination of different and often conflicting behavioral patterns. Motor learning theories are most often applied to explain the acquisition of speech skills in the areas of phonology, voice, and fluency.

Learning Theory and Procedural Planning.   Four categories of learning theories have been identified and described with reference to what each theory says about what can be learned and how learning takes place. Box 1–6 presents salient features of each theory and how the theories compare with one another. These features are organized according to a set of considerations that are useful for procedure planning. Those considerations are (a) the nature of the information to be learned, (b) the action of the learner, (c) the action of the teacher, and (d) the conditions preceding and following the action of the learner.

The information in Box 1–6 can be used as a basis for deriving principles of learning. Consider the nature of information to be learned and the action of the learner associated with constructivist-cognitive learning theory in Box 1–6: Individuals learn about the content of language (ideas about the world). They do so by engaging in constructive activity, which includes setting goals, organizing and coordinating actions, reflecting on actions and environmental events with reference to the success or failure of goal achievement, selecting information from feedback from goal-directed behavior, and projecting that information to higher levels of thought and reorganizing information. We can derive a number of principles from these components of the theory: (a) goal orientation is necessary for learning; (b) sensory stimulation (i.e, sensory feedback) from the manipulation of concrete objects, and from other forms of personal behavior, facilitates awareness and

BOX 1-6. A COMPARATIVE SUMMARY OF FOUR LANGUAGE-LEARNING THEORIES

Components	Language Learning Theory			
	Operant	Constructivist-Cognitive	Social-Cognitive	Motor
Aspects of language to be learned	Any observable behavior	Developmental aspects of speech and language, including ideas about the world that constitute content categories(e.g., time, causality), syntactic rules, the symbols, rules, and metalinguistic ability to use knowledge about phonology, prosody, voice characteristics, and fluency	Relations among symbols and their referents Content-form-use interactions Metalinguistic and meta-cognitive strategies for processing information (e.g., for remembering, sequencing, and problem solving)	Articulatory gestures related to sound production and fluency patterns Laryngeal adjustments related to voice production
Action of the learner	Produce a target response Discriminate among stimuli	Engage in constructive activities (setting goals, identifying problems, devising and modifying problem-solving procedures, making distinctions and relations among actions and objects in the environment, reflecting upon actions and environmental events, making inferences, evaluating behavior with reference to the success or failure of goal achievement)	Observe, imitate, internalize information (problem-solving procedures, strategies, and associations and distinctions demonstrated by others) Learn to use language internally to direct problem-solving procedures and to stop and redirect behavior	Execute and practice sensorimotor procedures (self-generated or modeled by others)
Action of the teacher	Evoke target response Follow target	Create an environment that permits constructive activity (i.e., manipulable, patterned,	Direct the learner's attention to relevant environmental stimuli	Engage child in activities that evoke sensorimotor act

(continued)

BOX 1-6 *(continued)*

	responses with scheduled reinforcement	developmentally appropriate) Interact with client in ways that stimulate constructive activity (permit goal setting, errors, the manipulation of concrete objects) Facilitate problem identification Provoke inference making, evaluations of success and failure Response to child's communications with reference to the child's intents in a way that is meaningful to the child Expand upon the child's efforts to use language	Present rules and direct and model linguistic structures and problem-solving procedures (i.e., provide a scaffold for language learning) Present problems and information that are developmentally appropriate and attainable within the zone of proximal development (i.e., that are consistent with the learner's development level)	Model or physically shape sensorimotor act
Conditions preceding action of the learner	Stimuli that evoke target response	A manipulable environment that permits the child to set goals, identify and solve problems	Readiness for learning The presentation of a behavioral model or directions	An activity that provokes the child to execute the target sensorimotor act
Conditions following the successful achievement of target by learner	Scheduled reinforcement	Feedback from personal behavior and the environment Self-evaluation	Praise or other forms of socially mediated feedback Conscious self-evaluation	Sensorimotor feedback
Conditions following error	Nomresponse or punishment	Conflicting feedback from self and the environment Self-evaluation Behavioral variation	Feedback from others indicating error Conscious self-evaluation	Sensorimotor feedback Further modeling of appropriate behavior

understanding; (c) reflection upon personal behavior and the environment facilitates mental representation.

Extracting such principles provides a way to make learning theories accessible for clinical decision making. We can focus on these major principles to understand the relatedness and distinctiveness of the various theory categories. More important to the task at hand, we can use these principles to generate specific procedures of therapy and rationales for the procedures we generate. For example, knowing that locative action—a content category at Lahey (1988) Phase 2—has been targeted for a child might lead us to think about the constructivist principles cited above (since the content of language is an aspect of language learning to which constructivist theories apply). These principles would guide us in creating procedures that would encourage the child to set goals, manipulate objects, and reflect on his or her actions. One such procedure could involve baking cookies. We further develop the idea of how principles from learning theories can guide procedure planning below and throughout the book.

Drawing relations among theories. Our claim that it is possible to identify relations as well as distinctions among different learning-theory categories is somewhat nontraditional. The theories that constitute each of the categories, and the categories themselves, are often treated as differing in content and application and as mutually exclusive. Recently, both Carrow-Woolfolk (1988) and Nelson (1993) organized principles abstracted from a variety of language theories and formulated an integrated approach to assessment and intervention in language disorders.

Our orientation concurs with these authors. We do not view learning theories as mutually exclusive or universal in their explanatory power. On the one hand, learning theories belonging to different categories embody similar principles. For example, operant, motor, and constructivist-cognitive learning theories account for much learning through the learner's physical actions (Piaget, 1977; Mounoud & Hauert, 1982; Inhelder, Sinclair, & Bovet 1974; Skinner, 1989). On the other hand, principles embodied in different learning theories *do* differ in significant ways. Some cognitive and motor theories may be distinguished from others on the basis of whether conscious reflection is necessary for learning (for example, compare Leith, 1984; and Pressley, Forrest-Pressley, Elliot-Faust, & Miller, 1985). Learning theories may be distinguished from one another according to their domain of applicability. For example, articulation skills may be most sensitive to motor-learning and operant processes, whereas the development of language content may be influenced more by cognitive processes.

Thus, it is our position that procedural planning does not involve committing to any single theory to the exclusion of others. Procedural planning requires selecting principles from theories relevant to a particular client's language problem and differentially applying these principles to design comprehensive therapeutic contexts (i.e., clinician-child interactions and materials; see Kamhi, 1993, who points out how the clinical use of learning theories differs from the use of theory in research, which is usually guided by adherence to a single theoretical position). Figure 1–5 illustrates the idea that all four categories of learning theory can be useful in intervention planning. Each type of theory guides the planning of clinician-child interactions and the selection of appropriate materials.

Essentially, then, principles from learning theories are most useful for procedural planning because they suggest procedures and rationales. We will make this utility explicit in subsequent chapters detailing the three phases of clinical decision making. Box 1–7 presents principles of learning, the theories from which they derive, and the domains of speech and language to which they apply.

The Clinician's Conceptual Framework. Box 1–7 contains a rather lengthy list of learning principles. Given all these principles, how does one go about selecting principles in procedural planning? We see two issues influencing the selection process.

The first issue is the relation between the goal of the particular intervention and the learning principle. One should select principles of learning that apply to the behavior that needs to be learned by the client. One would not operate with reference to a learning principle that only explains the acquisition of linguistic content when phonology is the target of intervention. We develop this point in subsequent chapters.

FIGURE 1–5. Knowledge that guides intervention planning: Alternative theories to explain learning.

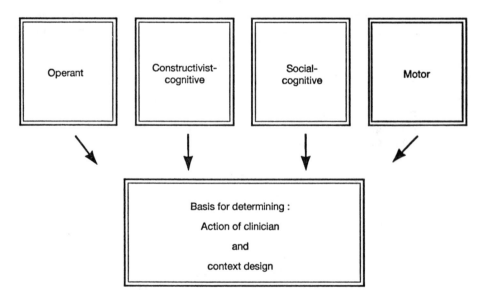

BOX 1–7.   PRINCIPLES OF LANGUAGE LEARNING
AND THEIR DOMAINS OF APPLICABILITY

Principles about Learning	*Learning Theories That Incorporate the Principle*	*Examples of Speech-Language Skill Potentially Affected by the Learning Process*
Learning is facilitated by:		
1. Events following a behavior, which can reinforce (strengthen) or extinguish (weaken) behavior	Operant (focus is on any type of consequence) Social-cognitive (focus is on social consequences)	Pragmatic skills (gaze, turn taking) Lexical acquisition Voice and fluency characteristics
2. Efforts to match models presented by the clinician	Social-cognitive	Form (speech sounds, suprasegmentals, lexicon, morphology, syntax) Voice and fluency characteristics
3. Noticing similarities and distinctions among actions and events mediated by adults	Social-cognitive	Concept formation, speech sounds, voice and fluency characteristics, morphology, syntax
4. The internalization of problem-solving strategies mediated by clinicians	Social-cognitive	Using language to self-monitor and solve problems (metalinguistics)— applied to the learning of voice and fluency characteristics, lexical retrieval
5. Interactions with materials and tasks commensurate with the child's past experience, present developmental level and interests	Constructivist	Language content, form, use
6. Efforts to convey meaning successfully and overcome the miscommunication of meaning	Constructivist Social-cognitive	Pragmatic skills (referent function), lexicon, speech sounds, concept development, content categories
7. Varying actions during problem solving (including the production of	Constructivist	Language content, form, use

(continued)

BOX 1–7 *(continued)*

erroneous behavior)		
8. Reflection upon personal behavior and the environment, inference making, inductive and deductive reasoning	Constructivist	Content categories, speech-sound production, pragmatic skills (referent function), metalinguistic skills
9. Sensory stimulation (i.e., sensory feedback) from movement, including movement involved in articulation	Constructivist Motor	Language content, speech-sound production, voice, and fluency characteristics

The second factor that we believe contributes to the clinician's selection of principles is *the clinician's own beliefs about language and language learning.* We believe that clinicians bring their own personal theories (i.e., belief systems) about language learning to clinical decision making, whether or not the clinician has formally studied learning theories (see Shapiro & Moses, 1989; also see Gentner & Stevens, 1983, for examples of "naive" theories in non–speech-language professional domains, such as physics). These personal belief systems—whether "expert" or "naive"—often correspond to aspects of classic linguistic theories. Clinicians' belief systems help direct clinical decision making.

Consider teaching vocabulary. One common belief is that adults direct language learning by making associations between objects and words for the child to observe and internalize (a belief that corresponds with principles of social-cognitive theory; e.g., Ninio & Bruner, 1978). Another, less common belief is that children facilitate their own learning of vocabulary by first constructing mental representations of sensorimotor activities in which they are engaged (a belief that corresponds with constructivist-cognitive theory; e.g., McCune, 1987; Piaget, 1962).

A clinician who holds the first belief might approach vocabulary teaching by focusing on Principle 3, Box 1–7, which states that learning is facilitated by the child's efforts to make associations among stimuli mediated by adults. Based on this principle, the clinician might create procedures to model associations between vocabulary words and pictures in a book.

A clinician who holds the second belief might focus on Principles 9 and 5, Box 1–7, which state that sensory stimulation (i.e, sensory feedback) from the manipulation of concrete objects facilitates language learning and that developmentally appropriate tasks are necessary for learning. (These two principles relate to the child's representation of a sensorimotor activity.) This clinician might create procedures to engage the child in play and might comment on the child's activity using targeted vocabulary.

These examples illustrate that personal beliefs about language learning interact with procedural planning. The clinician's personal beliefs will also affect goal setting. Bloom and Lahey (1978) have explained that the clinician's definition of language will determine aspects of language that are assessed and targeted for intervention.

Consider, for example, setting goals for a three-year-old child who comes to therapy using only single words. A clinician who views language as consisting only of phonology and syntax (i.e., form) might evaluate the child's articulation, vocabulary, and grammar. The clinician might then set out to expand the child's articulation, vocabulary, and syntactic repertoire. A clinician who views language as comprising interactions among content, form, and use—and as potentially affected by cognitive, sensorimotor, and psychosocial factors—would probably conduct a broader assessment. In addition to language form, that clinician would probably target developmental achievements relevant to language content and use as well as factors maintaining the disorder.

It goes without saying that the content of this book reflects the *authors'* conceptions about language, language learning, and the intervention process. We also believe that an important component of the intervention process for every clinician needs to be an ongoing *explicit* reassessment of *personal* beliefs about what behaviors constitute language, what behavioral systems interact with language, how particular aspects of speech and language are learned, why specific interventions succeed in particular cases, and why others fail. It is our intention throughout this book to stimulate such ongoing reassessments.

SUMMARY

In this chapter we introduced our conceptualization of the intervention-planning process. This process unfolds over three phases. Each phase involves decision making about goals and procedures. Three bodies of information—the nature of language, factors maintaining language problems, and theories regarding language learning—need to be considered at each phase of intervention planning. This intervention process, then, can be viewed as the progressive management of a complex body of information. In subsequent chapters we will detail each phase of this planning process.

2

History of Intervention Planning

It is 1958 and Sheila is enrolled in a Master's Degree Program in Speech Pathology. She has just been given her initial case load and has researched the popular texts of the time (i.e., Berry & Eisenson, 1956; Van Riper, 1954; West, Ansberry, & Carr, 1957). She explains to her supervisor that she read a book about techniques used to "train the child retarded in speech." She feels that she should "motivate" the children, "build a basic vocabulary," and "stimulate [them] to talk," but some major questions remain. She is unsure of the ultimate expectations for her client, what she can accomplish during one semester, and where she should begin.

Although our Sheila is fictitious, this particular scenario is realistic because the major texts of the fifties emphasized how to teach the child (procedures) but neglected what to teach (goals). Over the past four decades, approaches to therapy have undergone various modifications and shifts in focus. These changes may be traced to the prevailing views or belief systems about the nature of language, language learning, and language disorders.

The purpose of this chapter is to identify major theories of language and language learning that we have drawn upon to develop our model of the intervention planning process. We will explain how these theories affected our view of goal setting and procedural planning; more specifically, we will demonstrate how these theories affected our conceptualization of both the development of goals and procedures at each phase of intervention planning and the relationship between levels of decision making.

Numerous theories have been developed to explain the nature of language and the way in which language is acquired. Five of these theories, more than any others, influenced our model of intervention planning: behavioral, psycholinguistic, information-processing, cognitive, and pragmatic. The impact of these theories on our view of goal setting and procedural planning reflects their broad influence on the field of speech-language pathology over the last few decades (Carrow-Woolfolk, 1988; Launer & Lahey, 1981). Figure 2–1 is a graphic representation of the relative time periods during which the various theories emerged and maintained some influence on the profession.

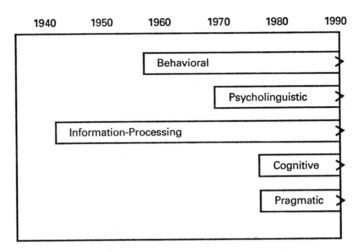

FIGURE 2–1.   Periods of influence of major theories on speech-language pathology.

During its period of influence, the popular theory of the day motivated changes in thinking about assessment as well as intervention planning. This dual influence of theory on assessment and intervention is not surprising, since decisions made about assessment and intervention are interdependent. Because of this close relation, we give some consideration to the effect of theory on both assessment and intervention in this chapter.

BEHAVIORAL THEORY

Behavioral theory is concerned with operant conditioning, the process of shaping observable behaviors by controlling the consequences of behavior (Glenn, Ellis, & Greenspoon, 1992). This theory did not emerge as a dominant paradigm in speech-language pathology until the 1960s. We begin with behaviorism because it, perhaps more than any other paradigm, motivated clinicians to reexamine the way intervention planning in speech-language pathology is conceived. Its far-reaching influence was seen in the popularity of operant-based language programs, such as Monterey (Sloane & McCauley, 1968) and DISTAR (Englemann & Osborn, 1972). Its continuing influence is seen in fluency-shaping programs (e.g., Nittrouer & Cheney, 1984; Shames & Florance, 1980); in three principal texts that treat intervention planning within an operant framework (Hegde, 1985; Leith, 1984; Mowrer, 1977); and in the application of PL 94–142 to special education (Benner, 1992; Cook, Tessier, & Klein, 1992).

PL 94–142.   The educational bill of rights for individuals with handicapping conditions—PL 94–142—was enacted in 1975. This legislation required that Individualized Educational Plans (IEPs) be developed for children with handicaps who receive federally subsidized services. It requires that educators and clinicians specify goals and procedures, criteria for assessing whether goals have been achieved, and the basis on which goals have been derived (assessment data). The IEP is a legal document. It functions as a management plan (Benner, 1992; Bigge, 1988; Cook, Tessier, & Klein, 1992; Reid & Hresko, 1981).

Behavioral theory has influenced how IEPs have been operationalized to meet the accountability requirements of PL 94–142 and subsequent legislation. Behavioral theory has especially influenced goal writing. The following are principles of IEP goal writing that have been influenced by behavioral theory:

1. Goals are to be written with reference to the performance of functional tasks (e.g., tooth brushing; talking in sentences).
2. In developing educational objectives, tasks should be analyzed and broken down into sequences of small, manageable skills. (These skills represent adults' perception of the steps required to perform the task.) The task to be learned represents one goal level; the steps leading to task achievement are a second goal level.
3. Goals are to be written in terms of observable behavior, and performance criteria for their achievement need to be specified.
4. Goal statements must indicate the context in which the target behavior is to be elicited.
5. Principles 1–4 apply to the formulation of goals regardless of the disorder under consideration.

In addition to influencing goal formulation, behaviorism, as a learning theory, comprised principles that influenced procedural planning. Those principles made clinicians aware of the need to address the critical issue of *how* children learn language. The major behavioral premise about language learning is that linguistic behavior is shaped and controlled by its consequences—i.e., environmental events that occur after the behavior is expressed (Skinner, 1957; Hayes & Hayes, 1992). Consequences that increase the probability that a behavior will be used again are *reinforcers*. Consequences that decrease the probability that a behavior will be expressed again are *extinguishers* or *punishments*. Thus, language learning from an operant perspective involves the shaping of observable behavior by the reactions of the environment. Procedural planning must involve planning a schedule of consequences that will follow desirable and undesirable behaviors (e.g., tokens, stickers, the comment, "good speaking").

These behavioral principles stand in marked contrast to the categorical orientation that guided intervention planning during the period before the emergence of behaviorism. This contrast will be explicated in the following section.

The categorical orientation. During the 1940s and 1950s, the focus of intervention planning was on the remediation of symptoms associated with major etiological categories (Launer & Lahey, 1981). Aram and Nation (1982) termed these decades the "era of etiologic typologies and differential diagnosis" (p. 15).

Etiology was determined through a differential diagnosis. Etiologic categories were specified and children were classified based on comparisons of case histories and presenting behaviors of children with speech-language disorders. These categories included deafness and hearing impairment, emotional disturbance and autism, mental retardation, and childhood aphasia. Unique constellations of behavioral symptomatology (characteristic cognitive, social, motor, and auditory behaviors) were designated for each category. Examples of such disorder categories and constituent behaviors appear in Table 2–1. (For seminal texts illustrating this position see Berry & Eisenson, 1956; Myklebust, 1954; Van Riper, 1954; West, Ansberry, & Carr, 1957.)

Information about etiologic categories provided the basis for formulating goals and procedures. Placing a child within an etiologic category was tantamount to describing the factors assumed to maintain his or her disorder. Goals, in turn, were directed toward eliminating or minimizing maintaining factors. For example, Berry and Eisenson (1956) suggested the following goals for "training the child 'retarded' in speech" (p. 135): (a) developing in the child an awareness of the environment and of him- or herself in relation to the environment, (b) developing auditory discrimination of speech sounds, (c) strengthening visual-kinesthetic cues, (d) increasing flexibility of the articulators. This example is representative of the textbook approach to "therapy" during the '40s and '50s (e.g., Berry & Eisenson, 1956; Van Riper, 1954; West, Ansberry, & Carr, 1957). This approach emphasized the identification of *specific areas of disability* that *require remediation.* Such an approach, however, neglected to address important issues. For example, the way in which speech-language behavior was expected to change when these areas were remediated was not considered. Furthermore, a sequence of steps that would lead to the achievement of these goals was not delineated, and the way in which children learned skills that resulted in the ameliorization of symptoms was not specified.

Behaviorism compared to the categorical orientation. As a reaction to the lack of objectivity and specificity that characterized the categorical orientation, principles of intervention planning derived from behavioral theory were introduced. This led to five significant changes in the conceptualization and formulation of therapy goals and procedures.

First, there was a move away from targeting nonobservable processes presumed to be disordered. For example, the goal "auditory discrimination of speech sounds," which was targeted in Berry and Eisenson (1956), is an internal process and not observable. In contrast, a session-goal statement related to auditory discrimination written in behavioral terms could read as follows: "Joanne will raise her hand in response to words beginning with /k/ when they are paired with words beginning with /g/."

Second, there was an effort to address context in formulating goal statements. Goal statements written prior to the behavioral period did not specify the task context in which the skill is to be learned. Goals written in behavioral

TABLE 2–1. The Characteristic Performance of Each Type on the Areas Evaluated in Making a Differential Diagnosis

Type of Disorder	History	Behavioral Symptomatology	Auditory Responses	Mental Capacity	Social Maturity	Motor Capacity	Language Functioning	Emotional Adjustment
					Test findings			
Peripheral deafness	Indicates alertness in general and often consistent response to loud sounds. Not bizarre or seriously retarded genetically.	Not bizarre. Compensatory use of other sensory avenues. Integrated and use environmental clues well.	Consistent and integrated. Good listening behavior. Use hearing projectively. Give scanning responses.	Cluster around average level. Little scatter. Integrated and consistent in performance on tests.	Good except for communication area. Average social quotient of approximately 90.	Good but balance may be disturbed. No generalized incoordination or retardation.	Good inner language. Good gesture. Use voice projectively. Behave symbolically.	Good responsiveness to people through vision. Social perception and contact with environment is good.
Aphasia	Indicates some retardation in development. Confusion regarding hearing. Lack of shyness but not bizarre.	Disinhibited, hyperactive and forced responsiveness. Not use other sensory avenues in compensatory way.	Inconsistent, erratic, cannot listen. Disturbed in auditory perception. Not use hearing projectively.	Inconsistent and much scatter. Perceptual disturbances improve with structuring.	Retarded in all areas but especially in communication, socialization and motor areas. Average social quotient of approximately 75.	Slightly delayed in sitting and walking. Generalized incoordination.	Poor inner language. Little or no use of gesture. Not use voice projectively. May unexpectedly use a word. May be echolalic.	Emotional expression lacks intensity. Try to relate to people. Are not oblivious or bizarre.

(continued)

TABLE 2-1 (continued)

Psychic deafness	Began using speech, then stopped. Many anxieties. Willfulness in rejection of environment. Withdrawn and in world of their own.	Bizarre, no compensatory use of senses. Not relate to people. Poor social perception. No projective use of hearing or voice and no gesture.	Seem to willfully reject sound, give indirect responses. No projective use of hearing. Not disturbed in auditory perception. May show fear of sound.	Not perceptually disturbed. May do well on formboards. Reject the test situation in total or in part. Behavior suggests good mental ability.	Deficient in all areas but notably in socialization. Average social quotient of approximately 80.	Stereotyped activity. Rigidity and random movements. Only slight retardation in sitting and walking.	Good inner language but used only for fantasy. No use of gesture and do not use voice projectively. May be mute.	Withdrawn in own world. Lacking in relationship to people. Stereotyped and bizarre.
Mental deficiency	Retardation in all development is most characteristic in history.	Responsive but in low genetic and concrete manner. Not bizarre.	Respond directly or indirectly to tests which are suitable genetically. Use hearing projectively.	Marked retardation in general.	Marked generalized retardation in all areas. Average social quotient of approximately 55.	Generalized retardation with incoordination. Marked delay in sitting and walking.	Language is deficient but not seriously discrepant with mental age. Retarded in all phases of language development.	Passive, phlegmatic, infantile and deficient in animation.

From Myklebust, H. R. (1954). *Auditory disorders in children: A manual for differential diagnosis.* New York: Grune and Stratton, Inc., pp. 352–353. Reprinted by permission of Grune and Stratton, Inc., and the author.

terms do. According to Bigge (1988), short-term and session-goal statements should include materials (e.g., the presence or absence of manipulables) and the teacher-child interaction aimed at provoking the behavior (e.g., gestural prompts, verbal cues).

Third, there was a change in the direction of differentiating levels of goal setting. During the etiological category period there was no clear-cut distinction between goal levels. In contrast, behavioral approaches to intervention planning distinguish short-term and session goals and circumscribe links between these goal levels.

Fourth, there was a change in the engineering of consequences aimed at shaping target behaviors. During the categorical period, procedural planning was not driven by established theories of learning. Principles based on behavioral (operant) theory, however, helped guide the clinician in planning responses to the client's efforts.

Finally, the behavioral movement promoted the application of a common set of intervention planning principles across disorder categories. These principles involved teaching observable skills in specific task contexts without regard to disorder. Thus, the behavioral approach represented a change from a mindset characteristic of the categorical orientation—that of addressing individuals belonging to different etiologic categories differently.

The Influence of Behaviorism on Our Model of Intervention Planning. Although our approach to intervention planning is not primarily behavioral, we have been influenced by behaviorism. A number of behavioral principles have been incorporated into our thinking about the construction of goal statements, especially writing session goals and relating session to short-term goals. In addition, behaviorism, as a learning theory, has influenced our thinking about procedural planning.

Influenced by behaviorism, our session goals are written in observable terms and include reference to the context in which the behavior is expressed. An example of a session goal written in observable terms and referencing context was cited above: "Joanne will raise her hand in response to words beginning with /k/ when they are paired with words beginning with /g/."

Influenced by behaviorism in planning intervention procedures, we give careful consideration to the issue of how children learn language. We consider the conditions under which the child is expected to respond as well as the potential effect of contingencies following behavior.

Guided by behavioral axioms, we apply a uniform set of principles to intervention planning across disorders. We emphasize the importance of describing behavior and the context in which it is expressed regardless of the disorder under consideration. We also agree that there must always be a specifiable connection between different goal levels (e.g., between session and short-term goals). Box 2–1 summarizes the influence of behavioral theory on intervention planning.

BOX 2–1. THE INFLUENCE OF BEHAVIORAL THEORY ON PHASES
OF INTERVENTION PLANNING

	Phases Influenced	
Influential Principles	*Goals*	*Procedures*
1. Target observable behavior	Session	
2. Address context in formulating goal statements	Session	All phases
3. Specify relationships among long-term, short-term, and session goals	Short-term Session	
4. Engineer consequences aimed at shaping target behaviors		Session

Departures from Behaviorism.   We depart from behaviorism, however, in the way that we define short-term goals and conceptualize the relation between session goals and short-term goals. Our approach to short-term goal setting reflects developmental psycholinguistic influences.

We also depart from behaviorism in terms of the factors we consider when we *formulate* session goals and procedures. Here, we have been influenced by information-processing and cognitive learning theories. The influence of psycholinguistic, information-processing, and cognitive learning theories on our intervention planning model will be discussed next.

DEVELOPMENTAL PSYCHOLINGUISTICS

Beginning in the late 1950s and burgeoning in the 1970s, a line of thinking developed that posed a major challenge to behaviorism. This was the developmental psycholinguistic movement. This movement, which continues to be highly influential, has more recently been incorporated into the discipline known as cognitive science.

The focus of developmental psycholinguistics has been *developmental sequences of behavior* and ways of describing the organization intrinsic to these sequences. Organization has been described as schemes and schema (influenced by Piaget, 1971), rules and parameters (influenced by Chomsky, 1957, 1982b), linguistic categories (e.g., content categories conceptualized by Bloom & Lahey, 1978), and phonological processes (introduced to child language by Stampe, 1969, 1972 and advanced by Ingram, 1974).

This concern with developmental sequences and underlying organization had a major impact on the conceptualization of short-term goal setting and the relationship between short- and long-term goals. The developmental psycholinguistic approach brought a child-centered perspective to the planning of goals and goal sequences. This approach is considered to be child centered because researchers writing from this perspective have recommended that data from normal language development be used as a basis for goal planning in a language intervention program (Bloom & Lahey, 1978; McLean & Snyder-McLean, 1978; Miller, 1984; Muma, 1978).

This child-centered orientation marked a departure from behaviorism's adult-centered focus. From a behavioral perspective, goals are based on adults' intuitions about the steps required for the performance of practical tasks (Lahey, 1988; Moses & Papish, 1984).

The Roots of Developmental Psycholinguists.   Jean Piaget, Noam Chomsky, and Lois Bloom were most influential in the evolution of developmental psycholinguistics.

Piaget. It was largely Piaget's influence that set the stage for the child-centered orientation that characterizes developmental psycholinguistics. For more than fifty years, Piaget conducted systematic observations of children as a means of understanding how they conceived of their world (Gallagher & Reid, 1984).

Equally influential was Piaget's conceptualization of cognitive development as proceeding in a stagelike fashion. Piaget's descriptions of cognitive stages brought to light the idea that observable behavior may be driven by an underlying organization (Piaget, 1971). These descriptions made child specialists aware that certain developmental achievements may be prerequisite for others.

Chomsky. Chomsky's major contribution to developmental psycholinguistics stems from his conceptualization of organization underlying linguistic behavior. His early works on syntactic structures (Chomsky, 1959, 1965) and the phonological system (Chomsky & Halle, 1968) introduced a generative approach to the study of language. The generative approach conceptualized language production as the product of innately delimited systems of rules for organizing linguistic behavior. These rule systems could yield an infinite number of possible observable linguistic forms on one hand, and restrict differences among languages and children's behavior on the other. This generative paradigm inspired much research in language acquisition (e.g., Bellugi, 1967; Brown, 1968; Bloom, 1970; Smith, 1973; Stampe, 1973) and language disorders (e.g., Compton, 1970; Menyuk, 1964). The concern with parameters of organization underlying linguistic behavior continues to be viable across the various areas of speech and language with reference to syntax (e.g., Chomsky, 1982b; Pinker, 1989; van Riemsdijk & Williams, 1986), semantics (Braine, 1990), pragmatics (Cheng & Holyoak, 1985), and phonology (Elbert & Gierut, 1986; Ingram, 1976, 1989).

Bloom. The early work of Lois Bloom reveals the integration of Piagetian and Chomskian influences (see especially Bloom, 1970). Bloom and her colleagues provided the major impetus for a child-centered orientation to the description of normal and disordered language (see Bloom & Lahey, 1978; Lahey, 1988.) The taxonomies of linguistic organization that Bloom and her colleagues used to describe child language were derived from observations of children learning to talk. These taxonomies differed significantly from those of other researchers because they reflected the way in which *children* organized language. This organization was captured by reference to the way in which form interacts with content and use in each utterance produced by a child. Until this point, investigators such as Lee (1974), Menyuk (1969), and Tyack and Gottsleben (1974) proposed taxonomies and learning sequences for children's language that were not driven by child data and made reference only to language form.

Developmental Categories of Behavior. Bloom and Lahey's *Language Development and Language Disorders* (1978) was the landmark work that introduced the psycholinguistic approach to speech-language pathology. A central feature of Bloom and Lahey's text was the description of language content, form, and use in terms of developmental categories of behavior. Content categories (e.g., existence, action, locative action) are an example of one set of such developmental categories. Appendices A–1 and A–2 present taxonomies of content, form, and use interactions originally formulated by Bloom and Lahey (1978) and later expanded by Lahey (1988) for planning language development goals.

Developmental categories have been described in other linguistic areas as well. Phonologic processes such as stopping, final consonant deletion, and voicing (Ingram, 1976) are categories of sound change. The functions that verbs and prepositions serve in the production of well-formed sentences (e.g., assigning case and theme) are categories of syntactic relations (Hsu, Cairns, Eisenberg, & Schlisselberg, 1989; Hyams, 1986; Pinker, 1989). Such categories are presumed to represent natural parameters of organization inherent in linguistic behavior. These categories are developmental in the following sense: It is believed that in the natural course of development or maturation they appear in children's behavioral repertoires or are eliminated in a specifiable sequence.

These developmental structures (e.g., phonological processes, content categories) have great explanatory power. Their very existence explains the child's tendency to generate a variety of utterances embodying a common set of features. This capacity for generating a variety of utterances embodying a common set of features is termed *generativity* (Chomsky, 1959).

Consider the content category *existence*. It stands for all utterances that signify that specific objects exist (e.g., "that's a cat," "this is a dog," "it's an elephant"). Similarly, the content category *action* is embodied in all utterances that encode the idea that somebody or something is moving (e.g., "mommy eat", "daddy is jumping"). Similarly, a child who exhibits use of the phonological process *stopping* would be producing fricative consonants (e.g., /f/, /s/) as stops ([p], [t]).

The Influence of Developmental Psycholinguistics on Our Model of Intervention Planning. The developmental psycholinguistic movement profoundly influenced the way in which we conceptualize and formulate long- and short-term goals and the way in which we view their relationship. We view the achievement of both long- and short-term goals as developmental accomplishments.

That is, in the course of intervention planning, we endeavor to facilitate the development of linguistic or neuromotor organization.

We write short-term goals in terms of developmental categories of behavior that reflect the influence of neuromotor or linguistic organization (e.g., content, form, use). The following are examples of short-term goals: "Stacey will code existence with two words" (form-content interaction goal), "Jason will eliminate the processes of fronting and stopping" (phonologic goal), "Peter will produce two word utterances fluently in response to what and where questions" (fluency goal), "Lisa will maintain appropriate volume for the production of complex sentences used for a variety of pragmatic functions" (voice goal). In order to realize long-term goals, we prioritize short-term goals based on sequences that have been observed in the development of children's linguistic and neuromotor organization (see Bloom & Lahey, 1978; Lahey, 1988; Andrews, 1986).

There is yet another way in which developmental psycholinguistics has influenced our intervention model. The principal concern of the psycholinguistic approach is with language *production* (Lahey, 1988). As a result, we write short-term goals in expressive-language terms (i.e., as acquisition of categories of behavior, such as the coding of content categories or the use of syntactic structures). Our reasons are best summarized by Lahey (1988), who wrote that "contrary to the expectations of many, comprehension does not always precede production. A sequence of development related to comprehension cannot yet even be approximated" (p. 182).

Although we do not write long- and short-term goals that target receptive language or comprehension, these modalities are stressed in procedural planning—particularly at the session level of intervention planning. Procedural planning involves designing a context in which language learning is facilitated. A preferred design is one in which the clinician codes content-form interactions that reflect the child's presumed intent. As Lahey pointed out, "Input is stressed throughout. Thus, comprehension is being facilitated at the same time as production" (p. 182). We concur. Comprehension and reception will

---

BOX 2-2. THE INFLUENCE OF PSYCHOLINGUISTIC THEORY ON PHASES OF INTERVENTION PLANNING

	Phases Influenced	
Influential Principles	*Goals*	*Procedures*
1. Formulate goals with reference to developmental or neuromotor categories of behavior	All phases	
2. Prioritize goals with reference to a developmental sequence	Short-term session	

again be discussed in the chapter on session goals. Box 2–2 summarizes the influence of psycholinguistic theory on intervention planning.

INFORMATION–PROCESSING THEORIES

The beginnings. Developmental psycholinguistic theory was not the only influence on speech-language intervention during the 1960s. An historical review of information-processing theory conducted by Wiederholt (cited by Reid & Hresko, 1981), traced a line of thinking that has its foundations in the works of Gall, Broca, Jackson, and Goldstein, dating back to the late nineteenth and early twentieth centuries. Broca and Gall were among the first researchers who attempted to find the location of language functions in the brain. Jackson (1915) and Goldstein (1948) were interested in the effect that traumatic war-related brain injury had on language functioning and how the brain compensated for such insult.

This interest in the relation between brain functioning and language behavior influenced a number of researchers working with children with language disorders in the late 1940s and 1950s. The influence of Goldstein and Jackson is especially obvious in the work of Cruickshank (1967), Myklebust and Johnson (1967), Strauss and Lehtinen (1947), and Orton (1937). These authors wrote about perceptual-motor aspects of language disorders in children who are now commonly described as exhibiting learning disabilities. (For detailed reviews of this historical progression, see Hammill & Bartel, 1985; Reid & Hresko, 1981.)

The ideas of Broca, Jackson, and Goldstein, their contemporaries and critics (e.g., Head, Marie, Wernicke), and those child-language specialists who were influenced by these pioneers motivated the formulation of a number of theories to explain how information is processed when people receive and express language. Models of information processing developed by Osgood and Miron (1963) and Wepman, Jones, Bock, and Van Pelt (1960) were particularly influential in the application of information-processing theories to assessment and intervention planning in speech-language pathology. These models identified modes of information processing as the bases of language functioning and language disorders. Modes of information-processing that were cited include visual and auditory memory, auditory discrimination, visual association, visual reception, and visual closure. Auditory processes, in particular, have received a great deal of attention in the speech-language literature (Aram & Nation, 1982). Table 2–2 exemplifies the variety of auditory processes that have been identified.

Osgood's model of information processing was the basis for a number of assessment formats that dominated the field of speech and language for more than a decade. The McCarthy Scales (McCarthy, 1974) and the Illinois Test of Psycholinguistic Abilities (Kirk, McCarthy, & Kirk, 1968) were among the most widely used. A second generation of assessment instruments continues to reflect

TABLE 2–2.   A Search for Auditory Processes

A major thrust of the writings relevant to the perceptual processing stage and child language disorders has been to search for and define a series of auditory processes. Following is a listing of auditory processes as viewed by several major professionals working in this area:

Sanders (1977) Aspects of Auditory Processing

1. Awareness of acoustic stimuli
2. Localization
3. Attention
4. Differentiation between speech and nonspeech
5. Auditory discrimination
   a. Suprasegmental discrimination
   b. Segmental discrimination
6. Auditory memory
7. Sequencing
8. Auditory synthesis

Weener (1974) Basic Components and Measurement Procedures of Auditory Processing

1. Echoic memory
   a. Duration
2. Discriminative filter
   a. Selective attention
   b. Phoneme and word discrimination
3. Structural analyzer
   a. Utilization of linguistic structure

Chalfant and Scheffelin (1969) Auditory Processing Tasks

1. Attention to auditory stimuli
2. Sound versus no sound
3. Sound localization
4. Discriminating sounds varying on one acoustic dimension
5. Discriminating sound sequences varying on several acoustic dimensions
6. Auditory figure-ground selection
7. Associating sounds with sound sources

Eisenson (1972) Perceptual Functions Underlying Language Acquisition

1. Selectivity
2. Discrimination
3. Categorization
4. Perceptual defense
5. Proximal and distance reception
6. Sequencing

Wiig and Semel (1976) Auditory-Perceptual Processing

1. Attention
2. Localization
3. Figure-ground
4. Discrimination of nonverbal stimuli
5. Discrimination of verbal stimuli

(continued)

TABLE 2–2   *(continued)*

6. Sequencing
7. Synthesis: resistance to distortion
8. Segmentation and syllabication

Butler (1975) Subcomponents of Auditory Perception

1. Auditory vigilance
2. Figure-ground
3. Auditory analysis
4. Auditory discrimination
5. Auditory sequencing
6. Sequencing unrelated speech sounds
7. Intonation patterns
8. Auditory closure
9. Auditory synthesis
10. Auditory memory (for nonsense multisyllable words)
11. Auditory association

Bangs (1968) Avenues of Learning

1. Sensation
2. Perception
3. Memory-retrieval
4. Attention
5. Integration

From Aram D. M., and Nation, J. E. (1982). *Child language disorders.* St. Louis: C. V. Mosby, p. 92. Reprinted by permission of C. V. Mosby and authors.

the influence of information-processing precepts—for instance, the CELF-R (Semel, Wiig, & Secord, 1987), TOLD (Newcomer & Hammill, 1982), and the Revised Detroit (Hammill, 1985).

On-going research. There are several areas of research in information processing that have been and continue to be pursued. One of these areas is the effect of impaired rapid processing of auditory information on the discrimination of linguistic stimuli (Tallal & Percy, 1978, Tallal; 1988). Another area involves the specification of cortical and subcortical locations of specific language processes, hemispheric asymmetries and right- versus left-brain functions (e.g., Geschwind, 1984; Kirk, 1983; Penfield & Roberts, 1959; Tallal, 1975, 1988).

A third area involves the development of theories of memory. These include multiple-store models (e.g., Atkinson & Shiffrin, 1971; Loftus & Loftus, 1976), depth-of-processing models (e.g., Craik & Lockhart, 1972; Craik & Tulving, 1975), and encoding-strategy models (e.g., Reiser, 1986; Shank & Abelson, 1977). These models of memory stress how individuals go about transferring material from short-term to long-term memory and retrieving information. These models also address what happens to material in the process. The retrieval of information from long-term memory storage has been attributed to specific strategies and procedures that individuals use to direct searches for information (Reiser, 1986). The transfer of information from short- to long-term memory has been attributed to the operation of knowledge structures on new information (e.g., Potter, 1990). Knowledge structures are essentially networks of ideas and expectations derived from past experiences (see Galambos, Abelson, & Block, 1986; Gentner & Stevens, 1983; Nelson, 1986; Reid, 1988). Examples of knowledge structures (also termed scripts, schema, schemata) include impressions about going to a restaurant, visiting the doctor, and how electricity moves through a wire. (Note the overlap in the use of terms such as *schema* in the developmental-psycholinguistic and information-processing literature.)

In addition to the traditional modes of information processing discussed above, researchers continue to identify still other modes, such as scanning, attentional, and motivational mechanisms (DeRuiter & Wansart, 1982; Sternberg, 1984).

Modern theories of memory have had significant influences on intervention planning—especially in the areas of specific language impairment and learning disabilities (e.g., see DeRuiter & Wansart, 1982; Reid, 1988; Reid & Hresko, 1981). The impact on intervention planning is evidenced by an emphasis on making material meaningful and relevant to children's experiences and on teaching children information-processing strategies. The clinical applicability of teaching children processing strategies has been demonstrated for articulation (see Shriberg & Kwiatkowski, 1990, for summary of this literature) and listening and reading comprehension (Dollaghan & Kaston, 1986; Pressley, Forrest-Pressley, Elliot-Faust, & Miller, 1985; Reid, 1988).

The influence of information-processing theories on our model of intervention planning. On one hand, the influence of information-processing theory to intervention planning is limited by the nonobservability of processes such as auditory discrimination and memory. We try to write goals in terms of behavior that can be observed and measured. On the other hand, it is generally accepted—and it makes sense—that children must process information if they are to learn from experience (Aram & Nation, 1982; Nation & Aram, 1984; Wiig & Semel, 1984). Thinking about information processes can be helpful in (a) identifying goals to target at the session phase of intervention planning that involve the processing of information and (b) designing contexts to facilitate learning—although session plans will necessarily be written in terms of observable performance.

The decision to write a session goal to target auditory discrimination exemplifies the first application of information-processing theory to intervention planning. Consider a child who regularly substitutes /t/ for /k/ and whose short-term goal is to eliminate the phonologic process of fronting (i.e., to produce the phoneme /k/ correctly and spontaneously in all appropriate linguistic contexts). It seems reasonable to expect that that child must learn to discriminate among sensorimotor features that contribute to producing the phonemes /t/ and /k/ in order to be able to produce /k/. This consideration of the process of discrimination can lead to a session goal targeting auditory discrimination and written in terms of observable performance: for example, "Stephanie will put a block in a bucket in response to words beginning with /k/, given the oral presentation of word pairs beginning with /t/ and /k/." (See Tallal, 1988, regarding information-processing mechanisms involved in making phoneme discriminations.)

Another application of information-processing theory is to goal and procedure planning at the session level. We believe that clinicians need to be concerned with factors that may have an impact upon the retention and recall of information and, in turn, upon communication *performance*. A clinician would want systematically to control such factors in intervention planning. The purpose is to facilitate the acquisition of new behaviors or to generalize these behaviors to new situations. These *performance factors*, which are discussed at length in Chapter 6, comprise a number of nonlinguistic and linguistic variables. Primary among the nonlinguistic factors are meaningfulness, functionality, and manipulability of material for children. For example, a consideration of such nonlinguistic factors could influence procedure planning for the session goal of using four different locative action and action verbs (involving word retrieval). We might attempt to achieve this goal in an action oriented context, such as making chocolate pudding.

A major linguistic factor affecting communication performance is the complexity of language expected of the child. For example, an early session goal directed toward fluent speech might target fluency in short phrases rather than complex sentences. The purpose would be to simplify the performance demands on the child.

In sum, the efficient processing of information appears to be an essential ingredient in language learning. Thus, we consider the modification of or compensation for impaired processing modes throughout intervention planning. Box 2–3 summarizes the influence of information-processing theories on intervention planning.

BOX 2–3. THE INFLUENCE OF INFORMATION-PROCESSING THEORY ON PHASES OF INTERVENTION PLANNING

	Influential Principles	Goals	Procedures
		Phases Influenced	
1.	Consider information processes such as perception, discrimination, and information retrieval in formulating goals and procedures	Session	Session
2.	Consider aspects of linguistic and nonlinguistic complexity that affect communicative performance in formulating goals and procedures	Session	Session

Departures from information-processing theories. Although we consider the processing of information in devising session goals, we do not write session goals in information-processing terms. That is because one cannot directly observe or quantify how information is being processed (i.e., perceived, remembered, sequenced, and discriminated; Chiesa, 1992). The law PL 94–142 and its ethic of accountability demand that session goals be written in terms of behavior that is observable and quantifiable. Thus, we write session goals in terms of observable behavior. A session goal that involves feature discrimination for the child with the articulation problem described above might read as follows: "Jose will group pictures representing words beginning with either a /t/ or a /k/ according to the initial phoneme after the examiner produces the words." Session goals involving memory are recast in terms of the spontaneous production or recall of information (vocabulary, semantic, or syntactic structures). For example, "Margaret will label foods in the context of play with toy foods." (See also our discussion above of writing goals in terms of production as opposed to reception.)

COGNITIVE LEARNING THEORIES

Both Carrow-Woolfolk (1988) and Nelson (1993) have argued that no single theory exists that accounts for all aspects of language learning (see also Kamhi, 1993). Our intervention-planning model supports the premise that various learning theories taken together provide an integrated view of language learning. We recognize the usefulness of different theoretical positions in accounting for the acquisition of different facets of language.

In the section on behaviorism, we described the way in which operant theory accounts for some aspects of language learning and thereby influences procedural planning. Operant techniques were viewed as applicable for strengthening or weakening observable behavior. However, language learning and use manifest a hierarchical complexity that lies beyond the scope of operant theory. More specifically, linguistic behavior involves ideation (Piaget, 1962; Sinclair, 1970) and language-specific organization (e.g., syntactic, semantic, pragmatic; Bloom & Lahey, 1978; Chomsky, 1965; Ingram, 1989)—which demand an alternative developmental explanation. Two types of cognitive learning theories (*constructivist* and *social*) provide such an explanation; they guide us both in goal and procedural planning.

1. *"Constructivist"* theories are based on the work of Piaget and Inhelder (e.g., Inhelder, Sinclair, & Bovet, 1974; Karmiloff-Smith & Inhelder, 1975; Piaget, 1985). These theories are identified by their emphasis on children's contributions to their own development. These contributions are through self-generated cognitive activities, such as setting goals, making distinctions and relations among objects and events, recognizing and solving problems, and inventing strategies and procedures to achieve goals. These same self-generated activities have been identified as contributing to language learning

(Bates et al., 1979; Bloom, Beckwith, Capatides, & Hafitz, 1988; Ferguson & Macken, 1980; Ingram, 1989; Klein, 1981b; Locke, 1983).

2. *Social-cognitive learning* theories emphasize how learning is embedded in a social matrix. The focus on learning in a social matrix has included (a) how caregivers (parents and teachers) mediate language learning in children and (b) how interactions among children themselves facilitate learning.

Mediation may range along a continuum from adult-directed to adult-responsive interactions (van Kleeck & Richardson, 1986). Adult-directed interactions encourage the child to attend to linguistic forms and relations modeled by the caregiver. Adult-responsive interactions reflect caregiver sensitivity to the child's endeavors to make social contact—for example, responsiveness to the child's gaze and communication intents. Vygotsky's (1987) concept of instruction within a *zone of proximal development,* Bruner's (1983) notion of *scaffolding,* and Nelson's (1986) ideas about the development of *event knowledge* endeavor to account for language acquisition within a social-learning framework. These concepts and their application to language learning will be explored below.

Interactions among children also serve to motivate and mediate language learning in a number of ways. Children pose problems for one another, serve as resources for one another, and engage one another in games and conversations (Duckworth, 1976; Farber, N. G., 1990; Forman & Hill, 1984).

The Influence of Cognitive Learning Theories on Our Model of Intervention Planning. We have derived a number of principles of intervention planning from the cognitive learning theories cited above.

1. *Constructivist theories.* Constructivist theories support the premise that children learn language best when intervention contexts and interactions are commensurate with their developmental level, experiences, and interests (Bloom & Lahey, 1978). Under these conditions a child is most likely to pay attention to, remember, and reflect on his or her activities (Duckworth, 1972). This premise applies to procedural planning with specific reference to the selection of materials and tasks.

A second constructivist principle is that language acquisition is facilitated by goals that children set for themselves and procedures (strategies) that they devise for accomplishing their goals. Children's goals may interact positively with speech-language goals that we set for them. For example, *a child's* goal of operating a mechanical toy police car can provide a context for the achievement of the *clinician's* goals of getting the child to code existence, action, and locative action. In procedural planning the clinician prepares to provoke children to set such goals as contexts for language learning. The clinician specifies the child's *anticipated activity* as the *context* in the session-goal statement. (See Chapter 6.)

The procedures or strategies that children devise for accomplishing speech-language goals have been described extensively in the literature. These strategies have been described in the area of phonology with reference to the simplification of word productions (e.g., Ferguson, 1978; Klein, 1981a; for reviews of major strategy types, see Edwards & Shriberg, 1983) and the selection of early lexical items (Klein, 1982; Stoel-Gammon & Cooper, 1984). Children's strategies in the area of single-word form-content interactions have been characterized as "over or under generalizations" (e.g., Kamhi, 1982; Rescorla, 1980). Particular preferences have also been observed for the syntactic expression of meaning relations (i.e., pronominal versus nominal reference; Bloom, Lightbown, & Hood, 1975) and for the arrangement of two-word combinations (Braine, 1963).

Strategies or preferences imply an active participation in speech and language learning on the part of the child (Carrow-Woolfolk, 1988; Ferguson, 1978; Ingram, 1989; Klein, 1981a, 1981b; Menyuk, Menn, & Silber, 1986; Shatz & Ebling, 1991). This leads us to conclude that the planning of intervention goals and procedures should take into account the child's own approach to language learning. For example, a child's preference for bilabials during babbling might suggest that the clinician introduce early lexical items with initial /b/ and /m/.

A third principle of constructivism concerns children's problem-solving activities. Children's efforts to resolve problems that interfere with their goals can advance language learning. While engaged in problem solving, children tend to notice information they may have overlooked before. In this way they become aware of objects, actions, attributes, events, and their relations—a foundation for language production. Furthermore, common language-learning challenges, such as pronouncing multisyllabic utterances (Klein, 1981a, 1982) or learning the names of things (Rescorla, 1980), may be impetus for devising the production strategies discussed above. Clinicians, therefore, need to consider designing procedures that permit children to take initiative in recognizing and resolving problems.

Finally, constructivist theories have drawn our attention to a fourth principle: Relationships exist between cognitive achievements and linguistic achievements (Rice & Kemper, 1984; also see Box 1–3, Chap. 1). For example, much has been written about one major cognitive milestone, object permanence, as a prerequisite for the onset of language (e.g., Gopnik, 1984; Gopnick & Meltzoff, 1984; Tomasello & Fararr, 1984). Other cognitive achievements have also been cited as precursory to the acquisition of later-occurring linguistic structures, such as two-word utterances (McCune-Nicolich, 1981), conditionals (Byrnes, 1988; Braine, 1990; Moses, Klein, & Altman, 1990; van Kleeck, 1984), and parameters of government and binding syntax (Pinker, 1990).

We do not maintain that there is a causal relation between the achievement of a cognitive stage (in the traditional Piagetian sense) and the acquisition of specific linguistic structures. Instead, we take the position that there is a more general relation between cognition and language. We believe that children need to be aware of—and attach meaning to—objects, actions, attributes, events, and their relations in order to talk about them (Bloom & Lahey, 1978). Certain cognitive achievements may contribute to the development of this awareness and meaning. We summarized these achievements in Chapter 1, Box 1–3. They include the establishment of cause and effect relations, tool use, and pretend play.

Within our model of intervention planning, this fundamental relation between cognition and language influences both goal setting and procedural planning. Session goals leading to the accomplishment of early content-form interactions may need to address the cognitive skills associated with these linguistic structures. Furthermore, in the course of procedural planning the clinician will design interactions that promote the development of these cognitive skills. This will involve the selection of developmentally appropriate materials and tasks that stimulate constructive activity.

2. *Social learning theories.* The implications for intervention planning of social learning theories both parallel and depart from those of constructivist theories. The parallel implication is the need to consider a child's developmental level in goal and procedure planning. This construct follows from the work of Vygotsky, a seminal social-learning theorist. He proposed that the influence of caretakers on language learning occurs within a *zone of proximal development*–Wertsch, 1984). This zone is that area between the child's developmental level as manifested in spontaneous behavior and the level he or she can potentially achieve with adult guidance. Sensitivity to a child's developmental level is also implied in Bruner's conceptualization of *scaffolding.* This term describes how mothers manage communication episodes with their children. Mothers appear to be sensitive to their children's changing needs for communication supports (scaffolds). As children become more adept at initiating and maintaining communicative interchanges, mothers' interactive style is modified. Mothers allow children to initiate more frequently and, at the same time, expect more advanced linguistic skill.

Social learning theory departs from constructivist theory in the emphasis on the importance of adult modeling and verbal guidance as well as peer interactions in children's learning. The importance of the adult role is captured by van Kleeck and Richardson (1986) in their delineation of four key language-learning situations:

1. A positive and supportive relationship between the adult and child;
2. a willingness and skill in guiding and filling in for the child as learning occurs while simultaneously giving the child as much control as she or he is capable of handling;
3. skill at minimizing risk for the child until she or he has achieved some level of competence and confidence in task performance;
4. a gradual internalization by the child of the adult's thinking out loud about a specific task (p. 36).

The focus on modeling and adult guidance provides an orientation for procedural planning. It emphasizes the need for clinicians to reflect on the nature and consequences of an adult's (clinician's or caregiver's) input to a child. This complements the constructivist focus on the child's self-generated activities.

As noted above, social learning theories also highlight the importance for learning of children's interactions with their peers. In planning procedures, clinicians also need to become adept at designing contexts that promote interactions among children in pairs or small groups (Kamii & DeVries, 1993; Forman & Hill, 1984; Fosnot, 1991). The recent movement toward providing speech-language intervention in classroom contexts places special emphasis on this aspect of social learning theory (Moses & Siskin-Spector, 1991). The influence of cognitive learning theories on intervention planning is summarized in Box 2–4.

THE PRAGMATICS MOVEMENT

In the 1970s and 1980s, the pragmatics movement in the field of speech-language pathology, influenced by social-cognitive learning theory, reestablished the idea that language is embedded in a social matrix. This movement taught us that children do not talk about objects of interest in isolation. They

---

BOX 2–4.   THE INFLUENCE OF COGNITIVE LEARNING THEORY ON PHASES OF INTERVENTION PLANNING

| | Phases Influenced | |
Influential Principles	*Goals*	*Procedures*
Constructivist		
1. Formulate goals and procedures with reference to developmental level, experiences, and interests	All phases	All phases
2. Help children set goals for themselves to facilitate speech-language acquisition	Session	All phases
3. Encourage children to devise strategies for accomplishing their goals	Session	All phases
4. Address relevant cognitive achievements when targeting the development of meaning (or language content)	Short-term (prelinguistic) Session	All phases
Social Learning		
1. Formulate goals and procedures with reference to developmental level, experiences, and interests	All phases	All phases
2. Model target behavior	All phases	
3. Encourage children to interact with peers to facilitate goal achievement	All phases	

communicate in the context of social interactions, often for socially and emotionally driven reasons. This orientation underscored the importance of caregiver-child interactions for language development and broadened our awareness of the range of issues that need to be considered in language intervention.

The study of pragmatics in child language has been approached from two major perspectives: (a) the various purposes for using language and (b) the rules for engaging in conversation. The purposes of linguistic expression have been delineated in the writings of many child language experts with reference to *speech acts* (e.g., Dore, 1974) or functions (Halliday, 1975; Bloom & Lahey, 1978; Lund & Duchan, 1988). This area of pragmatics examines the reasons why children talk (e.g., to comment, request, respond, direct attention). A comprehensive list of these functions may be found in Lahey, 1988.

The pragmatics movement made us aware that language comprises rules for use as well as for form and content. Children need to learn the rules of language use in order to engage appropriately in conversation (i.e., discourse). Hymes (1971) aptly summarized the nature of these rules in his description of a competent language user as one who knows about "who can say what, in what way, where and when, by what means and to whom" (p. 15). In pragmatic assessments, rules underlying conversational competence may be evaluated with reference to (a) presupposition (i.e., being aware of the amount of information the listener has), (b) topic initiation and maintenance, (c) turn-taking behaviors and talking time, (d) deixis, and (e) repair of communication breakdown and failure (Lahey, 1988; Roth & Spekman, 1984a, 1984b).

With the pragmatics movement, two major factors influencing pragmatic performance were identified: (a) knowledge about self and others, including the ability to distinguish speaker from listener, to take others' perspectives, and to understand communicative roles; and (b) the nonlinguistic and linguistic context.

Schiff-Myers (1983) demonstrated one way that knowing about self and others affects pragmatic performance—the acquisition of pronominal deictic terms. Schiff-Myers's daughter learned the appropriate use of the pronouns *I, me,* and *you* only when she learned to role play with her doll. Her insight, related to a differentiation of the pronouns, was illustrated dramatically one morning at breakfast. While eating and referring to herself, Lauren said to her father, "You eating." Her father replied, "No, I'm not eating, you are." Lauren responded, "I eating. You am I" (p. 399). Similarly, the ability to take another's perspective was viewed as a basic skill in the acquisition of the contrast between *a* and *the* (Emslie & Stevenson, 1981; Karmiloff-Smith, 1979). Knowledge about self and others also influences presupposition, such as providing enough information in narrative presentations (Lahey, 1988).

Context can influence what a child says in a number of ways. Perhaps the best example of the influence of *nonlinguistic* context comes from Bloom & Lahey's (1978) description of their subject, Peter. Peter's spontaneous speaking in the context of play far exceeded his imitative ability when he was asked to reproduce the sentences that he, himself, had uttered while playing. He reduced these sentences considerably. The authors refer to an important difference between play and imitation to explain the discrepancy in Peter's productions. Play involves the intention to speak and the contextual support for the utterance, both of which are lacking in imitation. Further examples of the influence of nonlinguistic context on language production have been observed in children's modification of speech and voice registers. Children change registers as they engage in role playing, or as they talk to babies versus adults (Bloom & Lahey, 1978). In addition, Schiff (1979) reported that hearing children of deaf parents spoke differently to their parents than they did to hearing adults.

The *linguistic context* has been investigated in studies of discourse. Much research over the past decade into patterns of discourse between adult and child have revealed ways in which adult utterances influence children's linguistic behavior. The way children use adult utterances changes with development (Bloom, Miller, & Hood, 1975; Bloom, Rocissano, & Hood, 1976). Children become more adept at relating their comments to statements made by adults. They do so by making their comments contingent on adults' statements, adding information appropriately, and recoding (see Lahey, 1988, for a comprehensive guide to changes in language use). In addition, children learn that particular linguistic contexts obligate specific linguistic forms. For example, with reference to the linguistic context, children do not produce full sentences when the interlocutor's question requires a one-word response. Box 2–5 summarizes the influence of pragmatic theory on intervention planning.

The influence of the pragmatics movement on our model of intervention planning. The pragmatics movement has influenced our model in the areas of both goal and procedure planning. In terms of goal setting, the pragmatics movement suggests potential intervention targets at all three phases of the management plan (i.e., long-term, short-term, and session phases). Areas of consideration include the performance of a variety of language functions and the demonstration of discourse conventions.

Pragmatic considerations are also crucial in the development of intervention procedures. Pragmatic theory emphasizes the essential social ingredient of language learning. Social interactions require detailed planning. As noted above, it must be remembered that nonlinguistic and linguistic contexts influence or even determine a client's response. As a consequence, a clinician must be aware of the type of response that is likely to be evoked by his or her own actions. For example, a clinician interested in a complex utterance might interact with a child during play with toys as opposed to asking the child to imitate an utterance. Additionally, a clinician interested in a child's production of the auxiliary *is* would be inviting failure if the child was asked, "What is the lady in this picture doing?" Language conventions dictate that a response lacking an auxiliary is acceptable. The situation would be more optimistic if the clinician asked, "What is happening in this picture?" In the second case the auxiliary is obligatory.

Above all, a clinician must develop a relationship with the client that supports a nurturant communication environment. Two recent articles describe

---

BOX 2–5. THE INFLUENCE OF PRAGMATIC THEORY ON PHASES OF INTERVENTION PLANNING

| | Phases Influenced | |
Influential Principles	*Goals*	*Procedures*
1. Target language skills that affect communication success	All phases	
2. Target discourse skills that affect communication success	All phases	
3. Consider nonlinguistic and linguistic factors that may influence performance of target behavior	Session	All phases
4. Plan statements and questions that obligate specific forms or functions in the child's response	Session	Session
5. Provide communication environments that support the development of form-content-use interactions		All phases

---

the essence of such a relationship, how it fosters communication ease and differs from a more traditional, rigid environment (Cole & Dale, 1986; Duchan & Weitzner-Lin, 1987).

There is a final implication of pragmatic theory that may be drawn from the close relation between pragmatic and social learning theories. The development of pragmatic skills—as well as other aspects of language—may best be facilitated as children interact with one another and with caregivers. Thus, procedural planning often involves promoting interactions among children and between children and their parents. Such interactions are excellent contexts for achieving goals such as turn taking, topic sharing, and the establishment of reciprocal eye gaze.

SUMMARY

This chapter reviewed major theories of language and language learning that have contributed to our model of the intervention planning process: behavioral, psycholinguistic, information-processing, constructivist, social, and pragmatic. We demonstrated how these theories had differential effects on our view of the formulation of goals and procedures at each of the three levels of intervention planning.

Principles derived from behavioral theory and shaped by PL 94–142 provide a framework for the formulation of session goals and the conceptualization of the connection between session goals and the next step—short-term goals. Our session goals are written in observable terms and include reference to the context in which the behavior is expressed. We stress the importance of a speci-fied connection between different goal levels (i.e., the sequence of steps neces-sary to get from one level to the next). The influence of behaviorism is also felt in procedural planning. We consider the conditions under which the child is ex-pected to respond and the potential effect of alternative contingencies. Finally, as is consistent with a behavioral orientation, we apply a uniform set of princi-ples to guide intervention planning across disorders.

The developmental psycholinguistics movement influenced the way we conceptualize and formulate long- and short-term goals and the way in which we view their relationship. We view the achievement of long- and short-term goals as developmental accomplishments in linguistic organization. Thus, we write long- and short-term goals in terms of linguistic categories. To achieve long-term goals, short-term goals are prioritized according to a developmental sequence based on research with children learning to talk.

Aspects of information-processing and cognitive learning theories con-tribute to the formulation of session goals. It is at this phase that the main-taining factors of a child's communication disorder are targeted most directly. In attempting to achieve changes in linguistic organization (phase 1 and 2) we need to modify or compensate for presumed maintaining factors of the disor-der at phase 3. The domains of information processing (e.g., discrimination, retrieval, memory) and cognitive skills development have been identified as two of the areas of maintaining factors (also see Chapter 1).

Constructivist and social learning theories have primarily affected our view of procedural planning. In keeping with a constructivist approach, we believe that children learn language best when intervention contexts and in-teractions are commensurate with their development level, experiences, and interests. We also adhere to a second constructivist principle, which con-cerns children's problem-solving activities. As children work out solutions, they become aware of aspects of their environment and their own behav-ior—a foundation for language development. Social learning theory em-phasizes the impact of adults (therapists and caretakers) and children's peers on language acquisition. Consequently, we are reminded that clini-cians need to reflect on the nature of social contexts and the consequences of such contexts for the child.

The pragmatics movement has influenced our conceptualization of both goal and procedure planning. With reference to goal planning, language functions and conversational rules become potential intervention targets. In terms of procedural planning, interpersonal interactions and the effects of nonlinguistic and linguistic contexts become significant considerations.

In the next chapter we will introduce you to four children with different communication disorders. We will follow these children in subsequent chap-ters as we illustrate the three phases of intervention planning.

3

Baseline Data and Intervention Planning

In this chapter we introduce four children who require speech-language intervention: Darryl, Seth, Patty, and Alice. We describe these children with reference to a communicative profile generated from the results of their performance on a set of selected formal and informal procedures. In subsequent chapters, we will develop intervention plans for each of these children based on these data. In doing so, we will demonstrate the implementation of our intervention planning model. Before introducing the children we will discuss the relationship between assessment and intervention planning.

RELATIONS BETWEEN ASSESSMENT AND INTERVENTION PLANNING

We view the speech-language evaluation as preparation for intervention planning. Therefore, information needed to plan intervention should be anticipated when designing and interpreting a speech-language evaluation. Intervention planning relies on information about a child's (a) speech-language behavior and (b) performance in areas that may be maintaining a communication disorder. Information about current performance relevant to intervention planning may be termed *baseline data*. Baseline data will derive from formal testing and observation as well as background information from informants and referral sources.

Recall that our model of intervention planning represents speech-language functioning as a product of content, form, and use interactions, and that we think of content, form, and use in developmental terms (e.g., content categories, syntactic structures, phonological processes). Recall, too, that we consider deficits in the domain of language learnability and three nonlinguistic variables (cognitive, sensorimotor, and psychosocial behavioral systems) as potentially maintaining a speech-language dysfunction. The child's current functioning in each of these areas, therefore, represents the baseline data needed for intervention planning.

Ideally, an assessment would be organized by the clinician responsible for the intervention with reference to these data. Frequently, however, the speech-language pathologist assigned to carry out intervention has been given the results of an evaluation that do not include appropriate baseline data. In such cases, further assessment may be necessary to fill in the gaps.

We have developed three forms that can be used by the clinician to summarize the selection of assessment procedures and the application of results to intervention planning: (a) the diagnostic-procedure form, which outlines the procedures to be used in assessment (Form B-1); (b) the baseline data form, which presents the results of assessment (Form B-2); and (c) the management plan, which demonstrates the application of results to goal and procedure planning (Form B-3; for all three forms, See Appendix B). These forms will be discussed further as the data from the three cases are addressed.

Standardized and Nonstandardized Assessments

Assessment batteries generally comprise both standardized, norm-referenced and nonstandardized, criterion-referenced procedures. Information from each type of procedure serves a specific function relevant to intervention planning.

Standardized Instruments. We utilize standardized, norm-referenced measures primarily to document a speech-language disorder in need of intervention, as mandated by PL 94–142 and subsequent legislation. These public laws require that quantified data be the basis for the classification of children as speech and hearing handicapped for admission to intervention programs supported by public funds.

Standardized, norm-referenced assessments quantify linguistic performance: that is, they yield numerical data (e.g., percentiles and language ages) to be used to compare a child's performance on a set of tasks to the performance of his or her normally achieving peers. Such assessment instruments are aptly termed *standardized*, because they strictly control test-taking contexts (which are generally pictorial or verbal), the instructions clinicians present to clients, time constraints, and scoring procedures.

Standardized, norm-referenced instruments yield information about the mastery of particular linguistic skills, such as the ability to define vocabulary words. They do not provide ready insight into the developmental status of linguistic and nonlinguistic behavioral systems. Thus, we need to supplement information from standardized testing with information about the child's developmental status; such information is generally attainable through the administration of nonstandardized assessment procedures.

Nonstandardized Instruments. We rely on nonstandardized assessment procedures for much of the baseline data that will be used for intervention planning. That is because nonstandardized approaches to assessment (e.g.,

Lahey, 1988; McCune-Nicolich, 1981; Uzgiris & Hunt, 1978) permit us to iden-tify the developmental status of language content, form, and use interactions and the developmental status of behavioral systems that may be maintaining a speech-language disorder (e.g., cognitive, sensorimotor).

Nonstandardized assessments of language functioning generally involve the collection of data in relatively "naturalistic" contexts—typically, as chil-dren play with caregivers. These assessments, devoid of rigid procedural con-straints, allow children to demonstrate the ability to engage in conversation (Bloom & Lahey, 1978) and to produce numerous examples of specific lin-guistic structures (Ingram, 1976). Language generated during spontaneous interactions tends to be more representative of children's communicative per-formance than language evoked through standardized test probes. That is be-cause spontaneous productions involve intentionality and are supported by meaningful linguistic and nonlinguistic contexts.

Case History Data. We collect background information about a child's sus-pected disorder during an initial interview with the child's caretakers (which may involve the completion of a questionnaire). Although information gathered dur-ing this interview process eventually contributes to intervention planning, it is first utilized in the assessment process in three significant ways. First, information from the interview (or questionnaire) will help orient the evaluator to the area(s) of speech-language that will require assessment. Second, information from an infor-mant will supplement baseline data regarding maintaining factors (i.e., history in the areas of birth, early development, health, family, and psychosocial behavior). Third, information from caregivers may orient the clinician to the child's pre-ferred learning style as well as to the kinds of materials and interactions that are motivating and that promote optimal performance. These types of information ob-tained through the initial contact with an informant are clearly specified in many of the popular textbooks on diagnostic procedures (e.g., Meitus & Weinberg, 1983; Nation & Aram, 1984). It is the knowledge gained about maintaining factors and about facilitative learning styles, materials, and interactions that makes back-ground information so important for intervention planning.

Additional Assessment Considerations

There are two additional considerations in collecting baseline data for in-tervention: (a) the context in which assessment is carried out and (b) the type of collaboration that the speech-language pathologist engages in with allied professionals to solicit information about maintaining factors—interdiscipli-nary or transdisciplinary.

Contexts. Observations of a client in different types of assessment con-texts give us important information about environments that may facilitate or challenge linguistic performance. Such information will be especially useful in writing session goals and in planning procedures across all phases of intervention planning. Both standardized and nonstandardized assessment procedures give us information about contexts that may facilitate or challenge linguistic performance. In this respect, both types of assessments provide information relevant to intervention planning.

As noted above, standard assessments are carried out in directive, linguistically biased environments. That is, children are usually seated at a table, questioned or directed by an adult, and asked to respond to symbolic stimuli only (e.g., pictures, questions, written words). Nonstandardized assessments are generally carried out in less directive, more naturalistic settings (i.e., while children play with toys or converse with others; Cole & Dale, 1986; Lund & Duchan, 1988; Norris & Hoffman, 1990).

We find that we need information about a child's linguistic performance in both directive, linguistically biased and less directive, naturalistic settings for writing goals (especially session goals) and for procedural planning. Such information provides direction for the specification of contexts in which a child is expected to produce target behavior. The specification of context is part of the goal statement produced at the session phase of intervention planning. In terms of procedural planning, information about assessment environments provides a basis for designing appropriate, facilitative intervention contexts (i.e., the types of clinical interactions that the child will tolerate) at all phases of intervention planning.

Take, for example, six-year-old Tanya. Her baseline data indicated that when she was observed playing with concrete objects she produced complex content-form interactions (coding temporal, causal, and adversative semantic relations). However, results of standardized testing indicated that she only produced simple 3+ constituent utterances in response to directives and pictorial stimuli that obligated complex sentences. Based on these data, the production of complex sentences in all pragmatic contexts (including directive contexts) was targeted in a long-term goal statement. A related session-goal statement read, "Tanya will talk about three experiences from earlier in the school day using temporal-narrative structure in response to the teacher's directive, "Tell me about __ " Related procedural statements indicated that Tanya be engaged in concrete play-oriented interactions, followed, after a specified period of time, by directives to recall past events in the absence of related concrete objects.

Transdisciplinary (Collaborative) Assessments.   As mentioned above, our model of intervention planning directs us to the identification of possible maintaining factors. Consequently, assessment procedures must provide a mechanism for identification and in-depth testing of the maintaining factors. Possible maintaining factors may be identified during routine administration of assessment procedures—e.g., a peripheral speech-mechanism exam for assessment of sensorimotor behavior. When an area of impairment is suspected or not clearly described in available baseline data, further assessment is recommended. For example, a child suspected of having a developmental motor dysfunction affecting postural support required for efficient vocalization would require a thorough sensorimotor evaluation. Comprehensive testing in this area falls within the domain of the physical therapist, the occupational therapist, or both.

There are two approaches to assessment that would permit the speech-language pathologist to learn about maintaining factors. The first approach we term interdisciplinary. This approach involves referring the child for independent testing by an allied professional (e.g., the physical therapist). Following this format, the speech-language pathologist would receive a written report of test results and would take this information into consideration when planning goals and procedures (i.e., positioning a child in a way that is most facilitative for speech production).

The second approach is transdisciplinary (Connor, Williamson, & Siepp, 1978; Linder, 1990) or *collaborative* (Dyer, Williams, & Luce, 1991; Moses & Siskin-Spector, 1991). This involves the simultaneous evaluation of a child by allied professionals. Thus, in the case of a child suspected of cerebral palsy, the physical therapist would join the speech-language pathologist in selecting and administering a battery of tests.

From our perspective, the transdisciplinary or collaborative approach is ideal (although not always an option). It most closely mirrors our view that linguistic and nonlinguistic factors interact in the language-learning process. Therefore, the more holistic and integrated the assessment, the more adequate and complete the information available for intervention planning. We will discuss collaboration for intervention planning in Chapter 7.

RESULTS OF EVALUATIONS OF FOUR CHILDREN

In the second part of this chapter, we present the results of an evaluation of linguistic performance by four children with speech-language disorders: Darryl, a five-year-old who presents with a language problem; Patty, a five-year-old with a fluency disorder; Seth, a twelve-year-old who manifests a severe phonologic disability; and Alice, a six-year-old with a voice problem. These baseline data are provided as reference material for utilization in subsequent chapters, where we will develop and illustrate the three phases of intervention planning by developing goals and procedures for Darryl, Patty, Seth, and Alice. The reader may wish to scan the material below at this point, or proceed to Chapter 4 and return to the baseline data as intervention plans are developed for each child.

Darryl

Darryl is a five-year-old boy who was referred for a speech-language evaluation by his parents. A speech-language evaluation was necessary for appropriate public school placement.

Darryl was initially evaluated at three years and two months of age. His parents voiced concern that he had a very limited vocabulary, had not begun speaking in sentences, and relied primarily on gestures and one-word utterances to convey messages. Birth, medical, and developmental histories were uneventful.

Darryl's parents are divorced. His mother is the primary caretaker. The evaluator noticed that Darryl's mother spoke with very low intensity, did not establish eye contact when engaged in conversation, and was often unintelligible due to lack of intensity and apparently imprecise articulation.

Darryl attended two years of preschool for children with language impairment. At this placement he received individual speech-language therapy three days a week for thirty-minute sessions. The focus was on facilitating content-form interactions according to the Bloom and Lahey (1978) framework. According to his speech-language pathologist, Darryl exhibits separation difficulties and avoids playing with other children. He demonstrates good nonverbal play skills (with blocks, cars, trucks) and engages in script play with adults (e.g., at a barber shop, at a restaurant). Verbal output during play is usually very limited and consists of requesting additional toys or directing the clinician's role in the game. Spontaneous comments about ongoing activities during his play have begun to emerge. Darryl frequently withdraws from activities when the language level is too high.

Based on the client history and the presenting communication difficulties, assessment was directed to the areas summarized on the chart in Table 3–1. A summary of Darryl's baseline data is presented in Table 3–2.

Patty

Patty, a girl five years and eleven months of age, was brought to the clinic for a fluency evaluation. Patty's mother became aware of a problem when Patty was between two and three years of age. According to the mother, the problem has become worse in the past six months because facial grimaces and gestures have been added to her core pattern of dysfluencies. Stuttering appears to increase when Patty is trying to translate from English to Spanish.

One day after birth, Patty's breathing appeared rapid and required monitoring at the hospital. According to the mother, Patty suffers from a pollen allergy and exhibits "mouth breathing" at night and in cold weather. All other aspects of birth, health, and developmental history were reported to be normal. Patty's mother also noted that Patty is left handed.

Patty is an only child. Her parents are both college graduates. She speaks Spanish only at home. The mother reported that she has stopped requiring that Patty speak Spanish at home. Patty attends a Catholic school, where she is reportedly doing well. According to the mother, she is a happy, friendly child who works well independently and makes friends easily.

A summary of the areas assessed appears on the chart in Table 3–3. This is followed by a summary of Patty's baseline data in Table 3–4.

TABLE 3–1.   Areas of Assessment for Intervention Planning

Name: Darryl   **Age:** 5:0   **Primary Disorder:** language

Necessary Information	Source	Rationale
I. Language A. Content-Form	Lahey (1988) analysis	To obtain most representative measure of the developmental status of content-form interactions
	Additional syntactic analyses	To assess syntactic patterns not addressed by the Lahey format
	Test of Language Development (Primary) (Newcomer & Hammill, 1982)	To obtain a score from a standardized test as required for classification or school placement
	Preschool Language Assessment Instrument (PLAI; Blank, Rose, & Berlin, 1978)	To obtain information about complex semantic relations
B. Use	Lahey (1988) coding system for language use in a conversational context	To obtain most representative measure of developmental status of language function and influence of context
C. Phonology 1. Phonetic	Goldman Fristoe Test of Articulation (Goldman & Fristoe, 1986)	To obtain an inventory of phonemes and an estimate of phonetic ability in single-word productions
2. Phonological	Continuous speech sample	To obtain a measure of the developmental status of phonological process elimination in continuous speech
D. Fluency	Language sample	To obtain a sample of fluency in continuous speech
E. Voice	Language sample	To obtain a sample of vocal parameters in continuous speech

(continued)

73

TABLE 3–1 (*continued*)

Necessary Information	Source	Rationale
II. Maintaining Factors		
A. Cognitive	Bracken Basic Concept Scale (Bracken, 1965) Preschool Language Assessment Instrument (PLAI; Blank, Rose, & Berlin, 1978)	To obtain a measure of the child's developmental status in the area of cognition
	Wechsler Preschool and Primary Scale of Intelligence–Revised (WPPSI-R, Wechsler, 1967)	
B. Sensorimotor		
1. Peripheral Speech Mechanism	Oral Speech Mechanism Screening Examination (OSMSE-R; St. Louis & Ruscello, 1987)	To determine the structural and functional adequacy of the articulators and other points of valving
2. Body Stability	Assessment by the physical therapist	To obtain a measure of the developmental and functional status of the child's sensorimotor functioning in the area of locomotion and body stability
C. Psychosocial	Case history Observations of interactions with mother and examiners	To determine the nature of psychosocial behavior

TABLE 3–2. Summary of Baseline Data for Intervention Planning

Name: Darryl   **Age:** 5.0   **Primary Disorder:** Language

Area Assessed (include sources and results)

I. Language

  A. Content-Form

  Results of standardized testing suggest a syntactic problem with phonologic and semantic components.

	TOLD 2:	Picture vocabulary	50 %ile
		Oral vocabulary	37 %ile
		Sentence imitation	3 %ile
		Grammatic completion	25 %ile
		Word discrimination	37 %ile
		Word articulation	25 %ile

  PLAI   Strong on perceptually oriented items (Sections I & II)
  Weak on items requiring inference making and interpretation of complex sentences (Sections III & IV)

  Results of Lahey Content-Form analysis of language sample indicated:

  Achieved   —   All content-form interactions through phase 3
  Productive   —   Aspects of phases 4–6 content-form interactions

  Not productive or not achieved:

  Phase 4: Not productive — action + irregular past; temporal nondurative irregular past; habitual *s*; causal

  Not achieved — existence + article *a*; action + *ing*, + attribution, + place; locative state + prepositions *in* and *on*

  Phase 5: Not productive — existence + copula + *who* question, + multiple coordinations; locative action + possession, + non-existence, + infinitive complement; causal

  Not achieved — locative action + *ing*, + preposition; internal state or mood + attribution; possession; mood or internal state + *to*

  Phase 6: Not productive — locative action + attribution

  Not achieved — possession; causal; the (specification)

  Phase 7: Not productive — *what, how* questions; notice; VP + connective (when) + VP (simultaneous); causal; adversative

  Not achieved — VP + connective (*then*) + VP (sequential)

  Phase 8: Not productive — all phase-8, 8 + behaviors

  Narrative: Darryl can, while manipulating objects, retell a story that is characterized by additive and temporal chains

  (continued)

TABLE 3–2 *(continued)*

Area Assessed (include sources and results)

Additional syntactic analyses:

Verbs: Frequent verb phrases used: *put, got* (direct object + indirect object); *show* (direct object + indirect object); *finish* + V + *ing; go* + adverb; *keep* + direct object + *for*: indirect object; V + ing; *look* + *at* + indirect object + location

Regularly omits: copula, subject-verb agreement, to (with infinitival complement), for (assigning dative case).

Pron: Substitutions: objective/nominative (e.g., *him/he*), objective/possessive (e.g., *him/his*)

B. Use

Context:

- Produces most complex utterances and talks with greater frequency while engaged in play with objects
- In linguistic contexts, statements and responses to questions are generally contingent upon a prior utterance; does not extend topic beyond a single turn

Function:

- Uses language to comment, direct attention to self and events, obtain objects, obtain information, protest, engage in routine, pretend, inform
- When engaged in discourse, negates, initiates, and responds
- Attempts at repair limited to repetitions of prior utterances

C. Phonology

- Phonetic repertoire;
  Sounds not produced: tʃ, dʒ,
- Phonological processes not suppressed: liquid cluster simplification (gliding); deaffrication (partially suppressed); fronting (sensitive to assimilation, e.g., "Billy goat" = bIlidot)

II. Maintaining Factors

A. Cognitive

- Concept Development: Bracken Concept Ages:
  Colors, letter identification, numbers, comparisons, shape, 4.6; direction, position, 4.6; social, emotional 4.6; size, 4.10; texture, 3.10; quality, 4.2; time, sequence, 4.2; Total Test Score 4.4
- PLAI: Strong on perceptually oriented items (Sections I & II) Weak on items requiring interference making and interpretation of complex sentences (Sections III & V)
- WIPPSI-R: Performance IQ 93   Verbal IQ 90

B. Sensorimotor

- Peripheral speech mechanism - structure and function adequate for speech purposes
- Body stability - mild hypertonicity affecting stability; disassociation of oral-motor movements from fine-motor actions involving the extremities

C. Psychosocial

- Displays normal affect
- Interacts with adults in play contexts
- Engages in object play for extended period of time; does not remain engaged in language-oriented group activities such as story-telling
- Reticent to engage in play with peers

TABLE 3–3. Areas of Assessment for Intervention Planning

Name: Patty   **Age:** 5:11   **Primary Disorder:** fluency

Necessary Information	Source	Rationale
I. Language		
A. Content-Form	Evaluation of conversational speech with reference to Lahey's (1988) categories	To assess language performance
	Test of Language Development (Primary; Newcomer & Hammill, 1982)	To obtain a score from a standardized test as a measure of functioning compared with her peers
B. Use	Lahey (1988) coding system for language use in a conversational context	To obtain most representative measure of developmental status of language function and influence of context
C. Phonology		
1. Phonetic	Photo Articulation Test (PAT; Pendergast, Dickey, Selmer, & Soder, 1969)	To obtain an inventory of phonemes and an estimate of phonetic ability in single-word productions
2. Phonological	Continuous speech sample	To obtain a measure of the developmental status of phonological process elimination in continuous speech
D. Fluency	Continuous speech sample	To obtain a sample of fluency in continuous speech and to observe contextually based changes in fluency patterns
	Matrix of stuttering behaviors based on Wall & Myers (1984)	To serve as a framework for describing patterns of dysfluency
E. Voice	Language sample	To obtain a sample of vocal parameters in continuous speech

(continued)

TABLE 3–3 (continued)

Necessary Information	Source	Rationale
II. Maintaining Factors		
A. Cognitive	Background history Observation of play	To screen cognitive performance
B. Sensorimotor		
1. Peripheral Speech Mechanism	Oral Speech Mechanism Screening Examination (OSMSE-R; St. Louis & Ruscello, 1987)	To determine the structural and functional adequacy of the articulators and other points of valving
2. Body Stability	Informal evaluation of sitting, standing, gait, and movement	To obtain a measure of the developmental and functional status of the child's sensorimotor functioning in the area of locomotion and body stability
C. Psychosocial	Observation of interaction with mother and examiners Background history	To determine the nature of psychosocial behavior

TABLE 3–4. Summary of Baseline Data for Intervention Planning

Name: Patty **Age:** 5:11 **Primary Disorder:** fluency

Area Assessed (include sources and results)

I. Language

A. Content-Form

Results of standardized testing suggest normal functioning in semantics and syntax.

TOLD P:		
	Picture vocabulary	75 %ile
	Oral vocabulary	63 %ile
	Grammatical	85 %ile
	Sentence imitation	68 %ile
	Grammatic completion	63 %ile
	Word discrimination	91 %ile
	Word articulation	70 %ile

An assessment of content-form interactions suggested that simple sentences (3 + constituents, which constituted 43% of the utterances) covered a variety of content categories plus embedding and were coded with age-appropriate syntax. Complex sentences (26% of the utterances) were categorized as volitional-intentional (55%), causal (11%), epistemic (17%), adversative (11%), and communication (05%). No examples of notice or specification occurred. A variety of connectives were used. Single words and two-constituent utterances comprised 30% of all utterances.

B. Use

Linguistic Context: Patty's utterances were generally contingent on prior statements or questions. New information is usually added and topics are extended.

Function: Patty used language to respond (44%), obtain information (07%), comment (17%), obtain response (09%), inform (04%), routine (02%), direct action (06%), negate (04%), repair (03%), emote (01%), protest (01%), affirm (01%) and imitate (01%).

She initiated (36%) and responded (64%) appropriately and maintained eye contact. One striking response strategy noted was responding with a question, to a question. This response occurred primarily when the clinician asked Patty for directions (example: Clinician: "What can I make?"; Patty: "You wanna help me make a table?").

C. Phonology

Results of the PAT revealed only one phoneme substitution: dʒ/ʒ in *beige* and *measure*. A sample of continuous speech supported the findings for single words. This error is consistent with a Spanish influence on phoneme substitution.

(continued)

TABLE 3–4 *(continued)*

Area Assessed (include sources and results)

D. Fluency (framework for fluency analysis is based on Wall and Myers, 1984 matrix of stuttering behaviors)

Description of corpus

1. No. syllables: 365		4. No. utterances: 69
2. No. words: 316		5. Mean utterance length: 4.97
3. No. morphemes: 343		6. Percentage syllables stuttered: 10.1

Core behaviors of stuttering

1. Sound repetitions   (18.9%)
2. Syllable repetitions   (5.4%)
3. Word repetitions   (59.5%)
4. Phrase repetitions   (5.4%)
5. Sound prolongations   (2.7%)
6. Tense pauses or salient blocks   (8.1%)
7. Starters   (1.3%)

Accompanying features

1. Facial tension or struggle
2. Fixed articulatory postures
3. Pitch disruptions

Loci of stuttering

1. Beginning of utterance   (73%)
2. Beginning of clause   (19%)

Distribution of stuttering (% = proportion of utterances stuttered in specified category)

1. Utterance complexity

   Single word and two
   constituent utterances   (14%)
   3 + constituent utterance   (40%)
   Complex sentences   (67%)

2. Complex content-form interactions

   Conjunction: Causal   (50%)
                         Adversative   (50%)

   Complement: Epistemic   (67%)
                         Intention-volition (80%)
                         Communication   (0%; only one utterance appears in sample)

   Functions: Function categories with at least four tokens that manifested the greatest percentage of dysfluencies:

                     Obtain information (80%)
                     Obtain responses   (75%)

                     Function categories with at least four tokens that manifested the greatest percentage of fluencies:

                     Comment   (75%)
                     Direct action   (75%)

(continued)

TABLE 3–4 *(continued)*

Area Assessed (include sources and results)

II. Maintaining Factors

A. Cognitive: Age-appropriate cognitive functions. Parental reports revealed no learning problems at home or in school. Informal observation of play revealed age-appropriate behaviors and interactions.

B. Sensorimotor

- OSMSE-R revealed normal structure and function of the speech mechanism.
- Body stability and small and gross motor movements appear intact.

C. Psychosocial

- Interacts appropriately with mother and examiners
- Described as a friendly, happy, affectionate child who interacts well at home and in school with adults and peers.
- Mother reports that Patty becomes "anxious and frustrated" when dysfluencies occur, and is aware of her stuttering.

Seth

Seth, a boy of eleven years and eleven months of age, was brought to the clinic for a reevaluation and possible treatment. He was seen here initially when he was three years, four months. At that time he was essentially unintelligible due to a severe articulation problem marked by an unusually high degree of homonymy. Language content, form, and use interactions were also below age expectancy. Speech-language delay was associated primarily with impaired sensorimotor functioning. A psychological report highlighted considerable difficulty in the spatial motor area (i.e., judging where his body is in space and interpreting feedback from his actions). He was described as frequently bumping into things, occasionally falling, and demonstrating imprecision in manipulating blocks and pegs. Reports from the occupational therapist and psychologist revealed deficits in sensorimotor and cognitive functioning.

Speech and language intervention at that time, which commenced at our center, focused on the elimination of backing (he produced no alveolar consonants), stopping of /f/, and final consonant deletion. Phonological goals were embedded in Bloom and Lahey (1978) Phase 3 content-form interaction goals. Three constituent utterances were targeted. After approximately two years of treatment, therapy was terminated at the parent's request. At this point Seth was at Bloom and Lahey's Phase 5 and had begun to suppress the phonological processes targeted as goals. Least success was achieved with the elimination of backing.

For the past six years he has been receiving speech-language therapy from a speech-language pathologist in private practice. In addition, he sees a speech-language pathologist at his school. The primary focus of private therapy has been the phonological problem, while in school the focus has been "language reception and expression."

He is currently in a special school program for children with communication and behavior problems, receives speech-language intervention at the school, and has private treatment by an occupational therapist once weekly.

A summary of areas assessed appears on the chart in Table 3–5. This is followed by a summary of Seth's baseline data in Table 3–6.

Alice

Alice, a girl four years and three months of age, was brought to the center for a voice evaluation and treatment. Her birth and early development were reported to be unremarkable. However, when Alice was about one year of age her parents noticed that her voice was "low pitched" and "hoarse." No evaluation or treatment was initiated until four years of age, when Alice was seen by an otolaryngologist. The otolaryngologist's report indicated the presence of vocal nodules and recommended voice therapy.

Alice lives with her parents and three-year-old sister. Both parents are university professors. Alice's parents describe Alice as functioning at the lower end of normal in terms of speech and language.

Alice currently attends a preschool program. She is reported to be friendly and pleasant with teachers and children. Although she is generally cooperative, attentional problems involving visual and auditory modalities have been reported.

A summary of areas assessed appears on the chart in Table 3–7. This is followed by a summary of Alice's baseline data in Table 3–8.

TABLE 3–5. Areas of Assessment for Intervention Planning

Name: Seth **Age:** 11:11 **Primary Disorder:** phonology

Necessary Information	Source	Rationale
I. Language		
A. Content-Form	Lahey (1988) analysis	To obtain most representative measure of the developmental status of complex sentence production
	Test of Language Development, Intermediate Edition (Hammill & Newcomer, 1982)	To obtain a score from a standardized test as required for school placement
	Peabody Picture Vocabulary Test (PPVT-L; Dunn & Dunn, 1981)	To obtain information about receptive vocabulary
	Expressive One-word Picture Vocabulary Test (EOWPVT; Gardner, 1983)	To obtain information about expressive vocabulary
	Additional syntactic analyses	To assess syntactic patterns not addressed by the Lahey format
B. Use	Lahey's (1988) coding system for language use in a conversational context	To obtain most representative measure of developmental status of language function and influence of context
C. Phonology		
1. Phonetic	Photo Articulation Test (PAT; Pendergast, Dickey, Selmer, & Soder, 1969)	To obtain an inventory of phonemes and an estimate of phonetic ability in single-word productions
2. Phonological	Continuous speech sample	To obtain a measure of the developmental status of phonological process elimination in continuous speech
D. Fluency	Language sample	To obtain a sample of fluency in continuous speech
E. Voice	Language sample	To obtain a sample of vocal production in continuous speech

(continued)

TABLE 3–5 *(continued)*

Necessary Information	Source	Rationale
II. Maintaining Factors		
A. Cognitive	Wechsler Intelligence Scale for Children–Revised (WISC-R; Wechsler, 1974). Administered by a psychologist	To obtain a standardized measure of intelligence
B. Sensorimotor		
1. Peripheral Speech Mechanism	Oral Speech Mechanism Screening Examination (OSMSE-R; St. Louis & Ruscello, 1987)	To determine the structural and functional adequacy of the articulators and other points of valving
2. Body Stability	Observation of occupational therapist	To determine the developmental status of the child's sensorimotor functioning in the area of locomotion and body stability
C. Psychosocial	Case history Observations of interactions with examiners and family	To determine the nature of psychosocial behavior

TABLE 3–6. Summary of Baseline Data for Intervention Planning

Name: Seth   **Age:** 11:11   **Primary Disorder:** _____

Area Assessed (include sources and results)

I. Language

A. Content-Form

Standardized Testing:

TOLD	Was not testable. Did not appear to understand requirements of the first two subtests and refused to continue.
PPVT-R	Raw score 91; Standard Score Equivalent 69; % rank 2; Stanine 1
EOWPVT	Raw score 78; Language Age 8–6; % rank 5; Stanine 2

Complex Sentence Analysis:

Evidence of volition-intention, additive, temporal, causality, specification, notice, communication, internal state
Connectives produced: *and, when,*
and *how*

Narratives:

Attempts consisted of two to three-utterance samples. Unintelligibility of utterances and necessity for continuous probing for the continuation of a sequence of ideas interfered with the completion of an adequate narrative sample.

Additional Syntactic Data: Errors with the following syntactic structures may have been phonologically based (marked by word endings):

1. Copula—"What's this," [wa dl]; "who's there," [hu gɛə]
2. Third person singular— "my mother knows" [ma mʌno:]
3. Possessive—"brothers room," [bʌə wum]
4. Past irregular—"made" [meI]
5. Past regular—"wanted" [wʌd]

B. Use

Linguistic Context: Questions and responses generally contingent on prior statements or questions. Topics are typically extended by not more than two statements.
Function: Seth uses language to comment, direct action, obtain responses, routine, inform, protest, negate, amuse.
Discourse skills include acknowledgment of speaker's utterances, repair when not understood (primarily due to phonological impairment).
Initiates and responds to speaker appropriately.

C. Phonology

Single-word productions elicited by pictures from the PAT revealed the following:

(continued)

TABLE 3–6 *(continued)*

Area Assessed (include sources and results)

---

1. Consonants never produced as targets: tʃ, dʒ, θ, ʃ, ʒ, r, ŋ
2. Consonants produced only as substitutions: tʃ, r, θ, ŋ
3. Phonological processes and percentage of occurrence:

   Fronting of velars, k, g (43%)
   Backing, t, d (15%)
   Deaffrication, tʃ , dʒ, (60%)
   Stopping f, v (43%); θ, ð (33%); s, z (08%); ʃ, ʒ (60%)
   Gliding, l, r (44%)
   Vocalizing -l (100%)
   Final Consonant Deletion d, t, tʃ, g, z, s, l (27%)
   Weak Syllable Deletion, two-syllable (12%); three-syllable (25%)
   Cluster Reduction (90%)

4. Other processes and process combinations in which obligatory contexts are not readily specified:

   Assimilation "balloon" [bum]
   Stopping and backing "jar" [ga]
   Fronting of velars and stopping "shoe" [tu]

Continuous speech sample:

1. Phonological processes and percentage of occurrence:

Fronting of velars	(24%)
Backing	(38%)
Stopping	(77%)
Gliding	(100%)
Vocalizing	(100%)
Final consonant deletion	(74%)
Weak syllable deletion	(2-syll, 33%; 3-syll, 100%)
Cluster reduction	(100%)
Stopping plus backing	(5 instances)
Deaffrication plus backing	(50%)
Deaffrication plus fronting of palatals	(50%)

2. Contextual patterns:

   words omitted (generally monosyllable, weakly stressed functions words)
   neutralization of medial consonants "writer" [waljʌ], "Steven" [tijI]
   coalescence "brother"-"he" [bʌi]; "wanted" [wʌd]
   assimilation "to school" [səsu]; "ready" [wɛwi]
   /k/ becomes [t] after a front vowel "week" [wit]; "make" [met]

D. Fluency—within normal limits

E. Voice—variable denasality

II. Maintaining Factors

A. Cognitive: Report from psychologist

(continued)

TABLE 3–6 *(continued)*

Area Assessed (include sources and results)

Results on WISC-R

Verbal IQ	86
Performance IQ	68
Full Scale IQ	75

During the testing Seth occasionally stated "I can't do it," but it was possible to make him persevere. On the basis of much inter-intra subtest variability the psychologist concluded that results are believed to be a "minimal estimate" of his ability. Subtests ranged from far below average (areas assessed as "deficient" were block design and object assembly) to average (information, similarities, comprehension, and picture arrangement).

Low scores were obtained on tasks involving visualizing part-whole relationships, analyzing and synthesizing abstract designs, and matching symbols to numbers.

B. Sensorimotor

- Results on the OSMSE-R: appearance of lip, tongue, and palate was normal.
- Nonspeech functions not accomplished were puffing cheeks, directing tongue to alveolar ridge, and directing tongue tip left of lips (tongue deviated toward right during these tasks).
- Refused to imitate drawing tongue tip along hard palate.
- Results on tasks of diadochokinesis were below age expectancy. Repetitions were executed with spurts in speed and rhythmic changes. He refused to complete all tasks.

Reports of occupational therapist: Seth is viewed as presenting with a number of sensorimotor problems:

1. Low muscle tone: This affects posture, stability, and balance-related activity. This is believed to be associated with motor-planning problems. Low muscle tone is observed about his face. It is still difficult to determine whether tonal problems of the oral cavity are all low or mixed due to his tactile defensiveness (particularly about the head and shoulders).

2. Tactile defensiveness: He is reactive to being touched or handled, which interferes with oral and medical examinations. This behavior is being targeted indirectly with pushing and pulling exercises which require strong proprioceptive input.

3. Fatigue: He fatigues rapidly when standing, sitting, and moving. He appears exhausted after hammering nails into a board for 5 minutes. The appearance of fatigue may be confounded by his labored breathing. The appearance of breathing difficulty is believed to be result of allergies, anxiety and resistance, overweight, and low muscle tone. Breathing appears more labored when he is pushed to complete a task.

4. Incoordination and weakness: Seth has difficulty using the top part of his body against the lower part, and using the right side against the

(continued)

TABLE 3–6 *(continued)*

Area Assessed (include sources and results)

---

left side. Thus, he has problems using two arms in a coordinated manner, together or alternately. Part of the difficulty stems from the low muscle tone, which results in the general inability to pull into flexion against gravity. He compensates for postural instability by using a wide base of support when walking, standing, and sitting.

5. Immature hand function: Seth presents with a set of immature or primitive grasp-release patterns, which are related to muscle tone, motor planning, and incoordination. He demonstrates poor joint stability and an inability to use thumb in opposition to fingers. There is a lack of stability that affects finger movements, demonstrated when Seth grasps a pencil and tries to write. It also appears that Seth lacks motor memory for how to hold the pencil and succeed.

The occupational therapist's report was based on informal clinical observation rather than standardized testing. Seth is generally not cooperative in formal testing situations (Lefkofsky, personal communication, June, 1992).

C. Psychosocial

Rorschach result: Psychologist indicated that Seth's responses were perseverative, reporting the perception of "bat" on many of the cards. He named the color of the blots rather than integrating color and form; this was interpreted as evidence of a neurological problem.

Thematic Apperception Test: Responses to pictures revealed anxiety, sadness, vulnerability, and low self-esteem.

TABLE 3–7. Areas of Assessment for Intervention Planning

Name: Alice   **Age:** 4:3   **Primary Disorder:** voice

Necessary Information	Source	Rationale
I. Language		
A. Content-Form	Evaluation of conversational speech with reference to Lahey's (1988) framework	To assess language performance
	Test of Auditory Comprehension of Language (TACL-R; Carrow-Woolfolk, 1985)	To obtain a score from a standardized test as a measure of functioning compared with her peers (comprehension appeared somewhat impaired during spontaneous conversation)
B. Use	Lahey's (1988) coding system for language use in a conversational context	To obtain most representative measure of developmental status of language function and influence of context
C. Phonology		
1. Phonetic	Photo Articulation Test (PAT; Pendergast, Dickey, Selmer, & Soder, 1969)	To obtain an inventory of phonemes and an estimate of phonetic ability in single-word productions
2. Phonological	Continuous speech sample	To obtain a measure of the developmental status of phonological process elimination in continuous speech
D. Fluency	Informal observation	No problems with fluency were reported
E. Voice	Continuous speech sample	To obtain a sample of vocal parameters in continuous speech
	Respiration and phonation tasks (according to Andrews, 1986)	To assess factors associated with vocal production

(continued)

TABLE 3–7 (*continued*)

Necessary Information	Source	Rationale
II. Maintaining Factors		
A. Cognitive	Background history	Parents were concerned about development of cognitive and adaptive functions
	Wechsler Preschool and Primary Scale in Intelligence–Revised (WPPSI-R; Wechsler, 1967). Administered by psychologist	
	Vineland Adaptive Behavior Scales (Sparrow, Balla, & Cicchetti, 1985)	
B. Sensorimotor		
1. Peripheral Speech Mechanism	Oral Speech Mechanism Screening Examination (OSMSE-R; St. Louis & Ruscello, 1987)	To determine the structural and functional adequacy of the articulators and other points of valving
2. Body Stability	Informal evaluation of sitting, standing, gait, and movement	To obtain a measure of the developmental and functional status of the child's sensorimotor functioning in the area of locomotion and body stability
C. Psychosocial	Observations of interaction with mother and examiners	To obtain information about psychosocial functioning in interpersonal interactions
	Case history	

TABLE 3–8. Summary of Baseline Data for Intervention Planning

Name: Alice   **Age:** 4:3   **Primary Disorder:** Voice

Area Assessed (include sources and results)

I. Language

A. Content-Form

1. Results of TACL are within the normal range on all subtests.

2. MLU was 4.3 (low end of normal according to Miller & Chapman, 1981).

3. Simple sentences (3 + constituents) evidenced an expected range of content categories and coordinations.

4. Complex sentences are emerging with evidence of volition-intention, antithesis, epistemic, additive, temporal, and causal.
Connectives are frequently absent; those used are *and*, *because* (conjunction) and *what*, *where* (complementation).

5. Syntactic error forms include the following:

   omission of copula and auxiliary
   regular past, *paint/painted*
   irregular past, *ride/rode*
   third person singular, *use/uses* ("My mommy use this")
   pronominal use, *her/she; us/we; them/those*

6. Error patterns in the construction of or response to questions.

   Do omission from question forms: "Where this goes?"; "How get baby in there?" When questions demand a complex sentence response (two clauses) involving complementation, responses are reduced to simple sentence constructions.
   Examiner: "Why do we need clocks?"; Alice: "Because what time is it."

B. Use

Linguistic Context: Statements and questions were generally contingent on prior statement or question.

Function: Language was used to obtain information, comment, inform, obtain response, respond to questions, and direct action.

C. Phonology

1. Phonetic repertoire:

   Sounds never produced (in single-word responses): ð, r, dʒ , z
   Variable production: tʃ, θ, l, f, v
   Distortions: s, ʃ, lateral release
   Stimulable for ð, z, in isolation

(continued)

TABLE 3–8 *(continued)*

Area Assessed (include sources and results)

2. Phonological processes:

    Gliding - w/r (100%); w/l (40%)

    Stopping - d/z (100%); p/f (36%); b/v (38%); t/θ (80%); d/dʒ (100%); t/t∫ (75%); f/θ (10%) (place change)

D. Fluency—normal

E. Voice:

  1. Respiration-phonation:

- Infrequent replenishment of breath—talks until out of breath
- Short exhalation phase
- While blowing softly, maintained air stream for an average of 2.5 seconds (mean for preschool children = 4.5 seconds)
- Maintained production of /z/ for 2.3 seconds (mean for ages 3.0–4.8 = 4.15 seconds with S.D. of 2.08 seconds)
- Maintained production of /s/ for 4.4 seconds (mean for age = 3.7 seconds with S. D. of 1.99)
- Prolonged /a/ for 2.9 seconds (mean for age = 4.0–5.0 seconds)
- Some periods of aphonia
- Exhibits muscular tension in neck and shoulders during phonation

  2. Vocal parameters:

    Vocal quality:

      Hoarse

      Periods of aphonia

      Laryngeal hyperfunction

      Reduced nasal and oral resonance

    Loudness:

      Somewhat loud conversational tone

      Loudness is modifiable in game situation (i.e., fire engine moving closer, moving further away).

    Pitch:

      On production of vowel /i/ the average fundamental frequency was 238 Hz (on eight trials); was able to match clinicians' production of high and low contrast on 7:10 trials.

      On production of short phrases (two trials) fundamental frequency was 250 and 231 Hz respectively. Lowest pitch produced was 212 Hz and highest pitch was 287 Hz (acceptable range for four years old = 310–450 Hz).

(continued)

TABLE 3–8 *(continued)*

Area Assessed (include sources and results)

Fundamental frequency was determined to be 230–250 Hz (acceptable limits of fundamental frequency for age four = 310–450 Hz); pitch varies in spontaneous speech.

II. Maintaining Factors

  A. Cognitive:

    1. Wechsler Preschool and Primary Scale of Intelligence–Revised

Full Scale IQ	85
Performance IQ	80
Verbal IQ	92

Overall, the materials were handled well but she failed to remain focused on task. Attention to auditory and visual stimuli were observed to be inadequate.

    2. Vineland Adaptive Behavior Scales

Adaptive behavior composite is 96 ± 6, placing her at the 39th percentile in her age group. Performance in all four areas (communication, daily living skills, socialization, and motor skills) is adequate for her age.

  B. Sensorimotor

    1. OSMSE-R:

- Normal structures
- Diadochochinesis somewhat slow
- Tense jaw and laryngeal musculature
- Raises larynx and jaw when vocalizing

    2. Tonicity, body segmentation, coordination, and stability:

- Walks on toes
- Moderately elevated tonicity
- Inadequate body segmentation evident especially when kneeling, sitting from supine, standing up from a sitting position on floor, sitting from standing position; also evident in excessive oral movements when engaged in fine-motor prehensile activities.
- Some lack of coordination observed in handling small blocks and puzzle pieces

  C. Psychosocial

- Friendly and cooperative during testing
- Interacts appropriately with mother and examiners
- Motivation and attention are variable
- Appears to need approval after performance
- Observed to display an immature smile that is not always appropriate to situation
- Observed to display a blank look in eyes as though not participating in current event
- Has been described by parents as very competitive with younger, high-achieving sister
- Her frequent loud vocal volume appears to be associated with the need to engage others and compete with younger sister

4

Phase I of the Intervention Process

It is somewhat paradoxical that we begin intervention planning by thinking about its termination. Nevertheless, this is exactly what we do when we embark upon intervention planning with a new client. We predict outcomes and specify a likely time frame for intervention. Thinking about the end results of treatment cannot be avoided when a parent asks: "Will my child sound like other children his age when therapy is over?" or "How long will he need therapy?" The finite resources of families and public agencies is another factor that makes consideration of the termination of treatment—in terms of time frame and likely outcome—unavoidable. Answering questions regarding therapy outcomes is a professionally responsible and highly complex task. It is central to professional accountability.

In this chapter we elaborate on our conceptualization of the first phase of intervention planning. This first phase of intervention planning may be termed the *long-term phase*. The long-term phase of intervention planning involves the identification of both long-term goals and procedural approaches to treatment. In the course of this chapter we define long-term goals and procedural approaches. We then discuss decisions that need to be made in order to formulate these goals and procedural approaches. We illustrate this decision-making process as we formulate goals and procedures for the four children described in Chapter 3.

DEVELOPMENT OF LONG-TERM GOALS AND PROCEDURAL APPROACHES

Defining and Formulating Long-term Goals

We define a long-term goal as *a general statement about the best performance that can be expected of an individual in one or more targeted communication areas within a projected period of time.* This definition suggests that the formulation of long-term goals requires a set of decisions leading to (a) the identification of the communication area to be addressed, (b) the specification of "best performance," and (c) the projection of a time period.

The Identification of the Communication Area Targeted. There are two sources of information that contribute to the identification of communication areas that need to be addressed in the long-term goal: (a) the clinician's own point of view regarding the nature of language and (b) baseline data.

The clinician's point of view. In Chapter 1 we discussed the implications of differences among clinicians in their points of view regarding the nature of language. The impact of theoretical differences on intervention planning first becomes apparent in the conceptualization of long-term goals. Theoretical differences can lead to the targeting of different long-term goals by different clinicians for the same client. For example, a clinician who views the basic components of language as expressive and receptive will, given a child with a language delay, focus on the improvement of expressive and receptive language as an outcome of therapy. By contrast, a clinician who views language as the integration of content, form, and use will envision outcomes of treatment in terms of improvement in content, form, and use interactions. Within the domain of articulation and phonological disorders, a clinician using a traditional framework may project change in terms of the acquisition of age-appropriate speech sounds. Another clinician, using a more current linguistic framework, would describe change as the elimination of phonological processes. Regardless of the framework preferred, consistency must be maintained across the phases of intervention planning. We will return to the issue of theoretical consistency in subsequent chapters.

Baseline data. Baseline data represent a second source of information required by the clinician in order to plan long-term goals. Baseline data provide a point of reference for comparing the communication performance of a child suspected of having a speech-language disorder with the performance of normally developing children. An obvious discrepancy in a particular area of communicative functioning would direct us to target that area in a long-term goal statement.

Baseline data are particularly useful for goal planning when they are presented in terms of developmental categories of behavior (e.g., content-form-use, communicative functions, phonological processes, volume patterns associated with specific communication functions). These categories form the basis for long-term goal statements. In targeting a communication area in the long-term goal statement, we refer to selected categories of communication behaviors. Let us consider the following sample goal statements:

1. Owen will produce content-form-use interactions through all Lahey's (1988) phases. The data gathered from Owen at age four years, five months indicated that he had achieved Phases 5 and 6 content-form-use interactions. We know that a child of four years, five months should have achieved at least Phase 8

behaviors. Thus, using baseline data within a selected framework (Bloom & Lahey's), we have generated a long-term goal within linguistic categories (content-form-use interactions).

2. Rachel will eliminate phonological processes that are not age appropriate. The data gathered from Rachel at age six years, one month indicated that all common processes have begun dissolution. By this age she should have eliminated all processes except for weak syllable deletion in four and five syllable words and place changes for fricatives. Thus, using baseline data within a selected framework (phonological processes), we have generated a long-term goal within linguistic categories (phonological processes).

Referring to developmental categories in long-term goal statements provides a direction for further intervention planning. These categories will be helpful in the formulation of short-term goals, which will represent a hierarchy of steps that should lead to the achievement of the long-term goal. The relationship between long- and short-term goals will be discussed in Chapter 5.

The Specification of Best Performance and Time Duration. At this point, we have discussed the way in which a communication area is targeted in a long-term goal statement. The reader may have noticed in the long-term goal definition above that the long-term goal represents the *best performance* expected of the client. We now need to consider how to predict best performance and a time frame for achievement of this performance level. Hypotheses about best performance and time frame are initially formulated prior to the onset of treatment, but may be revised during the course of treatment (Kemp, 1983).

Prior to the commencement of therapy. Before beginning therapy, information about three interacting factors will be fundamental to making predictions about best performance: (a) the discrepancy between the child's current functioning and what is expected for his or her age, (b) the number of impaired behavioral systems maintaining the disorder, and (c) the degree to which each system is impaired. The greater the difference between the baseline performance and the mean level of performance of age-equivalent peers, the lower the probability that the child will eventually perform within the normal range. Differences in performance may be determined on the basis of (a) standardized scores obtainable from formal testing or (b) developmental profiles usually derivable from nonstandardized testing (e.g., Bloom & Lahey, 1978; Lahey, 1988; Grunwell, 1981). Chances of achieving linguistic performance within the normal range decrease as a greater number of behavioral systems are implicated in the disorder. The degree of disability associated with maintaining factors further diminishes the child's potential for normal communication functioning.

In addition to the two major factors influencing decisions about long-term goals, another issue must be considered. This is the child's rate and degree of change over the course of prior treatment. Past goal achievement is often a reliable predictor of present treatment outcomes. If progress in prior treatment was slow and inconsistent, a rapid change in a short period of time would not be expected.

In the course of therapy. The three factors just discussed are primary for making initial formulations of long-term goals. Intervention planning, however, is a fluid process. There are a number of factors that may cause the clinician to reevaluate and revise goals and procedures over the course of intervention. These factors, which become apparent with ongoing intervention, are (a) the commitment of the child's caregivers (e.g., regularity of attendance, follow-through, (b) developmental spurts, and (c) changes in clinician and in approaches to therapy over time.

Criteria for the Achievement of Long-Term Goals (Exit Criteria). The achievement of a long-term goal is equivalent to the termination of therapy. Therefore, the criteria that we set for such achievement are tantamount to *exit criteria* (Campbell & Bain, 1991). There is at present a growing concern regarding the determination of exit criteria (Eiger, 1988; Eiger, Chabon, Mient, & Cushman, 1986; Gantwerk, 1985). This concern is motivated in part by issues related to accountability, such as the documentation of cost effectiveness and treatment efficacy (Olswang, 1990).

Prognosis. In making a decision about exit criteria we are in essence making a prognosis—a well-founded hypothesis about the changes in speech-language behavior ultimately possible for a given client (Campbell & Bain, 1991; Rosen & Proctor, 1981). This prognosis is directly linked to the delivery of quality service, a major concern of speech-language pathologists and audiologists (Carney, 1991). Quality service must begin with a responsible prognosis based on firm knowledge of a child's current functioning and responses to prior treatment.

Exit criteria. In essence, the term *exit criteria* refers to a set of conditions that must be met in order to dismiss a client from treatment. The conditions are generally described with reference to an acceptable rate of performance of specified target behaviors. Rate of performance may be described in different ways. Rate may be stated as percentage of correct productions (e.g., Bloom & Lahey, 1978; Eiger, Chabon, Mient, & Cushman, 1986) or number of instances of a behavior within a particular time frame (frequency of occurrence; e.g., Bloom & Lahey, 1978; Lahey, 1988). Often these percentage or frequency criteria are specified within published assessment instruments used to obtain baseline data (e.g., Bloom & Lahey, 1978; Tyack & Gottsleben, 1974). When not specified in these instruments, percentage and frequency decisions for therapy termination can vary widely among clinicians. For example, in a study by Eiger et al. (1986) on articulation therapy for school-age children, participating clinicians viewed sound mastery as 90% to 100% proficiency in conversational speech. By contrast, Hodson and Paden (1991) terminate therapy when school-age children's phonological process percentage-of-occurrence scores are below 40%. (This is another way of saying that the children are not applying phonological processes—i.e., generating correct performance—60%

of the time.) It has also been suggested that performance criteria should be different for structured tasks than for tasks occurring in spontaneous contexts. For example, Fey (1986) suggests that one might expect 80% to 100% accuracy for targeted performance in clinician directed contexts before the achievement of 50% correct usage in naturalistic contexts.

Reaching a plateau. Related to dismissal criteria is the issue of reaching a plateau in treatment. Clinicians frequently describe a client who has plateaued (Eiger, 1988), as one whose "behavior has not changed over a predetermined amount of time" (Gantwerk, 1985, p. 45). Before a dismissal decision is made on the basis of arriving at a plateau, Gantwerk suggests that "there is documentation to show that the variables of frequency, intensity, type of service, intervention strategy, and service providers (parent, teacher, clinician) have been manipulated" (p. 45). For clients who plateau, it may be said that long-term goals have not been achieved within a projected period of time.

Differences between the long-term goal statement and statement of exit criteria. Let us return now to the long-term goal statement. The long-term goal statement is not isomorphic with a statement of exit criteria. To know exactly when to dismiss a client, an observable behavior that would signal achievement of the long-term goal must be described. It would also be necessary to specify the context in which that behavior would be expressed. This information would represent the "exit criteria." The long-term goal statement specifies one aspect of exit criteria—the expected terminal behavior within a designated taxonomy of communication behaviors. The exit criteria are specified during the course of therapy in session-goal statements (see Chapter 6).

Factors affecting prognosis. Differences in clients' current communication performance and maintaining factors will lead to differences in the degree to which predictions can be made about changes in behavior and duration of treatment (the content of long-term goals). With some clients, making predictions about outcomes may be straightforward. For example, a child who presents a few later-occurring phonological processes and intact associated behavioral systems is likely to achieve normal functioning within a determinable period of time.

It is also possible to make a relatively direct prognosis for some children with severe or profound disabilities affecting multiple behavioral systems. Consider an eight-year-old child with profound mental retardation and severe motor impairment who is at the single-word stage (using verbal and augmentative communication systems). We would anticipate that this child would achieve modest gains during the course of intervention—for example, an increased lexicon and spontaneous productions of two to three constituent utterances for a narrow range of communicative functions. It is likely that this child will require support in communication functioning across a lifetime.

Making long-term goal decisions for many clients, however, is much more complicated than the hypothetical cases presented above. Darryl is one such client. At age five, after some years of intervention, he continues to manifest deficits in all areas of language. Nonlinguistic behavioral systems appear to be relatively intact or manifest subtle deficiencies. In such cases, making decisions about change and duration of treatment is difficult.

Regardless of the nature and severity of the client's communication problem, there are certain questions that need to be answered before we can arrive at decisions about long-term goals. Answers to these questions lie in the data gathered during the assessment process. These answers and sources of information serve as rationales underlying the generation of long-term goals. Prototypical questions appear in Box 4–1. These questions will be applied to intervention planning with specific children later in this chapter.

Information Needed to Formulate a Procedural Approach

Procedures of therapy represent planned interactions and contexts which are designed to facilitate the achievement of desired linguistic goals.

BOX 4–1. QUESTIONS AND SOURCES OF INFORMATION THAT FACILITATE DECISION MAKING ABOUT LONG-TERM GOALS

Questions	*Aspect of Long-Term Goal Influenced*
1. What communication area do I want to target in my client before dismissal from treatment?	The communication area targeted in the long-term goal statement
2. Can I further delimit the area that requires change with reference to a taxonomy of communication behaviors?	The area of communication referred to in the long-term goal statement (e.g., content-form interactions, phonological processes)
3. How much change can I expect within targeted areas?	The level of performance targeted
4. How long should it take to make changes?	The time duration incorporated into the long-term goal statement

Sources of Information

A. Clinician's point of view on how to define and organize linguistic behavior (includes taxonomies used to conceptualize language)
B. Baseline data about communication function (including taxonomies used to organize information about communication)
C. Baseline data about maintaining factors (including information about current functioning and potential for modification)
D. Background information about the course of the problem to date, including prior treatment
E. Assessment instruments and research findings that report age-appropriate, culturally acceptable, physiologically efficient communication behavior

---

At the long-term phase of procedure planning we formulate a procedural approach. To accomplish this, we identify those sources of information that would be most helpful in designing interactions and contexts that will allow us to accomplish our long-term goal. Those sources of information, in addition to the long-term goal statement, itself, are (a) the maintaining factors that require modification and (b) principles from learning theories.

The Long-Term Goal Statement. The long-term goal statement for our client is the first source of information that we use to begin planning intervention procedures. The area of communication specified in the long-term goal statement (content, form, or use) will lead us to intervention approaches that we associate with remediation or facilitation of the problem. Different areas of communication may be associated with different intervention approaches. For example, it has been found that frequent, rapid productions of selected stimuli (drill) is most facilitative in cases of articulation intervention (Shriberg & Kwiatkowski, 1982b). In contrast, content-form goals are most readily achieved in the context of play with objects (Bloom & Lahey, 1978; Lahey, 1988; Lund & Duchan, 1988), and play at familiar routines, such as going to a restaurant or mothering a baby (Nelson, 1986). Certainly, in cases of pragmatic impairment, naturalistic social interactions would be incorporated into a procedural approach (Fey, 1986; Lund & Duchan, 1988).

Maintaining Factors. A second body of information that influences decisions about procedures at the long-term phase of intervention planning is data about factors maintaining the specific disorder. Knowledge of maintaining factors orients the clinician to speech- and language-related problems that the child needs to compensate for, modify, or eliminate in order to achieve the long-term goal. (See Chapter 1 and Lahey, 1988 for a discussion of different types of maintaining factors.) The decision to help the child eliminate or modify difficulties in these areas is a procedural decision, made explicit in the long-term procedural approach.

For example, most clinicians would agree that at least two major maintaining factors are associated with disorders of articulation or phonology (e.g., Bernthal & Bankson, 1988). These are sensorimotor (involving auditory discrimination and sound production) and cognitive-linguistic (involving rule induction). The decision to work with the child in the sensorimotor and cognitive areas would be captured in the long-term procedure approach.

Learning Theories. The intervention approaches that we "naturally" associate with particular speech-language disorders always reflect, to some extent, beliefs of the clinician regarding how children learn. As discussed in Chapter 1, these personal beliefs play an important role in the planning of procedural approaches. They help the clinician take a first step in making decisions about therapeutic environments and interactions that would facilitate speech-language learning.

Whether one is aware of this or not, such personal beliefs often derive from or correspond to theories of learning. Theories of learning that have been developed in the professional literature, however, serve as a more systematic approach for the planning of procedures than personal belief systems, alone. Language-learning theories comprise principles that can provide direction in the conceptualization of therapeutic environments and interactions. At the long-term planning phase we select learning principles in anticipation of their usefulness in designing therapeutic contexts at subsequent phases of procedure planning. Furthermore as noted in the introduction to this chapter, professional accountability requires that we be able to justify our therapeutic interventions. By citing learning principles the clinician is providing a justification for the procedure plan.

In Chapter 1, Boxes 1–6 and 1–7, we presented contrasting learning theories and their domains of applicability. The theories we focused on were behavioral, constructivist-cognitive, social-cognitive, and motor. A clinician may favor one of these over another to explain learning. We suggested, however, that the clinician need not choose only one theory as a basis for developing an approach to speech-language intervention. These approaches are neither mutually exclusive with reference to specific components nor universal in their explanatory power. It is important for the clinician to know how particular theories can shape what one does during the therapy session.

Several questions have been formulated that are intended to clarify what we mean when we say that principles of learning theories facilitate the development of procedural approaches. These questions are also intended to make the information on principles of learning theories displayed in Boxes 1–6 and 1–7 useful to the clinician in planning long-term procedural approaches. They direct the reader to the variety of principles that may be useful in procedural planning, and they suggest how principles drawn from different learning theories may help us devise an integrated procedural approach. These questions are as follows:

1. *What is the area of communication targeted?* This question is self-explanatory. The clinician chooses a principle that has been associated with learning in the area of communication targeted in the long-term goal.

2. *Is the child going to achieve change in the area targeted through self-directed efforts at problem solving or through imitating and otherwise internalizing information presented by others?* This question bears upon the distinction between constructivist- and social-cognitive learning theories.

Learning language through problem solving is a central tenet of constructivist-cognitive learning theories. Constructivist-cognitive theories suggest that, within certain domains of language, children learn best when they experience some kind of difficulty and when they respond by creating new structures and ideas without referring to past models (van Kleeck & Richardson, 1986). A clinician formulating a procedural approach according to this principle would envision possible problem situations and interactions that would allow for creative solutions on the part of the child.

The idea that children learn language by imitating and otherwise internalizing information presented by others is a central principle of social-cognitive learning theories. These theories suggest that language learning involves observing and replicating a model or internalizing rules about how to behave. Therefore, clinicians following these principles would focus on their role as providers of models and rules for children to observe in learning how to process and use language (Cole & Dale, 1986; Connell, 1987; Courtright & Courtright, 1976, 1979).

3. *What kinds of materials, tasks, and clinician-client interactions will encourage motivation and task orientation?* This question is intended to focus the clinician on the relevance of a distinction between interventions based on cognitive and behavioral learning theories.

In programs based on constructivist and social-cognitive learning theories, task orientation is viewed as interactive with the child's developmental characteristics and background (Poplin, 1988). Task orientation is not seen as a skill that has to be taught apart from target attainments. It is the meaningfulness of materials and tasks presented to the child that captures the child's attention and motivates the child to engage in activities that will facilitate speech-language learning. By contrast, behavioral programs treat task orientation in terms of observable behaviors, such as eye gaze (Guess, Sailor, & Baer, 1974). These behaviors are seen as discrete skills that must be trained before the attainment of other target behaviors is possible.

Planning a procedural approach with reference to cognitive learning theories would involve choosing materials for the therapeutic environment with the child's developmental level, social background, and family history in mind. Furthermore, the clinician would anticipate behaving in developmentally appropriate ways with the client. For example, the clinician might avoid asking questions as a primary way of stimulating language in a child who was at the one-word stage of language development; children do not respond well to questions until much later in their development (Brown, 1973). Focusing on behavioral concerns, exclusively, might lead the clinician to think about how to train attention without considering the connection between attention, the therapeutic context, and the child's cultural and developmental status.

In some social learning theories, task orientation is seen as governed by metacognitive rules that may be learned in the context of social interactions (e.g., self-directed comments such as "pay attention" and "listen to the teacher"; Reid, 1988). A clinician planning a procedural approach with reference to this theoretical model might develop materials and a therapeutic context that would facilitate the client's learning of such rules (e.g., see Reid, 1988).

4. *What type of reward system should be employed to strengthen target responses?* Behavioral theory directs us to ask this question, in relation to the principle that contingencies (events following a behavior) can serve to strengthen or weaken behavior. This behavioral principle applies to the development of procedural approaches regardless of the learning theory

most directly influencing a clinician's procedural planning. Whenever we develop procedural approaches, we need to think about what will be rewarding for a particular client.)

Different learning theories, however, lead us to look to different types of contingencies in devising reward systems. Behavioral and social-cognitive theories direct us to focus on two basic types of *external* reward systems: tangible and interpersonal. M & Ms, tokens, and stars are tangible rewards; a response to a question, a smile, a desired movement or reaction are interpersonal rewards. Constructivist-cognitive learning theories direct us to identify a third type of reward system: internal. Affects, such as personal satisfaction and feelings of success and accomplishment following the resolution of a problem, represent internal rewards. In planning a long-term procedural approach, the clinician will identify a reward system, which in turn will influence the design of clinical interactions and the selection of clinical materials.

As we noted above, Boxes 1–6 and 1–7 were designed to aid the clinician in identifying principles of learning theories that could be useful in planning and justifying procedural approaches. In Box 1–7, the clinician will be directed toward identifying (a) the speech-language domain (content, form, or use) in which change is targeted, (b) learning theories that address change in these areas, and (c) principles of learning that are derived from these theories. Box 1–6 provides more explicit information about procedural aspects (i.e., the action of the learner, the action of the teacher, conditions preceding and following the learner's response to the teacher).

In sum, at the long-term phase of intervention planning the task of the clinician is to develop a procedural approach. We have discussed three sources of information that are useful in establishing a procedural approach: (a) the long-term goal statement, (b) information about maintaining factors, and (c) principles of theories of language learning (including the clinician's own beliefs about language and language learning). In Box 4–2 we present a series of questions and corresponding sources of information that will help the clinician formulate long-term procedural approaches.

THE DERIVATION OF PHASE-1 LONG-TERM GOALS AND PROCEDURAL APPROACHES FOR SPECIFIC CHILDREN

In the remainder of this chapter, we will discuss how we arrived at Phase-1 goal and procedural statements for each child presented in Chapter 3. In this manner, we will illustrate the decision-making process at the long-term goal phase of intervention planning across disorder types. The four children we will follow are Darryl (content-form-use interactions), Patty (fluency), Seth (phonology), and Alice (voice). Our intent is not to present the "perfect" plan for these children; there are many possible plans that

---

**BOX 4–2. QUESTIONS AND SOURCES OF INFORMATION
FOR FORMULATING A PROCEDURAL APPROACH**

Questions	*Sources of Information*	*Aspect of Procedural Approach Influenced*
1. What area(s) of communication is (are) targeted in the long-term goal statement?	Long-term goal statement	All aspects
2. What maintaining factors are implicated in the communication problem?	Baseline data	Maintaining factors to be modified or eliminated
3. What theories about learning will influence decisions about contexts and interactions?	Theories about language learning, including personal beliefs	Principles from learning theories to be addressed
4. What reward system(s) would be useful in achieving the goal?	Theories about language learning Background information	Reward system to be implemented

---

could be developed that would be equally valid. Different plans would reflect different theoretical orientations and attention to different aspects of baseline data. To reiterate, our purpose is to illustrate the *decision-making process* that leads to the formulation of long-term goals and procedures.

In discussing the derivation of long-term goal statements and procedural approaches for the four children, we will adhere to the following format. We will first present the completed long-term goals and the procedural approaches. We will then detail the decision-making process involved in the derivation of these statements. Questions in Boxes 4–1 and 4–2 will be used to guide the decision-making process.

Darryl

The following are the long-term goals and procedural approach that were developed for Darryl, the first child we will consider at the long-term goal phase of intervention planning. Darryl presents with a developmental delay in the area of language.

Long-term goals:

1. Darryl will achieve content-form-use interactions through Lahey Phase 8+.
2. Darryl will increase number and variety of lexical items, coding all **Lahey** content categories through Phase 8+.

3. Darryl will produce multiple causal-chain narratives.
4. Darryl will initiate and maintain conversation in context of cooperative play.

Targeted attainments should be achieved within three years after the initiation of intervention.

Long-term procedural approach:

1. The achievement of all goals will be facilitated by modifying cognitive, sensorimotor, social-emotional, and linguistic maintaining factors.
2. The procedural approach has been influenced primarily by the following principles from constructivist-cognitive learning theory (selected from Box 1–7). Learning is facilitated by:
    —interactions with materials and tasks commensurate with the child's past experience, present developmental level, and interests;
    —efforts to convey meaning and repair communication breakdown successfully;
    —varying actions during problem solving;
    —reflection upon personal behavior and the environment, inference making, inductive and deductive reasoning;
    —sensory stimulation (i.e., sensory feedback) from movement, including movement involved in articulation or manipulating objects.
3. Internal and social rewards will be employed to facilitate the achievement of all goals.

The Derivation of Darryl's Long-Term Goals

Steps 1 and 2: Making decisions about areas of communication to address. The first step in developing a long-term goal statement involves determining (a) which communication area should be changed in the client before dismissal from therapy (i.e, what area of communication should be addressed in the long-term goal statement) and (b) whether the area that requires change can be delimited within a developmental taxonomy of behaviors. As noted above, baseline data are often presented with reference (explicit or implicit) to a taxonomy or framework. If this framework is consistent with the clinician's definition of how language is organized, it will be helpful in formulating the long-term goal statement. It will also provide direction for the formulation of short-term goals at the next phase of intervention planning. Information is provided about Darryl's current linguistic functioning in terms of Lahey's (1988) developmental framework. This taxonomy concurs with our understanding about how language is organized. As a consequence, we refer to this taxonomy in formulating a long-term goal statement.

The baseline data on Darryl indicate that he does not exhibit a number of semantic-syntactic categories that should be achieved between Lahey's Phases 6 and 8+. Although Lahey does not associate phase of development with expected ages, related research indicates that functioning at Phases 6, 7, and 8+ is generally achieved by three to four years of age. At this point, a decision is made to target form-content interactions that correspond to these phases in the long-term goal statement.

Related to this decision, we anticipate that as Darryl progresses in school he will be called upon to produce and process narratives of increasing complexity. Baseline data indicate that although Darryl is beginning to code content-form interactions that are transitional to complex narrative forms (e.g., additive semantic relations using conjunctions), he is manifesting some difficulty with more advanced structures expected for his age (e.g., he is not producing temporal or causal semantic relations, and he is generating few sentential complements and no forms of relativization). We think it would be functional and appropriate to target narrative structures in the long-term goal statement, and that Lahey's (1988) taxonomy of story-narratives would be helpful in delimiting a target achievement in this area.

Baseline data also indicate that Darryl exhibits lexical deficits—manifested especially in a restricted range of verb usage. We anticipate, however, that as Darryl achieves more complex content-form interactions, lexical problems become more obvious. It is possible in fact, that syntactic deficiencies, such as Darryl's failure to code articles and prepositions, may be related to the lexical problem. Thus, it would be beneficial to target lexical achievements into a long-term goal statement. Since the lexicon codes linguistic content, Lahey's taxonomy will be applicable to the formulation of a long-term goal that targets lexical items.

In the area of language use, Darryl manifests difficulties engaging in conversation with other children. He shows little evidence that he has acquired the pragmatic skills relevant to engaging in conversations appropriate for his age (Lahey, 1988; Lund & Duchan, 1988). Thus, a decision is made to target conversational skills in the long-term goal statement.

Steps 3 and 4: Determining level of attainment and time frame. So far, we have identified four areas of communication that we wish to target as long-term goals for Darryl, and we have specified developmental taxonomies that will be referenced in these goals. Next decisions must be made about a level of attainment that can be expected of Darryl in each area of communication that will be addressed (see Box 4–1, question 3). Furthermore, a time frame must be estimated for achievement of the targeted communication performance (see Box 4–1, question 4). Two sources of information will be useful in projecting levels of achievement and setting a reasonable time frame: prior therapists' reports of treatment results (background information) and baseline data about maintaining factors.

In reviewing Darryl's clinical history, we learn that, after two years of intervention, Darryl has expanded his use of single-verb constructions. He also has achieved some multiverb constructions and a greater variety of complement structures. However, it is also apparent that Darryl has shown limited progress in coordinating content categories in single verb constructions, and in the coding copula, noun-verb agreement, and certain pronominal forms. The evidence suggests, therefore, that progress in therapy has been slow.

As noted above, we need to consider baseline data relevant to cognitive, sensorimotor, and psychosocial functioning in order to make a prognosis about the course of intervention. In the cognitive domain, according to results achieved on the Bracken Test of Concept Development, Darryl appears to exhibit a mild delay in identifying colors, letters, numbers, shapes, directions, positions, social-emotional states, textures, quantity, and time sequences. His performance was weak on items from the Preschool Language Assessment Instrument (PLAI) that require inference making and interpretation of complex sentences. It must be kept in mind, however, that both the Bracken and PLAI assessments require the processing of linguistic information—especially lexical items. Therefore, linguistic factors may be depressing cognitive performance.

Although Darryl will need to continue to develop cognitively as a foundation for attaining the linguistic achievement we have targeted (e.g., causal narrative structures), it does not appear that mild delays in the area of cognition will interfere with the timely achievement of long-term goals. It is possible, however, that metalinguistic knowledge, which was not evaluated due to the child's chronological age, may become a maintaining factor that will have an impact upon goal achievement and that will have to be evaluated over the course of therapy.

In the psychosocial domain, Darryl manifests a reticence to engage in interpersonal interactions with peers. This behavior is certainly interactive with reported deficits in conversational skills. Social-emotional factors may affect progress in achieving long-term goals, but they do not seem to pose insurmountable problems.

In the sensorimotor domain, Darryl exhibits mild hypertonicity affecting body segmentation and disassociation of oral-motor movements from actions related to locomotion and body stabilization. Sensorimotor deficits will require collaboration with a physical or occupational therapist (or both), and are likely modifiable. (See Chapter 6 on session planning.) These difficulties may affect duration of intervention; however, they should not interfere with ultimate goal achievement.

To complete the long-term goal statement, it is necessary to specify a reasonable amount of time for the attainment of the levels of communication performance expected. A projection of time duration will be based on all the information reviewed to this point as well as our knowledge of frequency of intervention and intervention setting. Darryl will be receiving therapy two to three times weekly in a school setting. Taking these variables into consideration, three years is set as the expected duration of therapy.

Given this consideration of potential maintaining factors and the outcome of prior interventions, we are now prepared to complete the first part of the Long-Term Goals and Procedure section of the management plan (Form B–3 from Appendix B). The long-term goals, expected duration, and rationales are presented within this format in Table 4–1.

Darryl: The Derivation of a Procedural Approach Thus far, four areas of language have been targeted in a long-term goal statement for Darryl: content-form-use interactions through Lahey's (1988) Phase 8, lexicon, narrative structures, and conversational skills. At this point, a set of decisions needs to be made about a procedural approach. Recall that in thinking about procedures at the long-term phase of intervention planning we are concerned about general parameters of interactions and contexts that will allow us to accomplish our long-term goals. In making procedural decisions at Phase 1, it will be helpful to consider the set of questions, corresponding sources of information, and the format for developing a procedural approach presented in Box 4–2.

Step 1: Identifying maintaining factors that need to be addressed in order to reach the long-term goal. The first step in deriving a procedural approach involves the identification of behavioral systems that need to be modified or compensated for so that long-term goals may be achieved. Baseline data will provide relevant information in the areas of cognitive, sensorimotor, and

TABLE 4-1.   Management Plan: Long-Term Goals and Procedures

Client: Darryl_____	Clinician: _____
Supervisor: _____	Semester: _____

Long-Term Goals and Expected Duration:

1. Darryl will achieve content-form-use interactions through Lahey's Phase 8 +
2. Darryl will increase number and variety of lexical items, coding all Lahey content categories through Phase 8 +
3. Darryl will produce multiple causal-chain narratives
4. Darryl will initiate and maintain conversation in context of cooperative play

Rationales with reference to:

Baseline data (how current linguistic performance motivates goals):
1. Content-form interactions through Bloom and Lahey Phase 5 productive or achieved
2. Some content-form interactions between Phases 6 and 8+ are emerging (additive semantic relations using conjunctions and semantic relations using complementation. Darryl is not producing temporal or causal semantic relations or relative forms.)
3. Darryl exhibits a restricted range of verb usage
4. Darryl manifests difficulties engaging in conversation with other children

Maintaining factors (justification of long-term expectation and duration):
Mild cognitive, psychosocial, and sensorimotor involvements may affect duration of intervention but not ultimate goal achievement

psychosocial functioning. Maintaining factors that need to be addressed will be specified in the procedural approach statement.

We concluded above that Darryl's language difficulties are primarily linguistic in nature (as opposed to being primarily a consequence of deficits in nonlinguistic, behavioral systems, such as sensorimotor or cognitive). However, we also decided that Darryl's reticence to engage in interactions with his peers implicated psychosocial factors. We would expect children at age five to engage in cooperative play with others. Encouraging interactions with other children should facilitate language learning in all areas.

There are two additional behavioral systems that may be implicated in facilitating change in all the targeted areas of communication—cognition and sensorimotor. Although Darryl does not manifest a clear-cut cognitive dysfunction, it is reasonable to expect that cognitive functioning is involved in the attainment of the more complex content-form interactions (e.g., additive, temporal, and causal relations) and in the development of narratives (Moses, Klein, & Altman, 1990). Therefore, cognition will be addressed in the procedural approach.

As noted above, Darryl also manifests sensorimotor problems affecting the disassociation of oral-motor behavior from other body movements. This difficulty could be partially responsible for Darryl's tendency to omit function words of low phonetic substance. This deletion pattern is generally associated with auditory processing limitations (e.g., Leonard, 1989). It is possible, however, that deletions may also be influenced by difficulty in producing sounds in syllables of reduced duration (unstressed syllables). Mild hypertonicity may also affect Darryl's ability to process feedback from the environment during play. This could affect the development of language content.

At this point, it is possible to begin to formulate the first part of the procedural approach: the specification of maintaining factors that will need to be addressed in the course of intervention. The achievement of all goals will be facilitated by modifying cognitive, sensorimotor, psychosocial, and linguistic maintaining factors.

Step 2: Identifying principles from learning theories. The next step in the process of deriving a procedural approach involves identifying principles from learning theories that will guide procedure planning at subsequent phases. Box 1–7 (Chapter 1) is useful in this endeavor. These principles will suggest client-clinician interactions and materials that should facilitate achievement of the long-term goal specified. Clinician-child interactions and the design of the therapeutic environment will be elaborated at the short-term phase of procedure planning.

Recall that content-form-use interactions through Lahey Phase 8+, lexicon, and narrative structures were targeted in Darryl's long-term goal statement. In examining Box 1–7, we find that principles that derive from constructivist-cognitive theory best apply to the facilitation of language

TABLE 4–2.   Management Plan: Long-Term Goals and Procedures

Client: <u>Darryl</u>	Clinician: _____
Supervisor: _____	Semester: _____

Long-Term Goals and Expected Duration

1. Darryl will achieve content-form-use interactions through Lahey's Phase 8 +
2. Darryl will increase number and variety of lexical items, coding all Lahey content categories through Phase 8 +
3. Darryl will produce multiple causal-chain narratives
4. Darryl will initiate and maintain conversation in context of cooperative play

These goals will be achieved within three years

Rationales with reference to:

Baseline data (how current linguistic performance motivates goals):
1. Content-form interactions through Lahey Phase 5 productive or achieved
2. Some content-form interaction between Phases 6 and 8 are emerging (additive semantic relations using conjunctive form and semantic relations using complementation. Darryl is not producing temporal or causal semantic relations or relative forms)
3. Darryl exhibits a restricted range of verb usage
4. Darryl manifests difficulties engaging in conversation with other children

Maintaining factors (justification of long-term expectation and duration):
Mild cognitive, psychosocial, and sensorimotor involvements which may affect duration of intervention but not ultimate goal achievement

Procedural Approach:

Maintaining factors addressed:
Cognitive, sensorimotor, social-emotional, linguistic

Guiding principles (from learning theories, Box 1–7):
Learning is facilitated by:
5. interactions with materials and tasks commensurate with the child's past experience, present developmental level, and interests
6. efforts to convey meaning and repair communication breakdown successfully
7. varying actions during problem solving
8. reflection upon personal behavior and the environment, inference making, inductive and deductive reasoning
9. sensory stimulation (i.e., sensory feedback) from movement, including movement involved in articulation or manipulating objects

Reward system:
Internal and social

content-form interactions and most closely correspond with our orientation to development in the areas of communication under consideration. These principles will be listed in the procedural approach.

Step 3: Selecting a reward system. The final step in planning a procedural approach involves deciding upon a reward system. In a sense, this step reflects the application of the behavioral principle that contingencies following behavior serve to strengthen or weaken behavior.

In selecting a reward system, language-learning theories other than behaviorism can be useful sources of information. For example, constructivist-cognitive learning theory suggests that internal factors (e.g., the recognition of successful goal achievement, the formulation of wonderful ideas) represent a powerful system of rewards (Duckworth, 1972). We believe that internal rewards would be most applicable to the facilitation of all aspects of communication targeted for Darryl (content-form categories, lexicon, conversational skills). We also think that social factors such as adults' reactions to Darryl's successful communications will represent an effective reward system. Therefore, we add a statement to the formulation of a long-term procedural approach for Darryl: internal and social reward systems will be employed to facilitate the achievement of all goals.

Given of the above consideration of maintaining factors, learning principles, and reward systems we are now prepared to fill in the procedural approach section of the first management plan form (Form B–3 from Appendix B). The long-term procedural approach is presented within a completed Long-Term Goal and Procedure Form in Table 4–2.

Patty

Having completed the first phase of intervention planning for Darryl, a child whose primary disorder is in the area of language, we now turn to Patty. Patty presents with a fluency disorder. As with Darryl, the long-term goals and procedural approach that were developed for the client are listed. These are followed by a discussion of the decision-making process that led to these goals and procedures.

Long-term goal statements:

1. Patty will manifest fluent speech patterns while producing complex sentences for regulatory and discourse functions.
2. The targeted goal should be achieved within two years after the initiation of intervention.

Long-term procedural approach:

1. The achievement of fluent speech patterns will be facilitated by modifying sensorimotor, psychosocial, and linguistic maintaining factors.
2. The goal will be facilitated in contexts and interactions that maximize fluency.
3. The procedural approach is influenced primarily by principles from operant, motor, and social learning theories.

Learning is facilitated by:

—events following a behavior, which can reinforce (strengthen) or extinguish (weaken) the behavior;

—efforts to match models presented by the clinician;

—sensory stimulation (i.e., sensory feedback) from movement, including movement involved in articulation or manipulating objects.

4. Social rewards will be employed to facilitate the achievement of the long-term goal.

Patty: The Derivation of the Long-Term Goal.   We now refer to the questions and corresponding sources of information for planning long-term goals in Box 4–1.

Steps 1 and 2: Making decisions about areas of communication to target. To make a decision about the communication area to target (Box 4–1, question 1), we turn to baseline data about communication functioning (source B). Baseline data reveal that the primary disorder is in the area of fluency. With reference to Box 4–1, question 2, we need to delimit further the area of communication in order to formulate a manageable long-term goal statement. The baseline data in the area of fluency are organized with reference to three components of language: the dysfluency pattern, the way dysfluency interacts with content-form interactions, and the way dysfluency interacts with language functions. This organizational scheme is consistent with our view of language as an integration of three components: content, form, and use.

A review of Patty's baseline data suggests that the types of dysfluencies that occur most frequently are syllable and word repetitions. These occur primarily with the coding of 3+ constituent utterances and complex sentences. Dysfluencies occur less often in Patty's productions of single words and two-constituent utterances. In addition, fluency patterns appear to be differentially affected by categories of pragmatic functions. Consequently, the long-term goal statement will need to reflect the interaction among fluency, utterance complexity, and regulatory and discourse functions.

Steps 3 and 4: Determining level of attainment and time frame. To make decisions about levels of attainment and time frame we must utilize four sources of information: baseline data about communication functioning and maintaining factors, background information, and research findings regarding normal ranges of fluency (factors B, C, D, and E, Box 4–1). Baseline data that describe dysfluency patterns reveal an overall dysfluency rate of 10.1% syllables stuttered. According to some quantitative indices, this percentage would place Patty in the mild range (e.g., Wall & Myers, 1984; Wingate, 1988). In addition, the fact that Patty produces primarily syllable and word repetitions without much apparent struggle further supports the hypothesis that Patty is a mild stutterer (e.g., Starkweather, 1987).

Patty's apparently mild degree of dysfluency is one indication that she will achieve a high level of fluency over the course of intervention. Our optimism about Patty's prognosis is supported by relatively unimpaired nonlinguistic behavioral systems. There is no information in the case history that counterindicates targeting a high level of fluency in the long-term goal statement. Consequently, a decision is made to target fluent speech patterns across contexts. At this point, the long-term goal statement is formulated: Patty will manifest fluent speech patterns while producing complex sentences for regulatory and discourse functions.

Our projection of duration will be based on all the information we have reviewed already and our knowledge of the frequency of intervention. The bulk of the baseline data lead us to expect that our long-term goal would be achieved within a relatively short time duration. There are, however, two factors that have an impact on this prognosis. One is the bilingualism at home, which seems to affect fluency; the other is the pattern of increased dysfluency when it is necessary to obtain information from someone. This latter observation may implicate psychosocial variables. Taking all this information into consideration, we project that two years is a reasonable time duration. The long-term goal for Patty and the rationales for this goal appear on the Management Plan Form in Table 4–3 below.

Patty: The Derivation of a Procedural Approach.   Now that we have arrived at a long-term goal statement for Patty, we turn to the formulation of a procedural approach. We refer again to the questions and corresponding sources of information appearing in Box 4–2.

TABLE 4–3.   Management Plan: Long-Term Goals and Procedures

Client: Patty	**Clinician:**
Supervisor:	**Semester:**

Long-Term Goals and Expected Duration:
1. Patty will manifest fluent speech patterns while producing complex sentences for regulatory and discourse functions
2. The targeted goal should be achieved within two years after the initiation of intervention

Rationales with reference to:

Baseline data (how current linguistic performance motivates goals):
1. Baseline data reveal that the primary disorder is in the area of fluency
2. The most frequent types of dysfluencies are syllable and word repetitions
3. Dysfluencies occur primarily with the coding of 3 + constituent utterances and complex content-form interactions
4. Fluency patterns appear to be differentially affected by categories of pragmatic functions

Maintaining factors (justification of long-term expectation and duration):
1. Patty's apparently mild degree of dysfluency is one indication that she will achieve a high level of fluency over the course of intervention
2. Relatively unimpaired nonlinguistic behavioral systems
3. No information in the case history that counterindicates targeting a high level of fluency in the long-term goal statement

Step 1: Identifying maintaining factors that need to be addressed in order to reach the long-term goal. The identification of factors that need to be modified or compensated for will be the first step in the derivation of a procedural approach. There are a number of indicators in baseline data that suggest that sensorimotor, psychosocial, and linguistic factors need to be addressed in the course of therapy.

An examination of the distribution of stuttering reveals a marked increase in the proportion of utterances stuttered as utterance complexity increases; this indicates that linguistic factors are maintaining the disorder and need to be addressed in a procedural approach. The mother's report that stuttering increases in severity when Patty translates English into Spanish further supports the idea that linguistic factors are maintaining the problem.

The distributional frequencies reveal that stuttering increases in frequency when Patty is faced with two conversational demands: (a) the need to obtain information from another and (b) the need to obtain other types of responses from another. Furthermore, Patty's mother reported that Patty is becoming anxious about her speech. These trends suggest that there is a psychosocial contribution to the disorder.

Sensorimotor factors must also be considered as possible maintaining factors in cases of dysfluency. Dysfluency implies a disruption in the coordination of valvular functioning of the speech mechanism (Starkweather, 1987; Wall & Myers, 1984).

Having reached a set of conclusions about factors that may be maintaining Patty's dysfluencies, we formulate the first part of the procedural approach: The achievement of fluent speech patterns will be facilitated by modifying sensorimotor, psychosocial, and linguistic maintaining factors.

Step 2: Identifying principles from learning theories. The next step in the process of deriving a procedural approach involves identifying principles from learning theories that will guide procedure planning at subsequent phases. Again, Box 1–7 (Chapter 1) will be referenced.

Operant principles appear to be most directly applicable because most of Patty's speech is fluent. Behavioral principles suggest that we could shape fluent behavior in two ways: (a) by encouraging and reinforcing fluent behavior and (b) by removing stimuli and contingencies that promote dysfluent behavior. We are also interested in having Patty observe and imitate models of fluent speech. For this reason, we feel that principles derived from social-cognitive theory (involving modeling of behavior) and motor theory (involving movement and feedback) are also applicable.

Step 3: Selecting a reward system. The final component of the procedural approach will be the selection of a reward system that will be utilized in the course of therapy. Since psychosocial factors appear to be maintaining the dysfluency, modifying social contingencies that may be affecting the speech pattern would be most useful. We expect that family members and peers may be unintentionally reinforcing the dysfluent behavior. Thus, a decision is made to employ social rewards to facilitate the achievement of the long-term goal.

TABLE 4–4. Management Plan: Long-Term Goals and Procedures

Client: <u>Patty</u>	Clinician: _____
Supervisor: _____	Semester: _____

Long-Term Goals and Expected Duration:

Patty will manifest fluent speech patterns while producing complex sentences for regulatory and discourse functions

The targeted goal should be achieved within two years after the initiation of intervention

Rationales with reference to:

Baseline data (how current linguistic performance motivates goals):
1. Baseline data reveal that the primary disorder is in the area of fluency
2. The most frequent types of dysfluencies are syllable and word repetitions
3. Dysfluencies occur primarily with the coding of 3 + constituent utterances and complex content-form interactions
4. Fluency patterns appear to be differentially affected by categories of pragmatic functions

Maintaining factors (justification of long-term expectation and duration):
1. Patty's apparently mild degree of dysfluency is one indication that she will achieve a high level of fluency over the course of intervention
2. Relatively unimpaired nonlinguistic behavioral systems
3. No information in the case history that counterindicates targeting a high level of fluency in the long-term goal statement

Procedural Approach:

Maintaining factors addressed: sensorimotor, psychosocial, and linguistic

Guiding principles (from learning theories, Box 1–7):

Learning is facilitated by:
1 — events following a behavior, which can reinforce (strengthen) or extinguish (weaken) the behavior
2 — efforts to match models presented by the clinician
9 — sensory stimulation (i.e., sensory feedback) from movement, including movement involved in articulation

Reward system:
Social

These three components of the long-term procedural approach for Patty in Table 4–4 complete the first part of the Management Plan.

Seth

The following are the long-term goals and procedural approach that were developed for Seth, the third child we will consider at the long-term goal phase of intervention planning. Seth's primary problem is in the area of phonology.

Long-Term Goal Statements

1. Seth will decrease phonological process application across all categories to the point of intelligibility by people unaware of his speech pattern.
2. Seth will begin to suppress processes that have not begun dissolution (gliding and vocalization).
3. Seth will produce final consonants that code inflectional morphemes.
4. Seth will increase frequency and variety of multiverb content-form interactions and their associated connectives.
5. Seth will produce complex causal chain narratives.

Targeted attainments should be achieved within three to five years after the initiation of intervention.

Long-Term Procedural Approach

1. All long-term goals will be facilitated by modifying cognitive, sensorimotor, and psychosocial maintaining factors.
2. Language goals are expected to be facilitated with articulatory improvement.
3. The speech-language pathologist will collaborate with the occupational therapist to modify the following sensorimotor maintaining factors: (a) Seth's tactile defensiveness (in order to promote greater tolerance of phonetic placement techniques) and (b) stability and body segmentation (in order to promote independent oral motor movements for speech).
4. The long-term procedural approach for Seth is influenced primarily by the following principles from social-cognitive and motor learning theories (selected from Box 1–7).
   Learning is facilitated by:
   —efforts to match models presented by the clinician;
   —noticing similarities and distinctions among actions and events mediated by adults;
   —efforts to successfully convey meaning and overcome miscommunication;
   —reflection upon personal behavior;
   —sensory stimulation (i.e., sensory feedback) from movement involved in the performance of articulatory gestures.

Internal and social reward systems will be employed to facilitate the achievement of all goals.

Seth: The Derivation of the Long-Term Goals.   In discussing the derivation of the long-term goal statements for Seth, we again refer to the questions and corresponding sources of information that are presented in Box 4–1.
Steps 1 and 2: Making decisions about areas of communication to target. Baseline data for Seth indicate that the primary problem lies in the area of phonology. These data have been organized according to taxonomies of content,

form, and use and a taxonomy within form: phonological processes. A review of Seth's conversational-speech sample reveals a small percentage of complex sentences (21%). These are primarily volition-intention, additive, causality, and specification. Connectives are typically absent. Those that do appear are "and," "how," and "when." Juxtapositioning of clauses does suggest the beginnings of three structure types: conjunction, complementation, and relativization. Because Seth usually produces simple sentences and a narrow range of complex sentences without connectives, the content and form of complex sentences are targeted as a long-term goal.

During the assessment process it was observed that, although Seth enjoys informing the listener about his ideas and experiences, his narrative attempts do not persist beyond two or three utterances. These utterances are primitive additive and temporal chains. Seth also likes to tell jokes, and his jokes generally involve causality (i.e., "Why did the kid bring the ladder to school? Because he wanted to be in high school"). His knowledge of linguistic content appears to be ahead of his ability to execute complex linguistic forms. In other words, it appears that Seth's attempts at longer narratives are thwarted by difficulties in being understood. Until his speech-sound production improves it is difficult to determine how much of his problem with narrative has to do with the organization of ideas and how much has to do with the phonological production difficulty. Nevertheless, narrative production of causal chains has been selected as a goal because Seth is producing short narratives that demonstrate primarily additive and temporal sequences, and because he appears to be aware of cause-effect relations (underlying in complex sentences).

The baseline data on Seth's articulation-phonology have been presented in terms of phonetic-phonological aspects and contextual patterns (see Chapter 3, Table 3–1). Seth demonstrates the ability to produce the articulatory gestures for almost all sounds in the language (with the exception of /S/, /d$_3$/, and /ʒ/). He does, however, maintain a large number of processes that operate frequently and affect a wide range of speech sounds. By age eleven years, eleven months, all processes should have been eliminated. Seth, however, continues to use these processes from 15% to 100% in single-word contexts and from 24% to 100% in continuous speech contexts. Our long-term goals, therefore, reflect a consideration of the range and frequency of process application. Dissolution needs to be initiated for those processes applied in 100% of obligatory contexts. Others that have begun dissolution need to be targeted for reduction.

The baseline data on Seth's production of grammatical morphemes suggest that early developmental morphemes are generally absent from his productions in conversational speech. These are plural, copula, third person singular, possessive, past irregular, and past regular. All these morphemes are vulnerable to phonological processes of weak syllable deletion, final consonant deletion, and cluster reduction—all prominent in Seth's production pattern. Morpheme endings, therefore, will be targeted as a context for the reduction of final consonant deletion, cluster reduction, and weak syllable deletion.

Steps 3 and 4: Determining level of attainment and time frame. So far, we have identified five areas of communication that we wish to target in the long-term goal statement for Seth; we have also specified developmental taxonomies that we will reference in the statement. Next we need to make decisions about a level of attainment that we can expect of Seth in each area of communication that we wish to target (see Box 4–1, question 3). In addition, we need to arrive at some estimate of a time frame within which we can project achievement of the communication performance we target (Box 4–1, question 4). The sources of data that help us project levels of achievement and set a reasonable time frame are (a) the prior therapists' reports of their treatment results (a part of background information) and (b) maintaining factors.

In reviewing background information relevant to Seth's treatment history, we learn that Seth has received speech-language therapy since the age of three. Therapy has focused primarily on eliminating the processes of backing, stopping, and final consonant deletion. For these and other processes, progress in prior therapy suggests that achievements are slow and regression is frequent. Until now, treatment of his phonological impairment has been provided by a speech-language pathologist working independently. She has not collaborated with his school speech-language pathologist or his occupational therapist (see discussion of procedural approach, below). The school speech-language pathologist has focused primarily on syntactic errors and comprehension. Though a prognosis is still uncertain, collaboration between the occupational therapist and speech-language pathologist is expected to improve stability of performance. Based, however, on Seth's achievement history, it is not likely that we can expect the processes he now uses to be eliminated entirely. This projection is also made with reference to the factors believed to be maintaining Seth's speech-language problems.

Baseline data from assessment reports provide information about factors that may be maintaining Seth's speech-language disorder. Based on results achieved on WISC–R, Seth presents with much inter-intra subtest variability. Lowest scores were obtained on tasks involving the visualization of part-whole relationships, analyzing and synthesizing designs, and matching symbols to numbers. These tasks involve attention to detail and differentiation of similarities and differences among items. These difficulties may also be represented in attention to speech sounds, syllables, and syntactic elements. Therefore, cognitive factors may be depressing speech-language performance and affecting estimated time frame for achieving long-term goals.

The sensorimotor domain is perhaps the most problematic for Seth, and probably the primary maintaining factor of his severe phonological impairment. From the time of his first interview at three years of age, Seth was described by his mother as having coordination difficulty. Now, at eleven years, eleven months, he is described by the occupational therapist as having a number of sensorimotor difficulties, including low muscle tone, incoordination, and weakness in overall body movements (see Chapter 3, Table 3–6). These sensorimotor symptoms are likely to affect movement, coordination, and sensation associated with the production of speech sounds. This maintaining factor is perhaps the most influential in determining the level of goal achievement and expected time frame for the achievement of targeted goals.

Psychosocial factors may also be maintaining Seth's speech-language problem. Based on standardized tests administered by the psychologist, Seth is described as anxious, sad, vulnerable and low in self-esteem. A frequent response to a perceived challenge is "I can't do it." This behavior has also been observed by the speech-language pathologist and occupational therapist. While Seth can occasionally be encouraged to complete a task, the clinician will often need to end testing or task production because of his refusal to continue. Seth's psychosocial picture is further complicated by his tactile defensiveness (particularly around the mouth). This attitude poses a constraint on the clinician, who needs to touch him in order to demonstrate a motor action or phonetic placement. As we can see, psychosocial factors are additional maintaining factors that need to be considered in projecting long-term goals and time frames.

To complete the long-term goal statements, we need to approximate a reasonable amount of time for the attainment of the long-term goals. This is a difficult decision. The difficulty in making a specific projection about time has to do with Seth's inconsistent and slow progress in prior treatment, his age, the extent of involvement of those factors maintaining his speech-language problem, and the potential effect of speech-sound improvement on other areas of language targeted (inflectional morphemes, complex sentences, and narratives). These factors suggest that improvement will continue to be slow and inconsistent. However, the current plan includes treatment designed through collaboration between a speech-language pathologist and an occupational therapist. We also know that Seth will be receiving speech-language intervention with a more consistent approach by one speech-language pathologist three times weekly. (He had been receiving therapy from two different clinicians.) Given this information, we project that Seth will achieve the long-term goals we have set within five years.

Given the results of baseline data in speech and language, potential maintaining factors for a child Seth's age, and the outcome of prior interventions, we are prepared to fill out the first part of the Long-Term Goals and Procedures Form (Form B–3) for Seth (Table 4–5).

Seth: The Derivation of a Long-Term Procedural Approach. At this point, a set of decisions needs to be made about a procedural approach. We will again consider the questions and corresponding sources of information in Box 4–2 for developing a procedural approach.

Step 1: Identifying maintaining factors that need to be addressed in order to reach the long-term goal. In our earlier consideration of Seth's maintaining factors, we

TABLE 4-5.   Management Plan: Long-Term Goals and Procedures

Client: <u>Seth</u>	Clinician:
Supervisor:	Semester:

Long-Term Goals and Expected Duration:

1. Seth will decrease phonological process application across all categories to the point of intelligibility by people unaware of his speech pattern
2. Seth will begin to suppress processes that have not begun dissolution (gliding and vocalization)
3. Seth will produce final consonants that code inflectional morphemes
4. Seth will increase frequency and variety of multiverb content-form interactions and their associated connectives
5. Seth will produce complex causal-chain narratives

Targeted attainments should be achieved within three to five years after the initiation of intervention

Rationales with reference to:

Baseline data (how current linguistic performance motivates goals):
1. Seth typically produces simple sentences and a narrow range of complex sentences without connectives
2. His narrative attempts do not persist beyond two to three utterances. These utterances are primitive additive and temporal chains; attempts at longer narratives are thwarted by difficulties in being understood
3. He uses many developmental processes: from 15% to 100% in single-word contexts and from 24% to 100% in continuous-speech contexts
4. Early developmental morphemes are generally absent from his productions in conversational speech (plural, copula, third person singular, possessive, past irregular, and past regular)

Maintaining factors (justification of long-term expectation and duration):
Cognitive, psychosocial, and sensorimotor

concluded that Seth's production patterns were primarily maintained by his sensorimotor difficulty. Severely impaired articulation appears to be depressing the production of morphemes, complex sentences, and narratives. It is expected that procedures designed to facilitate the acquisition of speech sounds will also facilitate improvement in the other language areas. His baseline data further suggest that cognitive and psychosocial factors may play a role in the maintenance of impaired speech-language performance in all areas.

At this point, it is possible to begin to formulate the first part of the procedural approach, in which we specify the maintaining factors that will need to be addressed in the course of intervention and the related communication areas targeted in the long-term goal statement: All long-term goals will be facilitated by modifying sensorimotor, cognitive, and psychosocial maintaining factors.

Step 2: Identifying learning principles that will guide our procedural approach for Seth. Language-learning principles will be drawn from Box 1–7. In identifying

Table 4–6. Management Plan: Long-Term Goals and Procedures

Client: Seth	**Clinician:** _____
Supervisor: _____	**Semester:** _____

Long-Term Goals and Expected Duration:

1. Seth will decrease phonological process application across all categories to the point of intelligibility by people unaware of his speech pattern
2. Seth will begin to suppress processes that have not begun dissolution (gliding and vocalization)
3. Seth will produce final consonants that code inflectional morphemes
4. Seth will increase frequency and variety of multiverb content-form interactions and their associated connectives
5. Seth will produce complex causal-chain narratives

Targeted attainments should be achieved within three to five years after the initiation of intervention

Rationales with reference to:

Baseline data (how current linguistic performance motivates goals):
1. Seth typically produces simple sentences and a narrow range of complex sentences without connectives
2. His narrative attempts do not persist beyond two to three utterances. These utterances are primitive additive and temporal chains; attempts at longer narratives are thwarted by difficulties in being understood
3. He uses many developmental processes: from 15% to 100% in single-word contexts and from 24% to 100% in continuous-speech contexts
4. Early developmental morphemes are generally absent from his productions in conversational speech (plural, copula, third person singular, possessive, past irregular, and past regular)

Maintaining factors (justification of long-term expectation and duration):
Cognitive, psychosocial, and sensorimotor

Procedural Approach:

Maintaining factors addressed:
Cognitive, sensorimotor, and psychosocial

Guiding principles (from learning theories, Box 1–7):

Learning is facilitated by:
2 — efforts to match models presented by the clinician
3 — noticing similarities and distinctions among actions and events mediated by adults
6 — efforts to convey meaning and overcome miscommunication successfully
8 — reflection upon personal behavior
9 — sensory stimulation (i.e., sensory feedback) from movement involved in the performance of articulatory gestures

Reward system:
Internal and social

the principles that apply to the elimination of phonological processes, we find that the most appropriate derive from motor learning theory and social-cognitive theory. These principles appear at the beginning of the section on Seth. We will illustrate the way in which these principles affect planning a therapeutic context in Chapter 5.

Initial decisions about language-learning principles become the second part of the long-term procedural approach.

Step 3: Selecting a reward system. Seth, as a boy of nearly twelve, enjoys engaging in social interactions. The impact of improved intelligibility, which was targeted in the long-term goal statement, will be socially rewarding. Our focus on producing narratives as a long-term goal is also social in nature. It is for these reasons that we will employ a social reward system to facilitate the achievement of all goals.

A consideration of maintaining factors, principles from learning theories, and a reward system comprises the procedural approach in phase 1 of the management plan. The completed first part of the Management Plan for Seth appears in Table 4–6.

Alice

The following are the long-term goals and procedural approach that were developed for Alice, the fourth child we will consider at the long-term phase of intervention planning.

Long-term goals:

1. Alice will coordinate efficient respiratory and phonatory patterns while producing complex sentences in all pragmatic contexts.
2. Alice will eliminate phonological processes of stopping and gliding.
3. Alice will produce Lahey Phase 8 and 8+ verb inflections, subjective pronouns, and connectives in all pragmatic contexts. Targeted attainments should be achieved within three years after the initiation of intervention.

Long-term procedural approach:

1. All long-term goals will be facilitated by modifying sensorimotor, cognitive, and psychosocial maintaining factors.
2. It will be necessary for the speech-language pathologist to collaborate with an occupational or physical therapist (or both) on the modification of Alice's sensorimotor patterns related to tonicity and body segmentation. The clinician will use expansion and modeling techniques to encourage production of target behaviors.
3. The long-term procedural approach for Alice is influenced primarily by the following principles from social-cognitive learning theory and motor-learning theory (selected from Box 1–7).

Learning is facilitated by:

—efforts to match models presented by the clinician;

—noticing similarities and distinctions among actions and events mediated by adults;

—interactions and contexts commensurate with the child's past experience and present developmental level;

—sensory stimulation (i.e., sensory feedback) from movement involved in the performance of articulatory gestures.

Internal and social rewards will be employed to facilitate the achievement of all goals.

Alice: The Derivation of the Long-Term Goals. The questions and corresponding sources of information that are presented in Box 4–1 again served as a basis for the formulation of long-term goals.

Steps 1 and 2: Making decisions about areas of communication to target. As usual, baseline data direct us to areas of communication to target as long-term goals and to a format for organizing long-term goal statements. Baseline data for Alice have been organized according to taxonomies of vocal parameters, content-form interactions, and use. Alice was seen initially for the evaluation of a suspected voice problem. A vocal assessment revealed mild to moderate impairments in the coordination of respiratory, phonatory, and articulatory patterns. The outstanding vocal characteristics were low pitch and hoarseness. The otolaryngologist's report indicated the presence of vocal nodules and recommended voice therapy. Based on this information, one long-term goal statement will address achievement of efficient coordination of respiration and phonation for communication purposes.

A review of Alice's conversational-speech sample reveals that Alice is acquiring content-form-use interactions within normal developmental parameters, although several problems are evident. MLU is on the low side of the normal range. Alice produces a preponderance of simple sentences. A wide range of complex sentences are emerging. These are volition-intention, antithesis, epistemic, additive, temporal, and causality. Connectives are frequently absent, although Alice uses *and* and *because* to code conjunction and *what* and *where* to code complementation. In addition, the responses to questions that obligate the production of complex sentences are simplified. It is also noteworthy that Alice manifests a number of errors in verb tense inflections and in verb-subject agreement for number and person. She also exhibits pronominal substitutions: *her/she/us/we/them/those*. These problems will need to be addressed systematically in therapy. As such, we formulate a long-term goal: Alice will produce Phase 8 and 8+ verb inflections, subjective pronouns, and connectives in all pragmatic contexts.

Since we expect that Alice will produce content-form-use interactions by the termination of treatment this level of language production is targeted as the linguistic context for achieving efficient coordination of respiration and phonation for communication purposes. Consequently, the first long-term goal is formulated as follows: Alice will coordinate efficient respiratory and phonatory patterns while executing complex sentences in all pragmatic contexts.

A third area that appears to pose problems for Alice is phonology. Baseline data indicate that Alice never produces /ð/, /r/, /dʒ/, and /z/; expresses variable versions of /tʃ/, /ɵ/, /l/ /f/ and /v/; and distorts /s/ and /ʃ/ by producing them with a lateral release. These substitutions and distortions suggest that two phonological processes have yet to be suppressed: gliding and stopping. (We view the lateral emission on /s/ and /ʃ/ and the place change f/ɵ within the realm of the stopping process.) This information suggests that a long-term goal be formulated that targets the elimination of the phonological processes of stopping and gliding.

Steps 3 and 4: Determining level of attainment and time frame. The final decisions that must be made involve the specification of a time frame for the achievement of the goals set and the determination of a level of achievement that can be expected of the client. A consideration of maintaining factors and discrepancies between current functioning and age-expected behaviors will help us make these decisions.

We have already set a normal level of achievement in each of the areas of communication targeted as dismissal criteria. We did so for the following reasons. First, MLU data fall within the normal range of linguistic production (albeit on the low end) for a child Alice's age. Second, difficulties in the area of syntax involve structures that are achieved at the end of Lahey's developmental sequence—Phases 8 and 8+. This puts the language delay in the one-year range. In addition, phonologic processes not yet eliminated primarily affect later-developing sounds (e.g., sibilants and liquids; Prather, Hedrick, & Kern, 1975; Sander, 1972). The data suggest a mild to moderate developmental disability in the areas of content-form interactions and phonology.

In terms of maintaining factors, we need to consider three areas: cognition, sensorimotor functioning, and psychosocial functioning. Cognitive functioning was assessed on the Wechsler Preschool and Primary Scale of Intelligence–Revised. Performance on this instrument indicated a Full Scale IQ of 85 ± 3. This score is within one standard deviation of the mean. The examiner indicated that Alice "failed to remain focused on task." Administration of the Vineland Adaptive Behavior Scales revealed normal functioning in four areas: communication, daily living skills, socialization, and motor skills. Taken together, these results of formal testing suggest that cognitive and psychosocial functioning should not block the attainment of the linguistic structures targeted. However, weaknesses in some cognitive areas may have a negative impact upon the rate of achievement of some of the more subtle or complex syntactic and phonologic productions.

Although motor skills were assessed as normal on the Vineland, baseline data indicate that tonicity, body segmentation, and stability may be compromised.

These sensorimotor difficulties may very well be maintaining laryngeal tension and vocal harshness, respiratory inefficiency, the failure to suppress phonologic processes, and syntactic difficulties involving low stress or perceptually nonsalient structures. Our procedural approach calls for addressing the sensorimotor variables in collaboration with a physical or occupational therapist. We feel such collaboration will allow eventual attainment of the targeted communication behaviors. However, sensorimotor factors may delay rapid achievement of goals.

Taking all of the above factors into consideration—in addition to the knowledge that Alice will be receiving speech-language intervention three times weekly in a school setting—leads us to predict that Alice will attain the three long-term goals within three years of the initiation of therapy. This prognosis represents the second part of the long-term goal statement. Long-term goals for Alice appear as the first part of the Management Plan (Form B–3) in Table 4–7.

Table 4–7. Management Plan: Long-Term Goals and Procedures

Client: <u>Alice</u>	Clinician: _____
Supervisor: _____	Semester: _____

Long-Term Goals and Expected Duration:
1. Alice will coordinate efficient respiratory and phonatory patterns while producing complex sentences in all pragmatic contexts
2. Alice will eliminate phonological processes of stopping and gliding
3. Alice will produce Phase 8 and 8 + verb inflections, subjective pronouns, and connectives in all pragmatic contexts

Targeted attainments should be achieved within three years after the initiation of intervention

Rationales with reference to:

Baseline data (how current linguistic performance motivates goals):
1. Mild to moderate impairments in the coordination of respiratory, phonatory, and articulatory patterns
2. Low pitch and hoarseness
3. Vocal nodules
4. Mild delay in production of complex content-form interactions at Lahey Phase 8 (a preponderance of simple sentences and a wide range of emerging complex sentences: volition-intention, antithesis, epistemic, additive, temporal, and causality)
5. Simplification of syntax in response to questions
6. Never produces /ð/, /r/, /dʒ/, or /z/; expresses variable versions of /tʃ/, /ө/, /l/, /f/, and /v/; and distorts /s/ and /ʃ/ by producing them with a lateral release

Maintaining factors (justification of long-term expectation and duration):
Mild weakness in some cognitive areas should not block the attainment of the linguistic structures targeted, but may have an impact upon the rate of goal achievement
Mild sensorimotor impairment affecting tonicity, body segmentation, and stability may delay rate of goal achievement

Alice: The Derivation of a Long-Term Procedural Approach.   Once again a set of decisions needs to be made about a procedural approach, and again we will consider the set of questions and corresponding sources of information presented in Box 4–2.

Step 1: Identifying maintaining factors that need to be addressed in order to reach the long-term goal. In developing our prognosis for Alice, we concluded that sensorimotor difficulties in the areas of tonicity, body segmentation, and stability are likely maintaining voice, phonologic, and syntactic delays. Thus, we specify the need to address this set of variables in the achievement of all target behaviors in the procedural approach. Because planning for the modification of sensorimotor deficits lies outside the range of expertise of most speech-language pathologists, we note that it will be necessary for the speech-language pathologist to collaborate with an occupational or physical therapist (or both)on the modification of Alice's sensorimotor patterns related to tonicity and body segmentation.

Furthermore, as indicated above, although baseline data indicate that cognitive functioning is within normal limits, weaknesses are apparent in some areas. These weaknesses may be maintaining speech-language dysfunctions in all areas—for example, by affecting Alice's ability to discriminate among subtle or complex stimuli and by delaying the construction of rules related to voice, phonologic, and syntactic performance. Also, the stimulation of cognitive functioning may facilitate the production of complex content-form interactions. Thus, cognition is also included as a maintaining factor in formulating the procedural approach.

A review of the baseline data in the psychosocial area reveals a number of points that are likely to influence communication behaviors. These are (a) variable attention to and motivation for activities, (b) a strong need for approval, and (c) obvious competition with her younger sister. Because of these data, we must also address the psychosocial maintaining factor in formulating a procedural approach.

Step 2: Identifying principles of learning that will guide procedural planning. The next part of the procedural approach involves the identification of learning principles that will guide the selection of materials and design of client-clinician interactions at subsequent phases of procedure planning. Recall that we have targeted the coordination of efficient respiratory and vocal patterns for communication, the suppression of phonologic processes, and the production of syntactic forms in complex sentences and narratives as long-term goals. Recall, too, that we are planning for a four-year-old client. Referring to Box 1–7, we select a set of principles—primarily from social and motor learning theories—that complement our personal beliefs about language learning in these targeted areas. These principles are that learning is facilitated by (a) efforts to match models presented by the clinician, (b) noticing similarities and distinctions among actions and events mediated by adults, (c) interactions and contexts commensurate with the child's past experience and present developmental level, and (d) sensory stimulation (i.e., sensory feedback) from movement involved in the production of speech. Before these principles are entered on the Long-Term Goal and Procedure Form B (reproduced below), a system of rewards to be utilized in the course of therapy will be considered.

Step 3: Selecting a reward system. The procedural approach for Alice is concluded with the selection of a reward system for use in intervention. As in the case of Seth, each long-term goal (improved voice, speech sounds, and syntax), will have a social impact. In addition, baseline data on Alice suggest that she needs social rewards in the form of verbal approvals and praise in order to complete tasks. It is for these reasons that a social reward system will be employed to facilitate the achievement of all goals. A completed Long-Term Goal and Procedural Approach form for Alice is presented in Table 4–8.

Table 4–8. Management Plan: Long-Term Goals and Procedures

Client: Alice_____	Clinician: _____
Supervisor: _____	Semester: _____

Long-Term Goals and Expected Duration:

1. Alice will coordinate efficient respiratory and phonatory patterns while producing complex sentences in all pragmatic contexts
2. Alice will eliminate phonological processes of stopping and gliding
3. Alice will produce Phase 8 and 8 + verb inflections, subjective pronouns, and connectives in all pragmatic contexts

Targeted attainments should be achieved within three years after the initiation of intervention

Rationales with reference to:

Baseline data (how current linguistic performance motivates goals):
1. Mild to moderate impairments in the coordination of respiratory, phonatory, and articulatory patterns
2. Low pitch and hoarseness
3. Vocal nodules
4. Mild delay in production of complex content-form interactions at Lahey Phase 8 (a preponderance of simple sentences and a wide range of emerging complex sentences: volition-intention, antithesis, epistemic, additive, temporal, and causality)
5. Simplification of syntax in response to questions
6. Never produces /ð/, /r/, /dʒ/, or /z/; produces variable versions of /tʃ/, /ө/, /l/, /f/, and /v/; and distorts /s/ and /ʃ/ by producing them with a lateral release

Maintaining factors (justification of long-term expectation and duration):

Mild weakness in some cognitive areas should not block the attainment of the linguistic structures targeted, but may have an impact upon the rate of goal achievement

Mild sensorimotor impairment affecting tonicity, body segmentation, and stability may delay rate of goal achievement

(continued)

Table 4-8   *(continued)*

Procedural Approach:

Maintaining factors addressed:
  Cognitive, sensorimotor (collaboration with an occupational or physical therapist recommended)

Guiding principles (from learning theories, Box 1-7):

Learning is facilitated by:

2 — efforts to match models presented by the clinician

3 — noticing similarities and distinctions among actions and events mediated by adults

5 — interactions and contexts commensurate with the child's past experience and present developmental level

6 — sensory stimulation (i.e., sensory feedback) from movement involved in the performance of articulatory gestures

Reward system:
  Internal and social

SUMMARY

In Chapter 4, we developed a conceptualization of the long-term phase of intervention planning, and formulated long-term goals and procedural approaches for four children with speech-language disorders: Darryl, Patty, Seth, and Alice. In Chapter 5, we examine the short-term phase of intervention planning in a similar way—by defining short-term goals and procedures, and by detailing the decision-making process involved in their formulation. We also will derive short-term goals and procedures for each of the four children.

5

Phase 2 of Intervention Planning: The Identification of Short-Term Goals And Delineation of Procedural Contexts

Now that we have set our sights on the outcome of therapy (i.e., the formulation of long-term goals), we return to the nagging question, "What should I do first?" At this point in intervention planning we are not prepared to decide what to do first in terms of a first session; rather, we are ready to consider what to do first in a sequence of steps directed toward the attainment of our long-term goals. These steps within the sequence represent short-term goals, and during this second phase of intervention planning we focus on their formulation and prioritization. A complementary focus is the delineation of procedural contexts within which the short-term goals are addressed.

In this chapter we explicate the second phase of intervention planning. We define short-term goals and procedural contexts. We discuss the decisions that need to be made at this short-term planning phase, paying special attention to the developmental basis of short-term goals. We then continue to follow Darryl, Patty, Seth, and Alice in order to illustrate the decision-making process at Phase 2 of intervention planning.

DEFINING AND FORMULATING SHORT-TERM GOALS

Definitions

We define a *short-term goal* as a linguistic achievement that has been given priority within a hierarchy of achievements required for the realization of the long-term goal. The wording in this definition directs the clinician to the nature of decision making involved in the formulation of short-term goals. Decision making underlies (a) the formulation, in linguistic terms, of one or more speech-language achievements; (b) the projection of a hierarchy of target achievements that should lead to the attainment of long-term goals; and (c) the prioritization of one or more achievements. In addition, *short-term* implies a definitive period of time. Implicit in this definition is the central role that schedules of child language development play in the conceptualization of short-term goals. Below, we expand upon the significance of each of these components of our definition; we also identify sources of information that are relevant to each decision the clinician needs to make in formulating short-term goals.

A Linguistic Achievement.   The first part of the definition asserts that a short-term goal is a linguistic achievement. This signifies that the short-term goal be formulated with reference to linguistic (or prelinguistic) structures. As discussed in Chapters 1 and 2, linguistic structures are units or categories of speech and language that have a developmental or maturational basis; examples are form-content interactions, pragmatic functions, and phonological processes. Similarly, prelinguistic structures are categories of behaviors normally expressed by infants and toddlers that are presumed to provide a developmental foundation for speech and language; examples include babbling, prosodic variations, circular reactions with objects, and communicative acts. These behaviors may be viewed as precursors to linguistic categories of content, form, and use. An example of a short-term goal targeting a linguistic achievement for a child manifesting a severe phonological problem is: "The child will suppress the process of stopping in word-final position." An example of a short-term goal targeting prelinguistic structures for a one-year-old who is at risk for a language delay is: "Sean will communicate intentionally using gesture or vocalization for interactional or regulatory purposes."

Why we target linguistic structures as short-term goals. We have several reasons for formulating short-term goals in developmental and linguistic terms. The first concerns the child's role in the acquisition of behaviors that are developmental in nature. The developmental literature has taught us that the acquisition of linguistic structures does not involve simply the child's imitation of adult behaviors. The acquisition of such structures also requires active contributions from the child in relation to the child's intents, inferences, and organization of information. As a consequence of these internal mechanisms, normally achieving children and children with language-learning disabilities learn language by categorizing or organizing linguistic input (Bloom & Lahey, 1978; Ferguson & Macken, 1980; Leonard, 1989; Pinker, 1991). Each category that a child creates is foundational to the creation of more complex categories. For example, the process of abstracting and coordinating semantic categories such as agent, action, and object is foundational for the production of three-constituent utterances (Bloom, 1970; Bloom & Lahey, 1978). As speech-language clinicians, we have to factor in this natural tendency of children to be active in speech and language learning when we envision steps to the achievement of long-term goals.

The second reason that we always target linguistic structures in short-term goal statements is that we are speech-language pathologists. Our domain is language. Short-term goals are steps leading to the achievement of long-term *linguistic* goals. By targeting semantic, syntactic, phonologic, and morphologic structures at the short-term phase of intervention planning, we believe that we are appropriately oriented toward facilitating *the development of speech and language.*

The use of taxonomies in the formulation of short-term goals. Recall that, in formulating long-term goal statements, we anticipated the need to address the developmental nature of speech and language. We did so by specifying taxonomies of linguistic behavior that would provide direction in formulating short-term goals. It is with reference to the taxonomies cited in the long-term goal statement(s) that short-term goal statement(s) are formulated. For example, if a clinician set the achievement of Bloom and Lahey Phase 5 form-content interactions as a long-term goal, the short-term goal statement would need to be written in terms of one or more Bloom and Lahey form-content interactions: for example, "The child will coordinate locative action and attribution." Similarly, if the suppression of phonologic processes was targeted, short-term goals would be written in terms of phonological processes to be suppressed.

Implications of targeting linguistic structures as short-term goals. To elucidate the broad range of implications inherent in viewing short-term goals as targeted *linguistic structures* that are developmental in nature, let us consider some areas of language that at first glance may not appear to lend themselves to this type of treatment. Suppose that a clinician is planning for a seven-year-old child with a language delay, for whom English is a second language, and decides to target vocabulary. Traditionally, one might write a short-term goal with reference to a subject area that may be functional for the child. An example of such a goal might be, "Sandra will increase her English vocabulary relevant to cooking." Although cooking vocabulary may indeed prove useful for Sandra, cooking vocabulary is not a unit of language that has a developmental foundation. In the normal course of development, children do not learn *cooking* vocabulary as a basis for learning, say, *clothing* vocabulary. Indeed, when you think about what might constitute cooking vocabulary, you soon realize that there are all kinds of words that are relevant to cooking (e.g., *hot, cold, turn on, turn off, in, out, to, for, pot, microwave*). These words can be subcategorized with reference to a variety of linguistic units that are developmental in nature. For example, some cooking vocabulary words are verbs that code action or locative action. Other cooking vocabulary words are adjectives that code attribution. We maintain that short-term goals relevant to the acquisition of vocabulary, regardless of content, should be formulated in terms of such linguistic categories; e.g., "Sandra will produce English lexical items that code attributes and actions relevant to cooking."

Let us consider a second example of a speech-language dysfunction in which the linguistic basis for goal setting might be unclear: a voice problem. This voice problem is manifested by Sarah, a four-year-old with chronic hoarseness. In areas other than voice, Sarah's language functioning appears to be appropriate for her age. A speech-language clinician has established the following short-term goal: "Sarah will coordinate and sustain air flow and voicing to produce three-constituent utterances." This goal statement does have a developmental basis, although concepts such as *air flow* and *voicing* are not usually thought of as developmental or linguistic in nature. The co-ordination of respiration and phonation represented by these terms refers to a natural achievement that is necessary to code language and that under-goes transformations with growth (Kahane, 1983). Thus, sensorimotor achievements such as coordinated and sustained air flow and voicing may be viewed as developmental since they have a maturational component (i.e., naturally changing with growth). In addition, the production of three-con-stituent utterances targeted in Sarah's voice goal presented above also refers to a developmental achievement.

Nonlinguistic behaviors and short-term goals. We have been stressing the tar-geting of *linguistic* behaviors in the short-term goal. The reader may ask what could cause clinicians to target another behavioral system, instead. One moti-vation is often the clinician's hypotheses about nonlinguistic factors that are maintaining a linguistic problem. An example of such a factor is the cognitive function of *attention.* During an assessment, a child, Doris, flitted from one toy to another, never really focusing on any formal procedure that the examiner tried to present. Because of this behavior, the examiner hypothesized that one factor possibly maintaining Doris's language problem was her short attention span. As a consequence, the following short-term goal was formulated: "Doris will increase attention span." Although we recognize the need to address maintaining factors in the course of intervention, we do so in the short-term goal statement only if we can specify a category of linguistic behavior that in-corporates the maintaining factor (e.g., Doris's attention could be addressed through language use). Thus, the following short-term goal could be formu-lated: "Doris will demonstrate joint attention across a variety of play activities." This goal is directed toward the development of a category of language use (joint attention). In the process, attention is being addressed.

Not referring to nonlinguistic maintaining factors apart from linguistic structures in the short-term goal statement does not signify that we do not address these factors at the short-term phase of intervention planning. In this chapter we examine the way our knowledge of maintaining factors in-fluences the prioritization of a linguistic target. We also refer to these factors in delimiting a procedural approach. In Chapter 6 we refer to maintaining factors again in formulating session goals and procedures. Furthermore, in

Chapter 7 we discuss how maintaining factors may be addressed at the short-term phase of intervention planning through collaboration with allied professionals and the child's family.

Prioritization.   In our definition of a short-term goal, we stated that behavior targeted as the short-term goal is given priority within a hierarchy of achievements. "Given priority" means that, from a group of behaviors, one has been selected to be addressed first. Prioritization involves making three sets of decisions: (a) selecting long-term goal(s) to work toward first (if more than one long-term goal was set for the client), (b) identifying the hierarchy of short-term achievements necessary for reaching the long-term goals, and (c) selecting those short-term achievements to be targeted first. We will discuss these three aspects of the formulation of short-term goals in the next section.

Formulating Short-term Goals

Determining Which Long-Term Goals to Target First.   If more than one long-term goal was set for a child, we must decide which one(s) to target during the first contracted time period. This decision entails a number of considerations:

1. In the normal course of development, are any of the targeted goals under consideration achieved before any others?
2. Do the goals under consideration interact in such a way that they could be worked on simultaneously?
3. Does the achievement of any of the goals have more of an impact than others on the health or overall communicative success of the child?

The following two scenarios illustrate the utility of these questions. In the first scenario, three behaviors targeted as long-term goals are normally achieved at the same developmental phase and interact naturally in the course of development. As an example, consider the following three long-term goals which were formulated for a four-year-old: (a) to code content-form interactions at Lahey's Phase 8, (b) to use language to initiate conversations and regulate the environment, and (c) to increase lexical variety by extending the range of verbs and prepositions. In such a case, the answer to the first question cited above is "no," the answer to the second is "yes," and the answer to the third is "no." This indicates that we should develop short-term goals to address all the long-term goals.

   In other cases, targeted goals may be in different areas of language and interactions may not be immediately obvious. For example, a five-year-old with a voice problem may also have difficulties in syntax and phonology. Long-term goals for this child may include (a) the achievement of efficient coordination of respiration, phonation, and resonation in conversational speech; (b) the appropriate production of nominative case pronouns; and (c) the elimination of the phonological processes of gliding and cluster reduction. In this case we need to go beyond developmental considerations in making a prioritization decision. We are guided especially by the third question: "Does the achievement of any of the goals have more of an impact than others on the health or overall communicative success of the child?" In many cases of voice problems, immediate vocal intervention is recommended by the otolaryngologist. Therefore, the voice goal would take precedence (although other areas may be targeted in addition).

Information about interactions among components of language available in the literature on normal and disordered child language development will facilitate decisions about prioritization (e.g., Bloom & Lahey, 1978; Paul & Shriberg, 1982; Schwartz, Leonard, Folger, & Wilcox, 1980). Box 5–1 summarizes questions and sources of information for determining which long-term goal(s) to target first when prioritizing short-term goals.

Identifying a Hierarchy of Short-Term Goals.   Once long-term goals have been selected, it is necessary to identify one or more specific short-term goals with reference to the achievement of the long-term goal(s). This, again, involves prioritization. The short-term goal or goals will be drawn from a set of possible goals. This set of possible goals is referred to in the definition of short-term goals presented above as a *hierarchy of achievements*. This hierarchy of achievements has direction. It should lead to the attainment of the long-term goal(s) that have been targeted.

The term *hierarchy of achievements* has a number of implications. It suggests that the attainment of a long-term goal requires targeting a number of intermediate achievements or goals. It suggests, further, that

---

BOX 5–1.   QUESTIONS AND SOURCES OF INFORMATION
FOR DETERMINING WHICH LONG-TERM GOALS
TO TARGET FIRST

Question	*Sources of Information*
1. In the normal course of development, are any of the goals under consideration achieved before any others?	Developmental taxonomies
2. Do the goals under consideration interact in such a way that they could be worked on during one time period?	Research reports on language acquisition
3. Does the achievement of any of the goals have more of an impact than others on the health or overall communicative success of the child?	Baseline data

intermediate goals can be arranged in such a way that each success serves as a foundation for the achievement of subsequent goals. Furthermore, the term *hierarchy* implies that there may be a natural configuration and order to a set of achievements. The naturalness and order are associated with normal child development.

Sources of hierarchies. Proposed hierarchies for the development of certain speech-language behaviors appear in the literature and are most often based on research with normally developing children. Among these, one of the most frequently referenced is the sequence of content-form-use phases of Bloom and Lahey (1978; see also Lahey, 1988). Other sequences often referenced are found in the areas of prelinguistic cognitive achievements (Uzgiris & Hunt, 1978) and sound production (Proctor, 1989), phonology (Grunwell, 1981), and language functions (Halliday, 1975; Tough, 1977). These hierarchies may provide a beginning framework for prioritizing short-term goals. When there are no sequences of behavior summarized for a particular area of speech-language development, it may be necessary for the speech-language pathologist to review a number of articles in the specific speech-language area, such as the development of irregular verbs (Shipley, Maddox, & Driver, 1991), humor (Spector, 1992), and idioms (Nippold, 1985). These articles appear regularly in the publications of the American Speech-Language-Hearing Association and in related journals (e.g., *Journal of Child Language, Journal of Applied Linguistics, Child Language Teaching and Therapy*). We return to the issue of specifying sequences of behavior in the section on individual children later in this chapter.

The two-dimensional nature of the hierarchy. Within hierarchies, developmental achievements may be viewed as proceeding in two directions. In the normal course of development, some achievements may be higher-level and more challenging than others. Still other achievements may be of parallel difficulty or complexity. This distinction between parallel and higher-level complexity in child development is seen in Bloom and Lahey's (1978) description of phases in the development of content-form interactions. There are a number of linguistic structures that children achieve during a single phase (parallel achievements), and there are other sets of structures that are attained later in development (higher-level achievements). For example, during the first phase of development children use single words to code existence, recurrence, action, and negation (among others). In other words, a number of achievements occur at the same time (in a parallel manner). In contrast, single-word achievements occur at phase 1, before word combinations, which are a *higher level* achievement. Figure 5–1 depicts the relation between parallel achievements, hierarchic stages, and long-term goals.

Alternative approaches to developmental hierarchies. Some clinicians set goals that appear to be hierarchical in nature. These goals, however, do not imply any identifiable developmental sequence. For example, two frequently set goals for children with language-learning difficulties involve following multiple-step

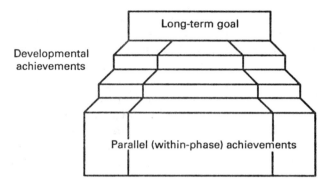

FIGURE 5–1.   Short-term goals (developmental achievements and parallel achievements) leading to the long-term goal.

commands and sequencing. Such goals may read "Jose will follow two-step commands" or "Miguele will correctly sequence activities represented in three pictures." These goals seem to fall within a clear-cut sequence of objectives; following two-step commands precedes following three-step commands, and seriating three pictures precedes seriating four pictures. Sequences like these, however, are generated intuitively rather than on the basis of developmental literature. In this case of sequencing goals, the clinician might consider targeting complex semantic relations or story grammars that are developmental in nature and relevant to sequencing, such as additive, temporal, and causal (e.g., see Lahey, 1988).

The projection of a hierarchy of achievements is a challenging undertaking due to the complex nature of speech-language disabilities and language learning. The clinician must sort through a great deal of information in order to answer the question, "What should be targeted first?" This question requires that thought be given to prioritization.

Selecting Short-Term Goals to Target First.   After projecting a sequence or hierarchy of linguistic achievements, one or more need(s) to be selected as targets for the initial short-term period. We will need to determine what represents a developmental step forward for the child and how many goals to target for the first short-term period. Once again, the decision-making process is enhanced by addressing a number of questions. Where is the child functioning now? Is the child capable of working on multiple achievements at one time? Which behaviors among a number of simultaneously occurring achievements (parallel achievements) may be facilitated most readily?

Where is the child functioning now? The major source of information that may be helpful in answering this question is baseline data about linguistic behavior. Recall that baseline data, available in a diagnostic report, represent information about a client's current level of functioning. The client's current level of functioning will be the starting point for targeting a linguistic achievement that is developmentally more advanced and a foundational step toward the long-term goal.

Is the child capable of working on multiple achievements during one time period? Making a decision to target a number of short-term goals simultaneously requires considering whether a child is capable of working on multiple achievements during one time period. Our knowledge of maintaining factors will influence such a decision. If a confluence of maintaining factors indicates that a child could not handle working on multiple achievements during such a limited amount of time, multiple goals should be avoided. Conversely, the absence of observable impairment in associated behavioral systems might suggest that multiple achievements would be feasible.

Another factor to consider here is the interaction among the goals (identified when we selected long-term goals). It might make sense to target multiple linguistic achievements during a single time period when one achievement may automatically influence functioning in other areas of language. For example, coding language content implies the use of syntax and the pragmatic function served by the utterance. Thus, a short-term goal could refer to more than one aspect of language (e.g., "Stacey will code locative action using two constituents to direct another's actions"). Consider a second example of a natural interaction among linguistic achievements: the impact that phonologic process suppression may have on morphology. A short-term goal targeting these two interactive achievements in a child with a phonological disorder might read: "Jennifer will suppress final consonant deletion of sibilants that serve the morphological function of coding plural, possession, and time."

Which behaviors among a number of simultaneously occurring achievements (parallel achievements) may be facilitated most readily? This is an optional question. It becomes necessary when a developmental taxonomy presents parallel goals to choose from (e.g., phases of the Bloom and Lahey framework; Lahey, 1988). Although a number of behaviors may be acquired simultaneously by normally developing children, it does not necessarily follow that language-impaired children will emulate this pattern. We know of no research evidence to support a different acquisition schedule for children who have difficulty learning language. However, it is our clinical experience that, among linguistic structures that appear at the same stage of development in normally achieving children, some may be more difficult to learn than others by children with language-learning disabilities (e.g., at Phase 2 of Bloom and Lahey, coding *existence* was found to be more difficult to facilitate than *action*).

Clinical experience suggests that certain structures are more crucial for communicative success than others. Such structures code information that, in a particular situation, must be included in order to transmit a meaningful message. These structures may be considered "pragmatically obligatory." For example, consider two possible short-term goals for a child with a language delay: coding action with two constituents and coding existence with two words. A child would be more successful persuading an adult to perform an action with the utterance "daddy jump" than with "jump" (if the mother and father are alternately jumping). The child's ability to control the environment does not suffer as much in expressions of existence. Existence serves more of a mathetic function. Therefore, a child can satisfy this function by producing an existence utterance with or without a demonstrative. Thus, given a child who is not producing two-word combinations, we might target a two-constituent action utterance before a two-word existence utterance— even though both are designated within the same developmental phase (Bloom & Lahey, 1978). This example illustrates the consideration of pragmatic saliency in making decisions about which content-form interactions to target as a short-term goal.

Consider, too, a child who manifests a problem in the area of syntax. Baseline data indicate that the child produces content categories through Bloom and Lahey Phase 6. However, there are noticeable gaps in production of function words: the child has not achieved consistent use of prepositions and articles. Evaluations of sensorimotor functioning and perception indicate deficits in these areas. The child's overall profile suggests that perception and production of linguistic forms with "low phonetic substance" (Leonard, 1989) may be a factor maintaining the syntactic problem. This variable becomes a factor in deciding which syntactic structures to target first. With reference to this child, perhaps the clinician should target first those function words that would receive stress in an utterance.

Box 5–2 summarizes questions and related sources of information that clinicians may refer to in deciding what linguistic achievement(s) to target first at the short-term phase of intervention planning.

BOX 5–2. QUESTIONS AND RELEVANT SOURCES OF INFORMATION FOR PRIORITIZING SHORT-TERM GOALS

Questions	*Sources of Information*
1. What is the client's current level of functioning?	Baseline data in speech and language
2. Is the child capable of working on multiple achievements during one time period?	Baseline data on maintaining factors
3. Which among a number of simultaneously occurring achievements (parallel achievements) may be facilitated most readily?	Baseline data on maintaining factors Baseline data in speech and language

Formulating Short-Term Goals for IEPs. Legislation such as PL 94–142 has mandated that, for the purposes of completing an individualized educational plan (IEP) for a child, short-term goal statements need to refer to observable behaviors and provide a criterion for measuring the child's achievement of this behavior. In actuality, the achievement of the short-term goal is measured during a specific session. Further consideration, therefore, is given to criteria for measuring short-term goal achievement at the third phase of intervention planning. For this reason, we specify the criteria for achieving short-term goals and create a criterion-goal statement for IEPs during the session-planning phase (Chapter 6). We present an IEP Conversion Form for developing short-term goals for IEPs in Appendix B, Form B–4. This will be discussed further in Chapter 6.

DEFINING AND DELINEATING
THE PROCEDURAL CONTEXTS

Definitions

Delineating Procedural Contexts. Having decided on which short-term goals to target, we turn our attention to augmenting the procedural approach that we introduced during the first phase of intervention planning. Recall that we defined therapy procedures in general as planned interactions and contexts that are designed to facilitate the achievement of desired speech and language goals. At the long-term phase of intervention planning, we were concerned with defining parameters of interactions and materials that will allow us to accomplish our long-term goal. In that procedural approach we referenced (a) the maintaining factors that require modification and (b) the principles from learning theories that guide the creation of an optimal learning environment.

At the short-term phase of intervention planning, therefore, we describe the linguistic and nonlinguistic contexts that will be created to facilitate achievement of the specified short-term goals. The description of these contexts will include reference to the types of materials, interactions, and elicitations that will be utilized.

The nonlinguistic context. The term *nonlinguistic context* refers to materials and activities that will be used with children during speech-language intervention to achieve targeted goals. Children learning language are especially sensitive to what surrounds them (Fischer, 1989; Muma, 1978). Consequently, designing an appropriate nonlinguistic context is an especially critical aspect of intervention planning. A number of child language specialists have suggested that the child's freedom to impose structure on the environment and the perceptual support available are the two principal components of the nonlinguistic context (Bloom & Lahey, 1978; Gallagher & Reid, 1984; Owens, 1992).

The environment may be more or less responsive to the child's effort to impose structure on it or control it. On one hand, a can of Play-Doh or a box of Legos may be manipulated by the child at will. On the other hand, a book of pictures or a card game may provide fewer alternatives for individual creations. People in the environment may be more or less intent on directing or imposing structure on the child. One adult may join in a child-initiated activity, while others may feel more comfortable telling children what to do.

Related to the child's imposition of structure on the environment is the matter of perceptual support. Perceptual support refers to the availability of visible or tangible referents for utterances. When a child talks about the ball he is bouncing or throwing, we can say that his actions with the object provide support for his utterances. When children tell their mothers what they did in school earlier that day, they are speaking without perceptual support. How the clinician designs the nonlinguistic therapeutic context with reference to the environment's malleability and the availability of perceptual support can have a significant influence on language learning in children. Therefore, delineating characteristics of the nonlinguistic therapeutic context is an important task at this second phase of intervention planning.

The linguistic context. The linguistic context comprises the utterances that surround the targeted utterances produced by the child. The surrounding utterances may be produced by the child, or they may be statements or questions produced by another. A great deal of variation within the linguistic behavior of individual children has been attributed to linguistic context. For example, children appear to generate more complex utterances following a statement by an adult about something the child is doing. They generate less complex utterances in response to questions (e.g., Hubbell, 1988; Shatz & Gelman, 1973). Phoneme production seems to be influenced by the phonetic, morphological, and syntactic environment surrounding the phoneme (e.g., Klein & Spector, 1985). Thus, the linguistic context is an important procedural concern; the language the clinician chooses to use—and the language the clinician chooses to provoke the child to use—will influence the child's linguistic behavior.

Delineating the Procedural Context

At this second phase of procedure planning, we refer to the short-term goal statement(s) and the two sources of information that were identified in the long-term procedural approach: maintaining factors and principles of language learning. These data will guide us in further delineating the environment in which we will do therapy. The short-term goal statement specifies the linguistic targets that the therapeutic context must facilitate. The maintaining factors identified, and baseline data relevant to these maintaining factors, will suggest materials and interactions. Learning principles will also bear on decisions about the nature of the nonlinguistic and linguistic therapeutic contexts.

We will first consider the three maintaining factors that most directly affect decisions about context: cognitive, sensorimotor, and psychosocial.

Maintaining Factors

Cognition. Information about the child's cognitive functioning will help us specify the kinds of materials we would want to have available for the intervention sessions. We want materials that are developmentally appropriate for language learning given the child's level of cognitive functioning.

The child's cognitive status interacts with the two features of nonlinguistic context discussed above: the degree of structure or control that the child is allowed to impose on the environment and the perceptual support available. How these environmental characteristics affect the child changes with development. Children first learning to talk produce more language when there are fewer constraints on their activities (Hubbell, 1988). Children also speak more when the environment provides perceptual support for their language. As children develop cognitively, their reliance on perceptual support decreases and they readily talk about objects and actions that are outside their perceptual field (Bloom & Lahey, 1978; Lahey, 1988). Also, as their cognitive and linguistic skills increase, children are able to converse within constraints imposed by others. After the clinician has consulted baseline data on the child's cognitive status, Box 1–3 (Chapter 1) may be a useful resource in delimiting a procedural approach. Information presented in this box indicates how cognition interacts with language acquisition at specified points in development.

Sensorimotor. The child's sensorimotor status represents an important consideration for the design of a therapeutic context. Knowledge about a child's tonicity, stability, body segmentation, and sensory status can affect the choice of furniture, play materials, and communication devices. An assessment of a child's sensorimotor status is usually conducted by a physical or occupational therapist. Having such an assessment will determine whether there is a need for collaboration in intervention planning. Recommendations by these professionals will guide client-clinician interactions (e.g., positioning, encouraging movement). Collaboration is discussed later in this chapter and in Chapters 6 and 7.

Psychosocial. The child's psychosocial history contains information useful for the delineation of a therapeutic context. Relevant psychosocial information includes what the child likes to play with, whether the child plays in a parallel fashion or cooperatively, and the nature of the child's responses to male and female figures. The clinician can apply knowledge of these variables in designing a context in which a child may comfortably work on linguistic achievements.

The inclusion of families in speech-language intervention is another psychosocial issue that needs to be addressed in delineating a procedural approach. Short-term goals targeting caretaker-child interactions are discussed in Chapter 7. Whether or not such goals are written, decisions concerning the delineation of a procedural approach should be made with the child's caretakers in mind.

Objects used in therapy should be replicated at home. Furthermore, linguistic and nonlinguistic clinician-child interactions should be designed so that their most essential characteristics are replicable by caretakers. Box 1–5 (Chapter 1) provides information about correspondences between psychosocial skills and language acquisition at specified points in development; thus, the information in Box 1–5 may be a useful resource in delimiting a procedural approach after the clinician has consulted baseline data on the child's psychosocial status.

Learning Theory.   At every phase of intervention planning, it is useful to further explicate personal beliefs about how children learn those aspects of language that have been targeted as goals. It also is useful to ground personal beliefs in principles derived from published learning theories. In the long-term procedural approach, the clinician cited those principles derived from learning theories that will guide the creation of a procedural approach. It would be worthwhile for the clinician to review these principles at this short-term phase of intervention planning—this time keeping the targeted short-term goals in mind. The clinician should ask, "Do these principles still account for the child's acquisition of targeted linguistic structures?" If so, continue to use the principle as guidance in further delineating the procedural context. If not, revise the list of principles until a satisfactory explanation of learning is available. In the section that follows we will illustrate how learning principles help us generate ideas for treatment contexts, for specific children.

Format for Describing a Delineated Procedural Context.   Let us now consider how a delineated procedural context might be described. As noted above, the short-term procedural approach will include a description of the contexts (linguistic and nonlinguistic) that will be created to facilitate achievement of the specified short-term goals. The description of these contexts will include reference to the types of materials, interactions, and elicitations that will be utilized. Box 5–3 presents questions and sources of information for delineating procedural contexts.

THE DERIVATION OF SHORT-TERM GOALS AND PROCEDURAL CONTEXTS FOR SPECIFIC CHILDREN

We will now continue intervention planning for the four children we met in Chapters 3 and 4. We will spend the rest of this chapter discussing how we arrived at Phase-2 goal and procedural plans for Darryl (content-form-use interactions), Patty (fluency), Seth (phonology), and Alice (voice). As in Chapter 4, this will allow us to illustrate the decision-making process for intervention planning across disorder types—this time as we plan short-term goals and procedural contexts. Again, we remind the reader that our

---

BOX 5–3.   QUESTIONS AND SOURCES OF INFORMATION FOR DELINEATING A PROCEDURAL APPROACH

Questions	*Sources of Information*
1. What linguistic structure is targeted as a short-term goal?	Short-term goal statement
2. What types of materials should be available for the child to facilitate achievement of the short-term goal targeted?	Theories about language learning Baseline data on maintaining factors
3. What types of elicitations will the clinician utilize when interacting with the child to facilitate the acquisition of the linguistic structure targeted in the short-term goal?	Theories about language learning Baseline data on maintaining factors

---

intent is not to present the perfect plan for these children; there are many possible plans that could be developed that would be equally valid. Different plans would reflect differen¬t theoretical orientations. Our purpose is to illustrate the *decision-making process* that leads to the formulation of short-term goals and procedures.

In deriving short-term goals and procedural contexts for the four children, we will continue to follow the format established in Chapter 4. First, completed short-term goals and procedural contexts will be presented for an individual child. Then the decision-making process involved in the derivation of these statements will be elaborated. Questions in Boxes 5–1, 5–2, and 5–3, as well as baseline data on individual children presented in Chapter 3, will be used to guide the decision-making process.

Darryl

Short-Term Goals and Procedural Context.   The following are the short-term goals and the procedural contexts that were developed for Darryl, a child who presents with a developmental language disorder:

Short-term goals:

1. Darryl will code locative action + prepositions *in* and *on.*
2. Darryl will code locative action + possession.
3. Darryl will state (modal form) + the preposition *to* + verb phrase.
4. Darryl will code the copula in existence and possessive state utterances.
5. Darryl will initiate conversation in context of cooperative play.

Delineated procedural context:

1. The nonlinguistic context will include manipulable toys that replicate real objects (e.g., toy cars, trucks, plates); less representational construction-objects (blocks, Legos, tubes); and books.
2. Linguistic contexts will be created that are obligatory for the targeted structures.
3. The clinician will elicit linguistic structures by:
    (a) modeling during conversations with Darryl in play activities.
    (b) enacting narratives with the support of manipulable toys.

The Derivation of Short-Term Goals. As we explained in the first part of this chapter, the derivation of short-term goals involves making two major decisions: determining (a) which long-term goals to address, and (b) a sequence of short-term advances. In deciding which long-term goals to address, we will refer to the three questions introduced above (see Box 5–1):

1. In the normal course of development, are any of the goals under consideration achieved before any others?
2. Do the goals under consideration interact in such a way that they could be worked on during one time period?
3. Does the achievement of any of the goals have more of an impact than others on the health or overall communicative success of the child?

The long-term goals that were formulated for Darryl are as follows: (a) the achievement of content-form-use interactions through Lahey's Phase 8, (b) acquisition of a lexicon for coding Lahey content categories through Phase 8, (c) production of multiple causal-chain narratives, and (d) initiation and maintenance of conversation in context of cooperative play.

To determine whether any of the long-term goals might naturally be achieved first (question 1) or at the same time (question 2), we refer to the relevant child-development literature. Developmental taxonomies that appear in Lahey (1988) indicate that the linguistic structures cited in long-term goals (a) and (b) (content-form-use interactions and supporting lexicon through Lahey Phase 8+) emerge before or at the same time as goal (c) (narratives). They also emerge simultaneously with the conversational skills targeted in goal (d). Moreover, goals (a) and (b) are naturally achieved within the same phase. Consequently, we will address long-term goals (a), (b), and (d).

The next step in formulating short-term goals for Darryl involves decisions about which linguistic structures we want Darryl to achieve by the end of the semester (the contracted time period in the preschool). As a guide for decision making we refer to questions and sources of information in Box 5–2. To answer question 1 ("What is Darryl's current level of functioning?") we turn to baseline data that relate to the long-term goals we have chosen to address (Chapter 3, Table 3–2). We need to know Darryl's functional status in the use of content-form-use interactions and lexicon through Lahey Phase 8+. Baseline data indicate that, on one hand, there are developmental gaps present from Phase 4 on; on the other hand, Darryl is producing some structures through Phase 7. Should we start at Phase 4 and fill in the missing structures, working first on all Phase 4 content-form interactions, then Phase 5, and so on? Or should we be more selective?

The fact that Darryl is producing linguistic structures through phase 7 suggests that (a) non-developmental factors may be affecting Darryl's performance, and (b) it is likely that he can achieve structures beyond phase 4. The next two questions will help us decide which structures to target.

Question 2 has to do with whether Darryl will be capable of working on more than one goal during a single time period. Baseline data on Darryl's cognitive functioning would give us some clues. These data indicate essentially normal intellectual functioning—with some weakness in inference making. Furthermore, these data indicate that Darryl has a language-learning disability. The data support targeting more than one linguistic structure at one time, but indicate that care must be taken with structures that may require Darryl to make subtle distinctions (e.g., perhaps distinguishing aspectual features of tenses, such as "habitual *s*" from present progressive *ing* tense markers).

We view question 3, the last question, as optional. It asks whether one linguistic structure at a given linguistic phase could be achieved more readily than another at that phase. The Lahey (1988) framework, which was used to organize Darryl's baseline data, describes the achievement of a number of structures during the same phase. Deciding which structure might be more easily achieved involves a consideration of the relative learnability of one structure as compared with others. To make this decision, it will be necessary to examine factors that may affect the learnability of possible target structures.

As noted earlier, baseline data on Darryl's cognitive and linguistic status indicate that Darryl may have special difficulty with structures that demand subtle discriminations, such as distinguishing morphemes that code the aspectual dimension of time (i.e., whether an action lasts over time, is momentary, or is habitual) or irregular tense markings. Additionally, baseline data on Darryl's sensorimotor functioning suggest that a sensorimotor problem may be contributing to gaps in Darryl's syntactic performance. Darryl exhibits mild hypertonicity with some lack of dissociation of oral motor movement from other actions. In the area of syntax, Darryl is omitting morphemes of low phonetic substance. Perhaps Darryl is having difficulty perceiving and producing linguistic structures of low phonetic substance as a result of his sensorimotor deficit.

Can this sensorimotor maintaining factor be addressed in the prioritization of short-term goals? Perhaps structures with more salient phonetic substance should be targeted first. An examination of Phase 4 and 5 morphemes not produced by Darryl reveals much variability in phonetic substance. Compare the preposition *in* or *on* with article *a* (*a* is typically produced with a schwa, associated with reduced stress). A decision is made to weigh phonetic substance in prioritizing linguistic achievements. We will target two structures of higher phonetic substance (in/ on and possession with locative action—goals 1 and 2), which should prove easier for Darryl to achieve. Two structures with lower substance (the copula, goal 4, and the preposition *to,* goal 3) will also be targeted. The latter structures were targeted because there were additional factors motivating their selection: Darryl's omission of the copula in "existence" utterances is particularly disconcerting for parents and teachers. Darryl has begun to produce modal + contracted *to* (e.g., "wanna," "have-ta") in some contexts.

At this point, short-term goals and rationales can be recorded on the Short-Term Goals and Procedures Form (Form B–3, Appendix B). This information is presented in Table 5–1.

Delineated Procedural Context. The clinician's next job at this second phase of intervention planning is to extend the procedural approach outlined at the long-term planning phase. This involves specifying the types of materials to be utilized (the nonlinguistic therapeutic context) and elicitation strategies (the linguistic context). These materials and interaction strategies will be aimed at helping the child achieve the targeted short-term goals. We refer to questions outlined in Box 5–3 for assistance. The questions contained in this box direct the clinician to consider short-term goals targeted and decisions already made at the long-term phase of intervention planning.

The nonlinguistic context. At the long-term phase of intervention planning, two preliminary procedural decisions were made to guide the delineation of the therapeutic context: (a) cognitive, sensorimotor, and psychosocial maintaining factors would be addressed in session; and (b) the procedural approach would be influenced primarily by principles from constructivist-cognitive learning theory (selected from Box 1–7). The influence of learning principles on procedural decisions will be considered first.

Three principles cited in the long-term procedural approach statement appear most helpful in procedure planning. They suggest that we:

> select materials and tasks commensurate with Darryl's past experience, present developmental level and interests;
> encourage Darryl to engage in problem solving;
> provide sensory stimulation (i.e., sensory feedback).

With reference to these guiding principles, we turn to the specific short-term goal statements. The first two involve coding locative action: locative action + prepositions *in* and *on* and locative action + possession. Two principles of learning guide us in specifying types of materials to use. First, materials and tasks should be commensurate with Darryl's interests and developmental level; baseline data indicate that Darryl needs perceptual support to facilitate

TABLE 5-1. Short-Term Goals and Procedures

Client: Darryl

Short-Term Goals	Long-Term Goals Addressed	Prioritization Source
1. Darryl will code locative action + prepositions *in* and *on*	1, 2	Lahey, 1988
2. Darryl will code locative action + possession	1, 2	Lahey, 1988
3. Darryl will code state (modal form) + *to* + verb phrase	1, 2	Lahey, 1988
4. Darryl will code the copula in existence and possessive state utterances	1, 2	Lahey, 1988
5. Darryl will initiate conversations in context of cooperative play	4	Westby, 1988

Procedural Contexts

Learning Principles

Maintaining Factors

Nonlinguistic Context (types of materials)

Linguistic Context

communication. Second, Darryl needs enhanced sensory feedback from his actions and from objects manipulated. Based on these principles, and with reference to coding locative action, we decide to provide objects that can be manipulated and that would lead Darryl physically to change the location of objects and himself. Furthermore, with reference to coordinating possession, objects that he could refer to as his or others' possessions would be useful. Toys, such as cars and trucks, would be consistent with the above principles. So would objects such as blocks or Legos or containers that are less iconic but that could be used in conjunction with toys suggestive of locative action.

Two other short-term goals were established for Darryl: to code state (modal form) + *to* + verb phrase ("I wanna eat") and to code copula in existence and possession statements ("This is a truck") and possessive state utterances ("This is mine"). The types of manipulable objects described above would also be facilitative of these goals.

As Table 5–3 suggests, information about nonlinguistic maintaining factors would also be useful in delineating a procedural approach. In the long-term procedural approach statement, it was noted that the achievement of all goals would be facilitated by modifying cognitive, sensorimotor, social-emotional, and linguistic maintaining factors.

The provision of manipulable, representational objects in therapy addresses, in part, cognitive functioning. These are perceptually salient objects that support conceptualization. As noted above, there are also sensorimotor issues to consider. Darryl is mildly hypertonic and demonstrates some difficulty stabilizing his body and dissociating oral motor movements from fine motor actions. These problems may be contributing to Darryl's failure to produce unstressed morphemes. Thus, it would be wise to consult with a movement specialist: the physical or occupational therapist. By engaging in such a collaboration, the speech-language pathologist could better specify types of materials and interactions that would address the body stability–body segmentation issues.

A consultation with Darryl's physical therapist revealed that she uses materials such as tricycles, balancing boards, and objects that provoke Darryl to pull against resistance. Perhaps some of these objects could, with the physical therapist's guidance, be integrated into the speech-language session.

At this point the nonlinguistic context can be delineated. It will include manipulable toys that replicate real objects (e.g., toy cars, trucks, plates); construction-objects (blocks, Legos, tubes); rideable tricycles, objects that can be pushed and pulled; and books. Now we turn to the linguistic context.

The linguistic context. In what kinds of communication interactions should the speech-language pathologist engage Darryl to facilitate achievement of the short-term goals? The learning principles identified in the procedural approach will be useful in delineating the linguistic context. The three most useful indicate that language learning is facilitated by:

efforts to convey meaning and repair communication breakdowns successfully
problem solving
reflection upon personal action
sensory feedback

It follows from the decisions made above that the clinician should create functional opportunities for Darryl to produce desired linguistic forms. These opportunities could involve problematic situations that promote reasoning, reflection, and the use of language to resolve problems. For example, in targeting locative action + preposition, the clinician might pretend to have difficulty getting a toy vehicle into a tube—provoking the child to reflect on spatial relations and to code locative action using a preposition (e.g., "get it in"). Or the clinician, targeting the modal intention, may initiate an activity in which necessary objects are missing. This should motivate comments such as "we're gonna get some blocks." The clinician might make ongoing comments about Darryl's activities or the clinician's own activities (e.g., talking to self about *intending* to go up the stairs while playing house).

The learning principles involving problem solving and sensory feedback are especially relevant to the production of the copula. Unless there is a clear-cut pragmatic reason to emphasize and produce the copula, a child with sensorimotor and linguistic involvement may choose to omit it and still successfully communicate an intended message. An interpersonal interaction in which emphasis of the copula could resolve a conflict or express a practical message would highlight the linguistic saliency of the copula and provide important sensorimotor feedback. An example might be an interaction in which Darryl had to emphasize that an object *"is* mine" to get the object.

An additional consideration in the designing of a linguistic context concerns the presentation of the target utterance. Modeling as Darryl is engaged in a meaningful related activity and expanding upon Darryl's spontaneous comments would be consistent with learning principles cited above.

At this point, the basic elements of nonlinguistic and linguistic therapeutic contexts have been defined with reference to the short-term goals that have been written for Darryl. Thus, we are now able to describe a delineated procedural context. We can now complete the Short-Term Goal and Procedure Form (Form B–3, Appendix B). This information is presented in Table 5–2.

Patty

Short-Term Goals and Delineated Procedural Context. The following are the short-term goals and the delineated procedural context that were developed for Patty, a child who presents with a fluency disorder.

TABLE 5–2. Short-Term Goals and Procedures

Client: Darryl

Short-Term Goals	Long-Term Goals Addressed	Prioritization Source
1. Darryl will code locative action + prepositions *in* and *on*	1, 2	Lahey, 1988
2. Darryl will code locative action + possession	1, 2	Lahey, 1988
3. Darryl will code state (modal form) + *to* + verb phrase	1, 2	Lahey, 1988
4. Darryl will code the copula in existence and possession utterances	1, 2	Lahey, 1988
5. Darryl will initiate conversations in context of cooperative play	4	Westby, 1988

Procedural Contexts	Learning Principles	Maintaining Factors
	5, 6, 7, 9	Cognitive, sensorimotor

Nonlinguistic Context (types of materials)

The nonlinguistic context will include manipulable toys that replicate real objects (e.g., toy cars, trucks, plates); less representational construction-objects (blocks, Legos, tubes); and books

Linguistic Context

The clinician will:

1. create a linguistic context that is obligatory for the targeted structures

2. elicit linguistic structures by modeling during conversations with Darryl in cooperative play activities

3. elicit linguistic structures by reenacting narratives with the support of manipulable toys

Short-term goals:

1. To respond to questions with 3+ constituent utterances that function to provide information.
2. To integrate respiration, phonation, and articulation ("easy speech") in words beginning 3+ constituent responses to questions.
3. To integrate respiration, phonation, and articulation ("easy speech") in coding the complex-sentence categories additive, causal, and epistemic.
4. To interact with parents in nonpropositional as well as conversational situations that increase fluent experiences.

Delineated procedural context:

1. The nonlinguistic context will include objects and pictures that can be used to support script play and narrative story-telling.
2. The clinician will promote fluent productions by:
   (a) modeling "easy speech" patterns,
   (b) modeling target structures in the context of script play and narrative story-telling,
   (c) reflecting upon differences between fluent and dysfluent productions,
   (d) rewarding fluent speech within pragmatically appropriate responses,
   (e) not reacting to dysfluent speech when produced in play and narrative story-telling.
3. Parents will provide home-speaking experiences that promote fluency.

Generally, the first step in the derivation of short-term goals is making a decision about which long-term goals to address during the first contracted time period (in this case a semester). As we can see in reviewing the long-term goal statement, only one long-term goal has been set for Patty. We can, therefore, move to the next step in decision making—a consideration of the steps necessary in achieving our long-term goal.

At this point we need to review the long-term goal proposed for Patty in Chapter 4 in relation to the questions in Box 5–1, "Patty will manifest fluent speech patterns while producing complex sentences for regulatory and discourse functions." This goal represents our conceptualization of the place of fluency within a language system. As discussed earlier (Chapter 1), fluency is viewed as an aspect of form (the rate and prosody with which utterance units are delivered). Thus, our approach to stuttering problems is essentially language based (similar to that of Wall & Myers, 1984). This approach requires a consideration of the child's fluency or dysfluency (as form) in relation to what is said (content-form) and why it is being said (use). At first glance, this long-term goal appears to be a unitary configuration, and in some ways it is. At the termination of therapy, we would like to see Patty achieving fluent speech in the context specified. The goal, however, may be viewed as an integration of the three components of language, which need to be considered separately during the short-term goal phase of intervention planning. With this view of fluency in mind, we turn to the second step in formulating short-term goals: prioritizing one or more linguistic structures to be targeted. In order to accomplish this, we must address questions that were formulated earlier (see Box 5–2).

Answering the first question, concerning where Patty is now, involves referring to baseline data (Chapter 3, Table 3–4). Baseline data that describe Patty's fluency are organized in terms of a *matrix of fluency behaviors* (modified from Wall & Myers, 1984). Semantic-syntactic and pragmatic performance is viewed within the framework of Lahey's developmental phases.

A review of Patty's fluency pattern in conversational speech reveals a 10% degree of stuttering. Since Patty stutters on only 10% of the syllables she utters, we need to examine some possible sources of variability (i.e., why she stutters more in some instances than in others). Three factors frequently referenced in explaining children's dysfluency variability are utterance position, complexity, and function (e.g., Bloodstein, 1981; Starkweather, 1987; Wall & Myers, 1984).

Patty's baseline data reveal some striking differences in percentages of dysfluency (of the overall 10% of dysfluencies) within these three variable categories. First, with reference to utterance position, we can see that dysfluencies occur more frequently at the beginning of utterances (73%) than at the beginning of clauses (19%). Second, as utterances increase in complexity from single-word and two-constituent to 3+ constituents and complex sentences, percentages of dysfluencies also increase from 14% to 67%. When we further peruse the complex-sentence content categories, we notice differences in percentages between the categories of causal and adversative (both at 50%) and epistemic (67%) and intention-volition (80%). Lastly, there are also obvious differences in the percentages of dysfluencies associated with different language functions. Dysfluencies were greatest when language was used to obtain information (80%) and to obtain a response (75%). In contrast, dysfluencies were reduced in the context of commenting and directing action (each 25%). It should also be noted that while she initiated, responded appropriately, and maintained eye contact, one striking response strategy was responding to a question, with a question.

Knowing the relationship between fluency patterns and linguistic contexts, we can begin to target linguistic contexts for the reduction of dysfluency. However, we need additional information about the status of Patty's nonlinguistic maintaining factors before formulating our short-term goals. Two of these factors (sensorimotor and psychosocial) warrant further scrutiny, because they are often implicated as causal factors in children who stutter (Gregory & Hill, 1980). Consequently, we may try to address these factors in the formulation of the short-term goal statements.

Checking baseline data, we can see that there are no obvious impairments in any of the three areas of possible maintaining factors: sensorimotor, psychosocial, and cognitive. Despite an evaluation of normal functioning on the PSM examination, Patty may still be viewed as a child with some difficulty in the sensorimotor domain—integrating mechanisms of respiration, phonation, and articulation. Children who demonstrate symptoms of repetitions and prolongations are often viewed as having difficulty in "control and regulation of the breath stream" (Adams, 1980, p. 291). Inability to control the breath stream implies some difficulty in the "speaker's execution of several complex motor behaviors, and in [his or her] ability to coordinate them" (Adams, 1980, p. 292). Wall and Myers (1984) also support the importance of considering the "synergism of respiration with phonation and coarticulation . . . especially . . . in reference to time because speech is an ongoing and relatively fleeting process" (p. 137). These are just a few examples from the literature that suggest that the sensorimotor maintaining factor needs to be considered simply on the basis of the stuttering symptoms.

   We also need to take a second look at the psychosocial maintaining factor. According to Wall and Myers (1984), "the focal points of the psychosocial factor consist of important individuals, both adults and peers, in the child's daily environment. Perhaps the most central figures are the child's parents" (p. 133). At this point in Patty's life she will be affected primarily by the responses she receives from her parents regarding her speech and language in general and her dysfluencies in particular. Scanning the background information, we note that the mother described Patty as most dysfluent when attempting to translate English into Spanish. (Although she comes from a bilingual home, Patty is English dominant.) The mother also reported that she has refrained from pressuring Patty to speak Spanish at home if this causes her to be more dysfluent. It seems reasonable to hypothesize that the parents need further clarification and direction in facilitating fluent experiences for their daughter.

   Given these baseline data in language and language-related systems, we are now at the point in decision making where we project where Patty should be linguistically at the end of her first therapy period (a semester). The goals we have targeted state that Patty should (a) respond appropriately to questions with 3+ constituent utterances, which function to provide information; (b) integrate respiration, phonation, and articulation ("easy speech") in words beginning 3+ constituent responses to questions; (c) integrate respiration, phonation, and articulation ("easy speech") in coding the complex-sentence categories additive, causal, and epistemic; and (d) interact with parents in nonpropositional as well as conversational situations that increase fluent experiences.

   Our rationales for these goals are based on developmental data, information about the phenomenon of stuttering, and Patty's baseline behavior regarding the interaction of fluency and language. First, we have decided to target appropriate responses to questions because Patty frequently responds to a question, with a question. We view this as an avoidance strategy. Second, we have selected to increase fluency in responses to questions with 3+ constituent utterances that function to provide information. We did so because Patty's dysfluencies increase when responding to requests for information. Third, we have chosen to increase fluency in coding complex sentences because this category of utterance complexity is associated with the greatest number of dysfluencies. Among the complex-sentence categories, we select additive because it is among the earliest for children to achieve (Bloom, Lahey, Hood, Lifter, & Fiess, 1980). We include causal and epistemic because they are the two categories in which dysfluencies were noted, but not with the frequency of intention-volition.

We have focused on increased fluency in *initiating* 3+ constituent utterances in responses to questions because the initial position of utterances produces the greatest percentage of stuttering. Again, by focusing on 3+ utterances (rather than complex sentences) we are reducing the complexity of response—and with it, perhaps, the anxiety related to beginning an utterance.

In an effort to increase fluency in selected linguistic contexts, we have targeted the integration of respiration, phonation, and articulation ("easy speech"). As we discussed above, fluency involves this developmental sensori-motor synergy, which is frequently conceptualized as "easy speech" (i.e., Van Riper, 1978; Wall & Myers, 1984).

The interaction with parents in nonpropositional and conversational situations that increase fluent experiences is essential for Patty's image of herself as a fluent speaker (e.g., Gregory & Hill, 1980).

We now need to determine how many goals to set for Patty during a single short-term phase. We are planning to set four goals. The number of goals that may be targeted at once is related to baseline data in language performance and maintaining factors and to the level of expectations for improvement across goals. If we review baseline data in content-form-use interactions, we find that she performs linguistically as a normally developing child. Her problem is not in learning such linguistic structures but in gradually extending the frequency of fluency across linguistic phases. The integration of respiration, phonation, and articulation essentially describes the accomplishment of fluency. We aim to achieve fluency on two complexity levels: 3+ constituent sentences and selected complex sentences that are well within her linguistic repertoire. Goals also include one communicative function: to provide information when responding to questions. The last goal, interacting with parents in situations that increase fluent experiences, is integrated with the others in that the more fluent speaking experiences Patty has, the more each of the other goals will be facilitated.

In deciding how many of these goals Patty may be able to accomplish during one short-term period, we also need to consider language-related systems such as cognitive, psychosocial, and sensorimotor. Patty demonstrates no evidence of impairment in any of these potential maintaining factors. The only basis for assuming problems in these areas are clinical data about stuttering. Moreover, the possible maintaining factors are addressed in her goals (integration of speech-mechanism components and guided parental interaction). Consequently, our decision to target four short-term goals appears appropriate. At this point, we can record short-term goals and rationales on the Short-Term Goals and Procedures Form (Form B–3, Appendix B). This information is presented in Table 5–3.

TABLE 5-3. Short-Term Goals and Procedures

Client: Patty

Short-Term Goals	Long-Term Goals Addressed	Prioritization Source
1. To respond to questions with 3 + constituent utterances that function to provide information	1	Lahey, 1988
2. To integrate respiration, phonation, and articulation ("easy speech") in words beginning 3 + constituent responses to questions	1	Wall & Myers, 1984; Starkweather & Gordon, 1983; Van Riper, 1978
3. To integrate respiration, phonation, and articulation ("easy speech") in coding the complex-sentence categories additive, causal, and epistemic	1	Wall & Myers, 1984; Starkweather & Gordon, 1983; Van Riper, 1978
4. To interact with parents in nonpropositional as well as conversational situations that increase fluent experiences	1	Wall & Myers, 1984; Starkweather & Gordon, 1983; Van Riper, 1978

Procedural Contexts	Learning Principles	Maintaining Factors

Nonlinguistic Context (types of materials)

Linguistic Context

Delineated Procedural Context.   We are now at the second part of the short-term phase of intervention planning for Patty. As with Darryl, we now must further develop the procedural approach outlined at the long-term planning phase. This involves specifying the types of materials and interactions that will comprise the nonlinguistic therapeutic context and the elicitation strategies that will characterize the linguistic context. We refer to questions outlined in Box 5–3 for assistance.

In addressing question 1 (the short-term goals targeted), we see that all the goals for Patty involve the increase or maintenance of fluency. They deal with promoting fluency in selected linguistic contexts. Next, we consider the maintaining factors of her dysfluencies. A careful scrutiny of her baseline data and the literature in childhood dysfluencies (described in prior sections of this chapter) highlights two major areas of concern: sensorimotor and psychosocial. Thus, our procedural approach is also directed towards elimination of inefficient sensorimotor patterns and disrupting environmental influences. These two areas of focus are major components of intervention approaches described in the literature (see, for example, Adams, 1980; Gregory & Hill, 1980; Shine, 1980; Starkweather, 1980; Van Riper, 1973; Wall & Myers, 1984).

A number of procedural decisions were made at the long-term phase that apply to the management of sensorimotor and psychosocial difficulties. The most significant of these decisions was the specification of principles from learning theories. These principles suggest that learning is facilitated by (a) events following a behavior, which can reinforce (strengthen) or extinguish (weaken) the behavior; (b) efforts to match models presented by the clinician; (c) sensory stimulation (i.e., sensory feedback) from movement, including movement involved in articulation or manipulating objects; (d) noticing similarities and distinctions among actions and events mediated by adults; and (e) interactions with materials and tasks commensurate with the child's developmental level. With our knowledge of Patty's short-term goals, her maintaining factors, and principles from learning theories, we are prepared to delineate a procedural approach with reference to the nonlinguistic and linguistic aspects of the therapeutic milieu.

The nonlinguistic context.   Again, based on our baseline data and the literature in treatment of fluency disorders, we opt for creating contexts that maximize fluency (see Phase 1 procedural approach and Wall & Myers, 1984). During the evaluation, Patty demonstrated a willingness to play and engage in verbal interactions with a clinician. Patty's behavior is consistent with learning principle 5 in Box 1–7, which suggests that the nonlinguistic context be developmentally appropriate for Patty. A context that would utilize play should facilitate fluency. This concept is supported by the literature on child language; this sort of environment is less intimidating and increases the types and frequencies of verbalizations children produce (Bloom & Lahey, 1978; Hubbell, 1988; Lahey, 1988; Lund & Duchan, 1988). In addition, many authorities on childhood dysfluencies suggest a minimally directive approach with children at the beginning stuttering stages. Since Patty is five years, eleven months, we must also consider those materials of greatest interest to her (i.e., toys, games, and books within her area of experience, cognitive level, and interest).

The linguistic context. We now turn to the linguistic interactions during treatment. Principles cited above from operant, motor, and social learning theories have guided us in our decision making about the nature of the clinician's speech and language (i.e., voice, fluency, and content and complexity of statements and questions). These principles have led to the following procedural guidelines:

(a) model "easy" speech patterns,

(b) model target structures in the context of script play and narrative story-telling,

(c) reflect upon differences between fluent ("easy") and dysfluent ("hard") productions,

(d) reward fluent speech within pragmatically appropriate responses,

(e) do not react to dysfluent speech when produced in play and narrative story-telling.

We can look at statements (a) and (b) together. Guideline (b) is actually a further delineation of (a). Social-cognitive theory suggests that children learn from caretakers about aspects of language (Fey, 1986; van Kleeck & Richardson, 1986). Modeling has been shown to be effective in the learning of linguistic structures by normally developing children (Cole & Dale, 1986; Connell, 1987; Courtright & Courtright, 1976, 1979). Furthermore, it has been argued by many experts in childhood stuttering that children who are dysfluent need to modify rate and prosody. Appropriate rate and prosody thus need to be modeled by the adult (clinician and parent; e.g., Adams, 1980; Shine, 1980; Starkweather, 1980).

Our specification of the context is based on our knowledge of the verbal scaffolds (props) that facilitate production of language in young children (Lund & Duchan, 1988; Ninio & Bruner, 1978). It has been demonstrated that children are likely to imitate the speech patterns of adults when they are involved in narrative play and story-telling (Ninio & Bruner, 1978). Social-cognitive theory further suggests that learning is facilitated by noticing similarities and distinctions among actions and events mediated by adults. This principle is operationally described for Patty with reference to her stuttering moments. We cannot say that Patty is unaware of her dysfluencies. Her mother stated that she becomes angry and frustrated when she stutters. We do not believe, however, that Patty fully differentiates between the way she feels during dysfluent and fluent conditions. For this reason we have decided to help Patty reflect on what she does and feels during difficult speech moments. We believe that this knowledge is important in order for her to be able to distinguish "easy" from "hard" speech and focus on "easy" speech (e.g., Wall & Myers, 1984).

The last two statements derive from operant theory. A major operant principle is that learning is facilitated by events following a behavior that can reinforce or extinguish the behavior. With Patty, we uphold the positive side of this principle. Since we are targeting fluent speech, we believe this behavior (fluent speech) should be reinforced (Starkweather, 1980). In addition, since Patty is a mild stutterer and a young child, we are not attempting to modify dysfluent moments. Overall, the procedural approach involves Patty's practicing new fluency patterns. This is consistent with motor learning theory, which requires sensory stimulation and feedback for learning, especially for sensorimotor learning (Kent & Lybolt, 1982).

Finally, for a young, beginning stutterer, it is most crucial that the parents be involved with the treatment (e.g., Bloodstein, 1981; Gregory & Hill, 1980; Luper & Mulder, 1964). Parents can also provide models of "easy speech." Most importantly, parents can insure that the child is given as many opportunities as possible for stutter-free speech (Bloodstein, 1981). A description of procedural contexts and rationales for these contexts completes the second part of Patty's Short-Term Goals and Procedures plan (Table 5–4).

Seth

Short-Term Goals and Delineated Procedural Context. The following are the short-term goals and the delineated procedural approach that were developed for Seth, a child who presents with a developmental phonological disorder.

Short-term goals:

1. Seth will reduce the phonological processes of fronting and backing in conversational speech.
2. Seth will reduce the stopping of /f/, /v/, and /ʃ/ in conversational speech.
3. Seth will begin the suppression of the process of gliding (i.e., the production of /l/ in initial position of words).
4. Seth will produce final /z/, and /s/, /z/ clusters coding plural copula, third person singular, and possessive.

Delineated procedural context:

1. The nonlinguistic context will involve: the participation of an occupational therapist, materials that will promote sensorimotor advancement, and materials on Seth's interest and experience level.
2. The clinician will elicit linguistic structures by:
   (a) modeling targeted sounds in words or sentences;
   (b) presenting comparisons between target and error sounds in minimal pairs;
   (c) creating situations in which Seth is faced with communicative breakdown due to mispronunciation;

TABLE 5–4. Short-Term Goals and Procedures

Client: Patty

Short-Term Goals	Long-Term Goals Addressed	Prioritization Source
1. To respond to questions with 3 + constituent utterances that function to provide information	1	Lahey, 1988
2. To integrate respiration, phonation, and articulation ("easy speech") in words beginning 3 + constituent responses to questions	1	Wall & Myers, 1984; Starkweather & Gordon, 1983; Van Riper, 1978
3. To integrate respiration, phonation, and articulation ("easy speech") in coding the complex-sentence categories additive, causal, and epistemic	1	Wall & Myers, 1984; Starkweather & Gordon, 1983; Van Riper, 1978
4. To interact with parents in nonpropositional as well as conversational situations that increase fluent experiences	1	Wall & Myers, 1984; Starkweather & Gordon, 1983; Van Riper, 1978

Procedural Contexts	Learning Principles	Maintaining Factors
Nonlinguistic Context (types of materials)		
Objects and pictures that can be used to support script play and narrative story-telling	5	
Linguistic Context		
The clinician will:		
1. model "easy speech" patterns	2	
2. model target structures in the context of script play and narrative story-telling	2	
3. reflect upon differences between fluent and dysfluent productions	8	
4. reward fluent speech within pragmatically appropriate responses	1	
5. not react to dysfluent speech when produced in play and narrative story-telling	1	Psychosocial
Parents will provide home speaking experiences that promote fluency	5	Psychosocial

(d) helping Seth to reflect on how phonetic gestures, sound, feel and look;
(e) reacting positively to Seth's efforts by maintaining communicative interaction.

The Derivation of Short-Term Goals. The first step in the derivation of short-term goals involves making a decision about which long-term goals to address during the first contracted time period (in this case, also, a semester). As we stated earlier, if more than one long-term goal was set, we are faced with a number of considerations presented in Box 5–1.

1. In the normal course of development, are any of the goals under consideration achieved before any others?
2. Do the goals under consideration interact in such a way that they could be worked on simultaneously?
3. Does the achievement of any of the goals have more of an impact than others on the health or overall communicative success of the child?

At this point we need to review the long-term goals proposed for Seth in Chapter 4 in relation to these questions.

1. Seth will decrease phonological process application across all categories to the point of intelligibility by people unaware of his speech pattern.
2. Seth will begin to suppress processes that have not begun dissolution (gliding and vocalization).
3. Seth will produce final consonants that code inflectional morphemes.
4. Seth will increase frequency and variety of multiverb content-form interactions and their associated connectives.
5. Seth will produce complex causal-chain narratives.

In order to answer question 1, we need to reference research data on normal development. The suppression and dissolution of most processes begin by the age of three (Grunwell, 1981), which is when children have begun to produce all of Brown's developmental morphemes (Owens, 1992) and a variety of multiverb connectives (Bloom & Lahey, 1978; Lahey, 1988). Goal 5, however, is a later development, located within Phase 8+ of Lahey (1988). It is built on the prior development of complex sentences and continues to develop throughout the early school years. Therefore, it is reasonable to target goals 1 through 4 during the same time period, postponing goal 5 until a later time. To answer question 2, we need to consult our baseline data in the areas of phonology and syntax (Chapter 3, Table 3–6). We can see that two of the most frequent processes operating during the production of conversational speech are final consonant deletion and cluster reduction. These two processes clearly affect the production of morphological endings, which are often missing in Seth's expressive language. In order to produce morpheme endings (i.e., /z/, consonant +/s/), and consonant + /z/, Seth must be able to produce final consonant singletons and clusters. Because of the interaction of these two levels of grammar, it appears most natural to target them together.

A review of Seth's baseline data suggests that question 3 should be answered in the affirmative. At this time, Seth's intelligibility interferes with his production of a sequence of ideas (i.e., narratives). His unintelligibility may be explained by the use of a large number of processes, the frequent use of processes, and the maintenance of unusual processes (i.e., backing) and very early processes (e.g., assimilation). What also adds to his unintelligibility is the use of process combinations (i.e., stopping and backing: "jar" = [ga]). The frequency of process application increases in conversational speech. Because Seth's unintelligibility may be a deterrent to the production of more complex linguistic structures, we decide that phonological goals should be among the first targeted. A consideration of the above questions results in the decision to target long-term goals 1 through 3 for the first semester of treatment.

The next step in formulating short-term goals for Seth involves prioritizing one or more linguistic structures to be targeted as short-term goals. In order to accomplish this, we must address questions that were formulated in Box 5–2:

1. What is the child's current level of functioning?
2. Is the child capable of working on multiple achievements during one time period?
3. Which behaviors among a number of simultaneously occurring achievements (parallel achievements) may be facilitated most readily?

To address question 1, we need to identify the taxonomies of linguistic behavior in which we view phonological and syntactic performance. We describe Seth's phonological performance in terms of phonological processes and his morphologic achievement within the framework of Bloom and Lahey's developmental phases.

A review of Seth's phonological patterns in conversational speech reveals the operation of a number of processes with a wide range of application. These include processes that should have been eliminated by three years of age as well as later-eliminated processes. Fronting and backing, which are applied less frequently than the others, continue to be evident after many years of treatment. Fronting should be eliminated by age three, and backing is an unusual process, infrequently used by normally developing children. Due to the reversibility of the processes (backing or fronting, with no identifiable contextual determiners) and the long duration of operation, sensorimotor involvement is postulated. This maintaining factor must be considered in our goal expectations. Thus, the expectation is to reduce the operation of the process still further without necessarily being able to eliminate it.

We can see that all processes except gliding and vocalization have begun dissolution in conversational speech. Although gliding is eliminated relatively later than other processes, dissolution is a lengthy procedure and begins as early as three years of age (Grunwell, 1981). Stopping is another process that is applied very frequently (77% of the time). Stopping most frequently affects /f/, /v/, /ʃ/, and /ʒ/. Clinical research with children suggests that processes applied more than 40% of the time should be targeted first to increase an individual's intelligibility (Hodson & Paden, 1991). For this reason, we have decided to target stopping and gliding as short-term goals in addition to other phonological goals. Since dissolution of the process of stopping has begun, our aim is to reduce its application. In the case of gliding, however, we aim to initiate the dissolution of the process since it operates 100% of the time in conversational speech.

Final consonant deletion is another process that should be eliminated by age three. It is used 74% of the time in conversational speech and affects a number of sounds, among them /d/, /t/, /s/, /z/ (associated with morphological endings). Because of the relationship between syntax and phonology and the knowledge that children tend to produce final consonants more readily in morphological endings than in noninflected contexts (Paul & Shriberg, 1982), the short-term goal for the elimination of final consonant deletion is integrated with the improvement of morpheme production.

At this point in our decision making we are considering targeting four short-term goals. These are (a) the reduction of fronting and backing in conversational speech, (b) the reduction of stopping of /f/ and /v/ in conversational speech and /ʃ/ in the initial position of words, (c) the suppression of the process of gliding (i.e., the production of /l/ in initial position of words), and (d) the production of final /z/, and /s/, /z/ clusters coding plural, copula, third person singular, and possessive.

Next we need to determine whether Seth can achieve all four goals simultaneously. The number of goals that may be targeted at once is related to baseline data in language performance and maintaining factors and to level of expectations for improvement across goals. If we review baseline data in phonology, we can see that the processes of fronting and backing, and stopping of /f/ and /v/ are used less frequently than gliding. For this reason, our expectations for advancement would be different for these two sets of processes. We would aim for reduced frequency of fronting, backing, and stopping of /f/ and /v/. At this time it would also be efficient to target the prodution of /ʃ/ the only fricative position not yet produced by Seth (palatal fricatives) and to aim for accurate single-word productions in this case. We are targeting the beginning of dissolution of gliding and would be satisfied with accurate single-word productions. Since our expectations for Seth are not uniform across processes, it is likely that he can manage intervention on these three processes. With reference to the fourth proposed goal, our baseline data inform us that dissolution has also begun with final consonant deletion. In this case, as with fronting, backing, and stopping of /f/ and /v/, we are interested in decreasing frequency of application. We have integrated the reduction of final consonant deletion with the production of certain morphological endings primarily because it has been shown that final consonants are produced more readily in inflected contexts (Paul & Shriberg, 1982). At the same time, we are interested in having Seth produce these morphemes to enhance his communicative interactions. It should be noted that the four goals proposed for Seth could be implemented efficiently within the framework of "cycles" (Hodson & Paden, 1991). Within a cycles approach each goal would be targeted intermittently for short periods during the semester.

In making decisions about how many goals to target, we also need to consider language-related systems such as cognitive, psychosocial, and sensorimotor. Although Seth's cognitive level is still questionable (on the basis of psychologist's report), he did receive average scores in information, similarities, and comprehension, which are language-based areas. Average cognitive performance is a positive prognosticator for the ability to handle more than one goal at a time. In addition, the psychologist's report indicated that it is often possible to encourage Seth to persevere when he feels he cannot do something. Although the baseline data indicate that Seth has many sensorimotor problems, the recent initiation of occupational therapy is a positive indicator for the management of the goals set for him.

With reference to question 3, in Box 5–2, we need again to reference developmental data. Processes have been categorized according to the time of their natural elimination: those disappearing by age three and those persisting after age three (Stoel-Gammon & Dunn, 1985). Although Seth is almost twelve years of age, he continues to maintain processes in both categories. Because Seth is well beyond the age at which these processes are normally eliminated, our selection of targets was based more on the frequency of occurrence than the developmental phase. After a careful consideration of baseline data and maintaining factors, the following short-term goals were formulated and stated in the second part of the Management Plan under Short-Term Goals, and Prioritization Source (Table 5–5).

Delineated Procedural Context. We are now at the second phase of intervention planning for Seth. As with the other cases, we must now specify the types of materials and interactions that will comprise the nonlinguistic therapeutic context and the elicitation strategies that will characterize the linguistic context. We refer to questions outlined in Box 5–3 for assistance.

In addressing question 1 (the short-term goals statement), we see that all the goals for Seth are phonological. They deal either with (a) further reducing the operation of processes by increasing the stability of sounds governed by a process (i.e., /f/, /v/, /s/, /z/) and establishing new sounds within a process (/ʃ/) or (b) initiating the suppression of a process (gliding). The materials chosen, therefore, should include opportunities for sound establishment and sound stabilization (Bernthal & Bankson, 1988).

TABLE 5–5. Short-Term Goals and Procedures

Client: Seth

Short-Term Goals	Long-Term Goals Addressed	Prioritization Source
1. Seth will reduce the phonological processes of fronting and backing in conversational speech	1	Grunwell, 1981; Stoel-Gammon & Dunn, 1985
2. Seth will reduce the stopping of /f/, /v/, and /ʃ/ in conversational speech	1	Grunwell, 1981; Stoel-Gammon & Dunn, 1985
3. Seth will begin the suppression of the process of gliding (the production of /l/ in initial position of words)	2	Grunwell, 1981; Stoel-Gammon & Dunn, 1985
4. Seth will produce final /z/, and /s/, /z/ clusters coding plural, copula, third person singular, and possessive	3	Brown, 1973; Paul & Shriberg, 1982

Procedural Contexts   *Learning Principles*   *Maintaining Factors*

Nonlinguistic Context (types of materials)

Linguistic Context

The nonlinguistic context. In order to plan appropriate procedures for Seth, we must first reference background information and baseline data in maintaining factors. One of the most salient points of information from background data (Chapter 3) is that Seth has been receiving phonological treatment for over eight years. Some of the sounds he started with are still problematic (backing, stopping of /f/, and final consonant deletion). The background data, as well as the baseline data on maintaining factors, indicate that Seth has a moderate to severe sensorimotor impairment. Tonicity, body stability and segmentation, and the processing of tactile-kinesthetic information appear to be compromised. It is likely that his difficulty in making adequate progress in phonological process dissolution is due to motor and sensory constraints. Because of the lack of progress and the presence of sensorimotor dysfunction, the nonlinguistic context must offer Seth the opportunity for the strengthening of tongue musculature and the heightening of sensory awareness. Collaboration with an occupational therapist should facilitate the movement and awareness necessary for anterior tongue articulation. This is required for alveolar sounds (/s/,/z/,/l/) and the differentiation between anterior and posterior sounds. The occupational therapist generally engages in tasks that decrease tactile defensiveness, increase muscle tone and tactile input, and differentiate motor movements of various parts of the body. These accomplishments are precursory to producing alveolar sounds and to differentiating them from more posterior articulation.

At this point, one aspect of the procedural approach can be delineated: the nonlinguistic context. It will include the collaboration of an occupational therapist who will work on the skills precursory to producing anterior sounds and differentiating them from posterior sounds.

The linguistic context. Having further defined the nonlinguistic therapeutic context, we turn to the linguistic context. At this point we need to decide about the kinds of interactions in which the speech-language pathologist engages the child to facilitate achievement of the short-term goals. We return again to the long-term goal statement. This statement should contain decisions bearing upon the linguistic context of therapy. In addition, a number of learning principles (derived from social-cognitive and learning theory) that were specified in Seth's long-term procedural approach (Chapter 4) appear to be helpful in defining the role of the clinician.

The clinician will elicit linguistic structures by:

modeling target sounds in words or sentences;
presenting comparisons between target and error sounds in minimal pairs;
creating situations in which Seth is faced with communicative breakdown due to mispronunciation;
helping Seth to reflect on how phonetic gestures sound, feel, and look;
reacting positively to Seth's efforts by maintaining communicative interaction.

Following these principles gives us direction in procedural planning for the facilitation of sound productions.

1. For all phonological targets it will be necessary to present models for Seth to imitate. The length (number of syllables) and complexity of the linguistic units presented as models will depend on the phase of process dissolution. For example, processes such as backing and fronting that have begun dissolution (i.e., sounds vulnerable to the process have been established) are targeted in conversational speech. In this case Seth will be engaged in activities that involve the embedding of alveolars, velars, and labiodental fricatives in sentences. These activities may be represented by minimal-pair card games such as "go fish," in which Seth must ask for a card the examiner is holding in order to complete a pair. It may also include the reading of short stories on Seth's interest and ability level. Seth views himself as a comic and enjoys telling jokes (see Chapter 3, Table 3–6, baseline data on Seth). Telling jokes would also be a vehicle for the stabilization of sounds in connected speech. In contrast, there are sounds within a process (/ʃ/ in stopping and /l/ within gliding) that have not yet been established. In these cases the clinician will need to model shorter, less complex units (sounds in isolation or in monosyllabic words). Activities may involve naming pictures or reading words with targeted sounds after the clinician.

2. A part of the treatment of phonological disorders has traditionally involved the differentiation of error from standard sound (see Mysak, 1966; Van Riper, 1978; and Winitz, 1969, as clinicians most often associated with this approach). For Seth this principle is particularly applicable, given his sensorimotor impairment. There are a number of techniques reported in the literature to make children aware of differences between their error sounds and the standard sounds (see Bernthal & Bankson, 1988, and Dickson, 1984, for reviews).

3. A more recent phonological intervention approach focuses on identifying meaning differences between target words and words created by the production of an error phoneme (replacement or absence of a phoneme). This approach aims to make children aware of the way in which sounds contrast in their language to affect meaning. The emphasis on meaning has been viewed as a cognitive-linguistic approach to remediation (Bernthal & Bankson, 1988) and is represented primarily by teaching contrasts between minimal word pairs (see Weiner, 1981, for a seminal article in this area). The identification of differences in meaning is most salient when a child is involved in a situation in which he must differentiate minimal pairs in order to get what he wants (a card for a match; a piece to complete a design or a puzzle). If a child cannot productively differentiate between the minimal pairs designed by the clinician, a communication breakdown occurs. Though this situation may initially appear cruel, it is one of the best ways we know of to make children aware of meaning differences created by error productions. Since Seth does not self-monitor well

(errors persist after articulations have been established), this approach should be efficient in increasing awareness on a cognitive-linguistic level.

4. Related to the cognitive-linguistic approach is the metalinguistic approach to sound learning. Children are encouraged to think about the characteristics of speech sounds in order to differentiate them perceptually and to produce them. A number of articles have been written recently promoting the use of metalinguistic techniques (Howell & Dean, 1987; Tomes & Shelton, 1989). These techniques, which involve tactile, proprioceptive, and auditory descriptions of the sounds, would also be likely to increase Seth's awareness of his own productions and how they compare with expectations. Attention to detail and differentiating similarities and differences among items should also help to improve the processing of forms with low phonetic substance (e.g., unstressed syllables, function words; Leonard, 1989).

5. Seth is aware of a communication breakdown and makes every effort to repair. He frequently gets closer to the articulatory target. When this is not possible, he tries other means of getting his message across by substituting words or by pantomime. For this reason, it is reasonable to assume that Seth is rewarded by success in communication as well. Thus, natural maintenance of communicative interaction with the occasional positive feedback for attempts to repair unintelligible utterances is sufficient reinforcement for Seth.

At this point, the basic elements of nonlinguistic and linguistic therapeutic contexts have been defined with reference to short-term goals that have been written for Seth. We are now able to formulate a delineated procedural context. This approach will have two parts: a description of (a) the nonlinguistic context and (b) the linguistic context. A summary of Seth's delineated procedural context appears in the second part of the Management Plan, Short-Term Goals and Procedures in Table 5–6.

Alice

Short-Term Goals and Delineated Procedural Context. The following are the short-term goals and the delineated procedural context that were developed for Alice, a five-year-old whose primary difficulty is in the area of voice:

Short-term goal statements:

1. Alice will coordinate and sustain airflow and voicing to produce 3 and 3+ constituent utterances.
2. Alice will reduce the process of stopping, targeting /z/ in single words and /f/ and /v/ in continuous speech.

Delineated procedural context:

1. The nonlinguistic context will comprise adaptive equipment prescribed by the occupational therapist that engages Alice in activities and positions the

TABLE 5-6. Short-Term Goals and Procedures

Client: Seth

Short-Term Goals	Long-Term Goals Addressed	Prioritization Source	Maintaining Factors
1. Seth will reduce the phonological processes of fronting and backing in conversational speech.	1	Grunwell, 1981; Stoel-Gammon & Dunn, 1985	Sensorimotor, cognitive
2. Seth will reduce the stopping of /f/, /v/, and /ʃ/ in conversational speech	1	Grunwell, 1981; Stoel-Gammon & Dunn, 1985	
3. Seth will begin the suppression of the process of gliding (the production of /l/ in initial position of words)	2	Grunwell, 1981; Stoel-Gammon & Dunn, 1985	
4. Seth will produce final /z/, and /s/, /z/ clusters coding plural, copula, third person singular, and possessive	3	Brown, 1973; Paul & Shriberg, 1982	

Procedural Contexts	Learning Principles	Maintaining Factors
Nonlinguistic Context will involve:		Sensorimotor, cognitive, psychosocial
1. the participation of an occupational therapist	9	
2. materials that will promote sensorimotor advancement	5	
3. materials on Seth's interest and experience level		
Linguistic Context		
The clinician will:		
1. model target sounds in words or sentences	2	
2. present comparisons between target and error sounds in minimal pairs	3	
3. create situations in which Seth is faced with communicative breakdown due to mispronunciation	6	
4. help Seth to reflect on how phonetic gestures sound, feel and look	8	
5. react positively to Seth's efforts by maintaining communicative interaction	1	

occupational therapist aimed at dissociating oral motor actions from other bodily actions.

2. Objects will be provided that represent characters (e.g., puppets, mechanical animals that vocalize) for modifying voice production in pretend play.
3. The clinician will elicit target speech sounds and parameters of voice production by modeling during play activities.

The Derivation of Short-Term Goals.   Three long-term goals were established for Alice (Chapter 4): (a) coordinate efficient respiratory and phonatory patterns while producing complex sentences in all pragmatic contexts, (b) eliminate phonological processes of stopping and gliding, and (c) produce Phase 8 and 8+ form-content-use interactions (verb inflections, nominative case pronouns, and connectives) in all pragmatic contexts.

As with the other children discussed above, the first decision to be made at this short-term phase of intervention planning involves determining which long-term goal to address first. Again, we will refer to questions in Box 5–1 as a guide to decision making. In answer to question 1 (are there developmental relations among the long-term goals), in Alice's case, there are none immediately apparent.

Question 2 concerns the possibility that there may be functional relations among the long-term goals. Would addressing any one of these goals automatically affect the others? There is no clear-cut dependency relationship among the long-term goals. However, there appears to be an underlying variable that connects the behaviors targeted. Voice and articulation are sensorimotor activities. At the long-term phase of planning, we concluded that difficulties in sensorimotor functioning may be maintaining both of these problems, as well as difficulties with verb inflections, connectives use, and production of the auxiliary form in questions.

Alice manifests a number of sensorimotor symptoms that may be related to her voice and phonology: tense jaw and laryngeal musculature, effortful movements of larynx and jaw when vocalizing, walking on toes, moderately elevated tonicity. These symptoms are consistent with a diagnosis of inadequate body segmentation and instability noted in baseline data. Adequate differentiation of oral motor actions from simultaneous actions involving other body segments is implied in normal voice functioning; such differentiation supports efficient respiration and valvular function underlying adequate subglottal pressure, resonation, and articulation for sustained linguistic productions (Davis, 1987).

With reference to the sensorimotor problem, it will be necessary to target body segmentation and stability at all phases of intervention planning. This is outside the expertise of most speech-language pathologists. It will be necessary to collaborate with an occupational or physical therapist. Given that sensorimotor dysfunctions may underlie both voice and articulation problems, we are inclined to develop short-term goals in phonology and voice for the same time period.

We next ask if any one of these problems requires attention before the others (question 3). We turn to baseline data relevant to Alice's linguistic and nonlinguistic functioning. Alice was referred for a voice problem, and this fact reinforces our decision to target voice at this short-term phase of planning. Alice's developmental history, which indicates that voice is an especially intractable problem, supports this decision.

We have not addressed the long-term goal involving complex content-form interactions. We do not think it is appropriate to do so at this time, because it is very possible that producing such structures would place undue stress on vocalization.

To summarize, we have decided to address two of the long-term goals at this point in intervention planning: (a) coordinate efficient respiratory and phonatory patterns while executing complex sentences in all pragmatic contexts and (b) eliminate phonological processes of stopping and gliding.

The next step in formulating short-term goals for Alice involves determining which structures to target during the initial intervention period. The primary source of information that we turn to at this point is baseline data on Alice's present linguistic status. With reference to the first long-term goal, we ask, "What would be a step forward in the achievement of efficient vocal production?" At this point it is necessary to note that the relationship of our baseline data to short-term goal planning is somewhat different from that of the other children. In this case baseline data are not presented with reference to developmental taxonomies. Instead, as is typical for voice assessments (Andrews, 1986), a number of symptoms within the vocal parameters are delineated: intermittent aphonia, muscular tension in neck and shoulders during phonation, hoarse voice quality, inappropriate variations in pitch (phonation), short exhalation phase and infrequent replenishment of breath (respiration), inadequate nasal and oral resonance (resonation). Even though our baseline data are not presented within a developmental framework, it is possible to approach the short-term goal from a developmental perspective. Information about the development of normal vocal functioning would guide us in planning the steps necessary to reach the long-term goal, which is "To coordinate efficient respiratory and phonatory patterns while executing complex sentences in all pragmatic contexts." A hierarchy is implied in this achievement. This hierarchy can be viewed with reference to the linguistic context in which this coordination of respiration and phonation develop. For example, the context in which appropriate voice production is expected may proceed as follows: phoneme, word, phrase, continuous speech (Andrews, 1986; Wilson, 1987). Symptomatically, achievement of the ability to sustain the coordination of respiration and phonation for language affects vocal quality, pitch, and the need to replenish breath.

One of Alice's symptoms that is not necessarily addressed in facilitating the coordination of respiration and laryngeal functioning is muscular tension in the neck area. One approach to Alice's muscular tension might be for the speech-language pathologist to focus on relaxation of the neck musculature (Andrews, 1986). However, our view is that language production is supported by sensorimotor functioning of the entire body. This leads us to take a more holistic and developmental view of the source of the problem. Facilitating body segmentation and stability would address factors maintaining muscular tension in the neck and shoulders during phonation. In order to implement a more holistic approach, we need to consult with a physical or occupational therapist. The physical or occupational therapist will develop short-term goals relative to body segmentation and stability. We should be able to work with reference to the motor goals in our efforts to facilitate voice production. (Appendix E presents forms for organizing transdisciplinary goals.) We will return to the occupational therapist's suggestions in delineating a procedural approach and again at the session phase of intervention planning.

Our premise that voice is a component of language implicates the interaction of content, use, and form throughout intervention planning. This premise colors our thinking about how to target further the exhalatory phase at the short-term planning stage. Traditionally, exercises are given for children to practice producing nonsense syllables (such as /a:/) for increasing periods of time (Andrews, 1986). Although this may be a useful exercise, in our view of intervention planning it represents a session goal. Over a period of time such as a school term, we would like to target sustained efficient voice production in a delimited but meaningful *linguistic* context. For Alice, 3 and 3+ constituent utterances would be reasonable.

The second long-term goal that we decided to address was phonology. Baseline data indicate that Alice still applies two major processes: stopping and gliding. According to data on phonological development, both these processes persist beyond the age of three (Stoel-Gammon & Dunn, 1985). These processes, however, begin dissolution earlier (stopping at two years of age and gliding at three years of age; Grunwell, 1981). Dissolution may be characterized by the differential application of the process to its vulnerable consonants. For example, we can see that Alice is beginning to produce those sounds that have been associated with the beginning of elimination of the stopping process (/s/, /f/, /v/). Of these sounds, /s/ is most consistently approximated, but it is lateralized. The phonemes /f/ and /v/ are stopped approximately 40% of the time, others over 60% of the time (see Chapter 3, baseline data). Because Alice's primary problem is voice, we have decided to minimize articulatory challenges. We have targeted /f/ and /v/ in conversational speech because these sounds have been established in her repertoire. We have targeted /z/ in single-word utterances because stopping occurs more than 65% of the time. In addition, the voiceless cognate /s/ is no longer vulnerable to stopping and, therefore, is expected to influence the correct production of /z/. Other sounds vulnerable to stopping generally emerge later and will not be targeted during the initial short-term period.

The dissolution of gliding also has begun with the variable production of /l /. Given Alice's tendency toward bodily tension and lack of stimulability for /r/ at this time, a decision was made to target gliding after some advances were made in the areas of voice and fricative production. It should be noted, however, that within a cycle approach (Hodson & Paden, 1991) we could also address gliding intermittently during one short-term period (a semester), depending on the child's tolerance for change in treatment objectives.

Baseline data on Alice's current levels of functioning in the area of cognition suggest that she should be able to handle intervention aimed at both voice and phonology. Short-term goals established for Alice and recorded on the Short-Term Goal and Procedure Form (Appendix B–3) are presented in Table 5–7.

Delineated Procedural Context.   The decision to prioritize voice and to address sensorimotor maintaining factors orients us in defining linguistic and nonlinguistic contexts that will comprise a delineated procedural approach for Alice. First, let us consider methods and materials that will comprise the nonlinguistic context.

Nonlinguistic context. An important decision was made for the speech-language pathologist to collaborate with an occupational or physical therapist on the modification of Alice's sensorimotor patterns related to tonicity and body segmentation. This decision is relevant to the delineation of the nonlinguistic therapeutic context. The occupational therapist is working on rotation, improved tonicity, and equilibrium reactions in sitting positions. As such, she has recommended that we have adaptive equipment such as a Rifton chair, a log, and scooters available.

The delineation of the nonlinguistic therapeutic context is also influenced by the decision that interactions and contexts be developmentally appropriate. Play would be a developmentally appropriate context for a child of Alice's age and level of cognitive functioning. Consequently, we will have objects available that will allow us to stimulate desired vocal productions during script play—for instance, puppets and dolls for play at familiar activities, such as reenacting a scene from a TV show, visits to a restaurant, or being a teacher. We will also use play to stimulate movement patterns specified by the occupational therapist.

The decision that Alice needs feedback from behavior, made at the long-term planning phase, has implications for designing the nonlinguistic context. There are computer programs that concretize voice qualities by presenting visual images of the voice. These programs allow children to compare visual images of their vocal production with target productions. Such programs would be developmentally appropriate for a child Alice's age and would provide an extra dimension of feedback for Alice to utilize. Therefore, we plan to use computer programs with Alice.

The linguistic context. Having further delineated therapy materials we focus our attention on the kinds of interactions we will engage in with Alice. Guided by

TABLE 5–7. Short-Term Goals and Procedures

Client: Alice

Short-Term Goals	Long-Term Goals Addressed	Prioritization Source
1. Alice will coordinate and sustain airflow and voicing to produce 3 and 3 + constituent utterances	1	Andrews, 1986; Wilson, 1987
2. Alice will reduce the process of stopping, targeting /z/ in single words and /f/ and /v/ in continuous speech	2	Stoel-Gammon & Dunn, 1985

Procedural Contexts	Learning Principles	Maintaining Factors

Nonlinguistic Context (types of materials)

Linguistic Context

173

TABLE 5–8. Short-Term Goals and Procedures

Client: Alice

	Short-Term Goals	Long-Term Goals Addressed	Prioritization Source
1.	Alice will coordinate and sustain airflow and voice to produce 3 and 3 + constituent utterances	1	Andrews, 1986; Wilson, 1987
2.	Alice will reduce the process of stopping, targeting /z/ in final word position and /f/ and /v/ in continuous speech	2	Stoel-Gammon & Dunn, 1985

Procedural Contexts	Learning Principles	Maintaining Factors

Nonlinguistic Context will involve:

1.	Adaptive equipment prescribed by the occupational therapist aimed at dissociating oral motor actions from other bodily actions		Sensorimotor
2.	Objects that represent characters (e.g., puppets, mechanical animals that vocalize) for modifying voice production in pretend play	5	Psychosocial

Linguistic Context

1.	The clinician will model target speech sounds and parameters of voice production during play activities	2	Sensorimotor

principles from social-cognitive learning theory and motor-learning theory identified at the long-term planning phase, the clinician will: (a) model voice productions and encourage imitation and (b) provoke Alice to distinguish among vocal pitches and qualities during play with dolls and puppets. At this point, it is possible to formulate a delineated procedural approach for Alice. This appears in a completed Short-Term Goal and Procedure Form in Table 5–8.

SUMMARY

The focus of this chapter has been decision making at the short-term phase of intervention planning. Special attention was paid to the use of developmental and maturational information in formulating short-term goals and the application of learning principles to the delineation of linguistic and nonlinguistic therapeutic contexts. We will now turn to the third phase of intervention planning—the derivation of session goals and procedures. In the process, we will finally resolve the issue of what to do first in a treatment session.

6

Phase 3: Planning Session Goals and Procedures

We have now arrived at the final phase of intervention planning. We are ready to plan for a session. Paradoxically, it is only at this last phase of intervention planning that we are prepared to answer the question "What do I do first?" We will answer this question by specifying the behaviors we wish the client to exhibit during a session and the specific procedures (materials and interactions) that we will employ during that session.

There are two important influences on our intervention planning during the session phase. The first involves requirements of PL 94–142 and subsequent legislation (e.g., PL 99–457 and PL 101–476). This legislation, influenced by behavioral learning theory, indicates that we should formulate goal statements that delineate, in observable and measurable terms, the targeted behavior and the context in which it is expressed. In our model of intervention planning, the foundation for deriving such goals is prepared at the long-term and short-term planning phases. Goals are actually written in observable and measurable terms at the session phase planning.

The second influence on session planning concerns how we conceptualize the child's behavior that we target in session-goal statements. We see this behavior as an act of learning that will lead to the acquisition of a linguistic structure targeted as a short-term goal. This conceptualization of a session goal as an act of learning is different from our conceptualization of long- and short-term goals. Long- and short-term goals were viewed as outcomes of treatment. These outcomes or achievements were linguistic structures, such as the /r/ phoneme or the content category *locative action*, which would be acquired as a result of activities carried out during clinical sessions. At these earlier phases, acts of learning were addressed only in planning *procedures*.

The view of a session goal is an act of learning, and the requirement that the session-goal statement include a description of the context in which the act of learning takes place, has a significant implication for decision making at this session phase of intervention planning. This implication distinguishes planning at the session phase from planning at earlier phases: At the session phase, virtually all decisions about intervention apply to both the formulation of the goal and the procedure statements. Both the session goal and procedure will be influenced by information about: (a) how and in what order children learn particular linguistic structures, (b) factors maintaining problematic behavior, and (c) the demands that particular tasks make on the child's performance. Consequently, the session goal and procedure will be complementary in nature: The session-goal statement will describe a clinical interaction with reference to the child; the procedural statement will describe the same interaction with reference to the clinician.

DEFINING AND FORMULATING SESSION GOALS AND PROCEDURES

Definitions

We will depart from the format we followed in Chapters 4 and 5 in defining goals and procedures and discussing their derivations. We derived goals and procedures in separate sections of the previous two chapters (which dealt with long-term and short-term planning phases). In this chapter, we will define session goals and procedures and then treat their formulation as a unitary decision-making process.

Definition of a Session Goal.   A session goal is an observable behavior, expressed in a specified context, that represents an act of learning that will lead to the acquisition of a linguistic structure targeted as a short-term goal. As was the case with all the definitions we have offered, the wording in this definition is designed to inform the clinician about the nature of decision making and the relevant time frame involved at this phase of intervention planning.

Time frame. The term *session goal* indicates that the time frame we are working with is one session. Depending on the setting, a session may comprise fifteen minutes (e.g., in a preschool serving infants and toddlers) to forty-five minutes (e.g., with older clients in a school or hospital setting). Given that so short a period of time is allotted for intervention, a session goal is by nature a small, immediate accomplishment or step forward for the client.

Observable behavior. In the definition under consideration, a session goal is characterized as an "observable behavior." The depiction of a session goal as an observable behavior is in keeping with mandates of PL 94–142 for writing Individualized Educational Plans (IEPs), required in all settings that receive state and federal funding for serving children with handicapping conditions. It also is consistent with PL 99–457 and PL 101–476, which make similar requirements for developing Individualized Family Service Plans (IFSPs). It means that the targeted behavior should be overtly physical and measurable (e.g., countable).

Context. Our definition of a session goal stipulates next that the clinician specify the context in which the target behavior is expected to be achieved.

Again, this is in keeping with mandates of PL 94–142 and subsequent legislation. As we explained in Chapters 1 and 5, the term *context* refers to the environment that surrounds a particular behavior. In Chapter 5 we distinguished between linguistic and nonlinguistic aspects of the environment surrounding a behavior. We said that the linguistic context was the linguistic environment surrounding a behavior. We outlined the nature of the linguistic context in the short-term *procedural* statement. In formulating session goals, the characteristics of the surrounding linguistic environment should be described in the *goal* statement, itself. An example is seen in the following session goal: "Bobby will raise his hand in response to CVC words beginning with /k/ when the clinician presents minimal pairs of CVC words beginning with /k/ or /t/ phonemes." The linguistic context in which Bobby is expected to express the targeted behaviors is the clinician's verbal presentation of minimal pairs of CVC words distinguishable by the presence of /k/ and/t/ phonemes.

It is important to note that *linguistic context* of an utterance may refer either to the language produced by the child in which the target behavior is embedded or to the language produced by the clinician (or any other individual interacting with the child). A session goal that refers to the clinician's behavior as the linguistic context was offered immediately above. An example of a session goal that makes reference to the language of the child surrounding the target behavior is as follows: "Peter will produce /r/ in stop-liquid clusters in the initial position of words when naming objects associated with Christmas." The phrase "stop-liquid clusters in the initial position of words when naming objects" represents the linguistic context—produced by the child—that surrounds the target behavior "producing /r/."

The nonlinguistic context comprises the materials and interactions that are not linguistic in nature. A session–goal statement specifies this aspect of context, too, if it is central to the expression of the target behavior. For example, the nonlinguistic context is specified in the session-goal statement, "Liv will code state + attribution using 3+ constituent utterances to describe dolls in context of play." "Play" (with dolls) is the nonlinguistic context. This goal could be expanded to include the linguistic context as well: for instance, Liv will code state + attribution in 3+ constituent utterances to describe dolls in context of play following the clinician's modeling of state + attribution structures."

A step toward achievement of the short-term goal. The next portion of the definition indicates that the behavior targeted as a session goal is an act of learning believed to be a step toward the acquisition of a linguistic structure that was targeted as a short-term goal. That it is a step toward the achievement of a short-term goal indicates that the behavior has a purpose and a direction—it should facilitate the acquisition of a linguistic structure that represents the short-term goal. Planning these steps entails a complex decision-making process.

This characterization of a target behavior represents a shift in focus from the long and short-term phases of goal planning. At these earlier phases, we wrote goals in terms of *linguistic* achievements. However, a session goal need not be formulated in linguistic terms, since a session goal represents a small step in the acquisition of linguistic structures. Consequently, a nonlinguistic behavior, such as a hand movement or a turn of the body in recognition of a sound difference or word, may be indicative of such a step. If this is so, we may target this type of behavior in a session goal (e.g., "Marianna will raise her hand when the clinician presents a sound beginning with /r/"). It should be noted that a session goal *may* be formulated in terms of a linguistic structure—as long as that structure is observable and its frequency of expression is measurable (e.g., "John will code action + attribution (three times) in telling a story about 'Little Red Ridinghood?' ").

In the next section we will define session procedures. We will then discuss three useful sources of information in the decision-making process underlying the derivation of session goals and procedures: (a) factors believed to be maintaining the disorder, (b) principles of language-learning theories, and (c) conditions that make demands on the child's effort to perform the target behavior (performance demands).

A note about terminology. As you can see, we have been referring to observable behaviors targeted at the session phase of intervention planning as session *goals.* There are some authors who term these behaviors "target behaviors" (Hegde, 1985). In the allied field of special education (Bigge, 1988; Cook, Tessier, & Klein, 1992) these behaviors are called "objectives." We have chosen to use the term *goal* at all phases of intervention planning to highlight continuity across these phases.

Defining Session Procedures.   We define a session procedure as the clinician's actions and the materials used to facilitate the expression of the behavior targeted in the session goal. This definition of a session procedure focuses on two critical variables that will have an impact upon the client's responses in a clinical session: clinician's actions and available materials. The clinician's actions are all those nonverbal and verbal behaviors in which the clinician engages in order to facilitate the child's achievement of the session goal. The clinician must be aware of the potential impact of these actions on the client.

The session procedure also describes those materials with which the child will engage to achieve the session goal. These may include toys, games, books, flash cards, word lists, a basin of water. As with the clinician's actions, the materials can have a significant impact on the client's achievement of desired responses.

The definition of a session procedure emphasizes that the clinician's actions and material available to the child have a specific aim: They should be designed to facilitate the behaviors targeted in the session goal. The wording of the definition recognizes the importance of conceiving the procedure as embedded within a clinical interaction. The term *interaction* implies a close, mutual, potentially changing relationship between client and clinician during each session. Subtle shifts in the behavior of each of the participants can influence the behavior of the other. Subtle changes in other types of environmental conditions (such as objects being manipulated) can have consequences on the behavior of the participants in the clinical interaction. This mutual sensitivity of clinician and client to one another's behavior and to conditions in which the clinical interaction is embedded becomes an important organizing force in the formulation of session procedures. (For further discussion of this concept, see Bateson, 1980; Ozer, 1979; Pickering, 1987; Watzlawick, Beavin, & Jackson, 1967).

A Comparison of Session Goals and Procedures. Let us consider, now, the close and complementary nature of the session goal and procedure. Compare the following goal and procedure. The session goal is "Maria will code the prepositions *in, on,* and *under* in locative action statements to direct the clinician and other children to hide toys and to move through a maze." The corresponding procedure states that "The clinician will model the prepositions *in, on,* and *under* in locative action statements and direct Maria and other children to move through a maze." The complementary nature of these statements is immediately apparent. The goal cites the child's production of the targeted behavior and the context in which it will be produced in terms of the child's participation in the clinical interaction. The session procedure describes the clinician's efforts to provoke those same client actions in the same context. Because of the complementary nature of session goal and procedure, we will discuss decisions involved in determining session goals and procedures and relevant sources of information for making these decisions in a single section, below.

Deciding Which Short-term Goals to Target During Sessions

There is a set of preliminary decisions that must be made at the session phase of intervention planning if more than one short-term goal was targeted for the term. The clinician must decide whether to address one or more short-term goals during individual sessions and in what order to address short-term goals. We have formulated a set of questions and sources of information that may be useful in making these decisions. These appear in Box 6–1.

Can the Short-Term Goals Be Ordered According to a Developmental Hierarchy?
Developmental hierarchies can be useful in deciding which short-term goals to address first in session planning. If the linguistic structures under consideration emerge in a particular order in the normal course of language development, it may be advisable to address these structures in the same order over a term. If these structures emerge during the same developmental phase, it might be expedient to target such structures during the same period of time. It is possible,

---

**BOX 6–1.   QUESTIONS AND SOURCES OF INFORMATION
FOR DECIDING HOW TO SEQUENCE SHORT-TERM GOALS**

Questions	*Sources of Information*	*Relevant Decision*
1. Can the short-term goals be ordered according to a maturational or developmental hierarchy?	Scales from the literature on child development	If "yes": consider sequencing session goals according to this developmental hierarchy
2. Is the client already producing the target structure in some contexts?	Baseline data in speech and language	If "yes": consider targeting the short-term goal during initial sessions
3. Are there separate skills that could be addressed in initial sessions that are foundational to the achievement of multiple short-term goals?		If "yes": consider targeting those short-term goals facilitated by similar skills during a single time period

---

however, that other factors would influence this decision (e.g., semantic and phonetic saliency of structures relative to one another). Recall that we made decisions relevant to this issue during the short-term phase of goal planning.

Is the Client Already Producing the Target Structure in Some Contexts?
A second question is whether the client is already producing the linguistic structures under consideration. It may be appropriate to target structures which are just emerging and promote increased frequency during initial sessions (Bloom & Lahey, 1978; Lahey, 1988). The use of these structures might be generalized to the contexts cited in the short-term goal statement over the course of the term. Information about the child's production of linguistic structures should be available in baseline data.

It is interesting to note that there is some controversy in the literature about whether to target structures that are *already* in the child's repertoire. Some researchers in the field of clinical phonology have recommended that early phonological targets should be selected from among those sounds that the child is not producing under any conditions. These researchers believe that those sounds that are stimulable will be acquired spontaneously by the child without the aid of intervention (e.g., Elbert, 1992; Gierut, Elbert, & Dinnsen, 1987; Powell, 1991).

Are There Individual Skills That Could Be Addressed in Initial Sessions That Are Foundational to the Achievement of Multiple Short-Term Goals?   Often the child will have to master a set of prerequisite skills in order to achieve a short-term goal. For example, a child with a fluency problem might have to learn to discriminate fluent from dysfluent speech productions and to articulate initial sounds in words with reduced tension in order to reach the short-term goal of coordinating articulation, phonation, and respiration in the production of 3+ constituent utterances. If such prerequisite skills are common to other short-term goals, it might be advisable to target all these short-term goals during the same time period. Thus, with reference to the child with the fluency problem, it might make sense to recognize that the discrimination and articulation exercises would be foundational to a second short-term goal: for example, coordinating articulation, phonation, and respiration in responding to requests for information. Thus, the clinician would, in essence, be working on these two short-term goals simultaneously.

Categories of Information for Formulating Session Goals and Procedures

Once a decision is made about the order in which to address short-term goals, we turn to the formulation of session goals and procedures. There are several categories of information that will be useful in this task. These are (a) factors maintaining the speech-language disorder under consideration, (b) principles of language learning, and (c) performance demands. Up to this point we have tended to associate this information with procedure planning. At this session phase of intervention, each of these categories of information contributes to the planning of both goals and procedures.

Maintaining Factors.   Our knowledge about factors maintaining a speech-language disorder is an important source of information for planning session goals. When we talk about maintaining factors, we are referring to those language-related behaviors that have not progressed according to developmental expectations. It is at this phase of intervention planning that we attempt to modify these factors in an effort to facilitate the acquisition of the short-term goal. In other words, we will help the child acquire those skills he lacks in order to make language learning possible.

During the first two phases of intervention planning, we used information about maintaining factors to make very general *procedural* decisions (see Chapters 4 and 5). That is to say, we identified those behavioral systems that appeared to account most directly for communication problems. This information provided direction for making general decisions about treatment *contexts* and allied professional services that would be required to effect change in these behavioral systems.

Consider the case of Seth. Knowing that he had a sensorimotor problem led us to formulate a procedural approach that included attention to sensory factors (auditory, tactile, and kinesthetic) associated with articulatory gestures. Similarly, knowing that we had to address cognition in the case of Darryl led us to focus on play and the use of manipulable toys in the design of the context.

Now, at the session phase, a knowledge of maintaining factors will direct the planning of session goals as well as session procedures. Skills within each behavioral category identified as a maintaining factor will be targeted within session-goal statements. Information about correspondences between developmental achievements in nonlinguistic and linguistic behavioral systems, which appears in Boxes 1–3 through 1–5, will guide these decisions.

Utilizing Boxes 1–3 through 1–5. Sensorimotor, cognitive, and psychosocial skills that support the development of language were identified in Chapter 1, Boxes 1–3 through 1–5. We will refer to these skills now, at the session phase of intervention planning, to specify behaviors that will be targeted in session goals.

To illustrate the use of Boxes 1–3 through 1–5 we will look at the hypothetical case of Jerry, a three-year-old boy with delayed language development. One of the short-term goals set was to coordinate attribution with existence. In long-term and short-term procedural statements cognition was identified as a maintaining factor to be addressed through the manipulation of concrete objects. At the session phase, cognitive skills related to the coding of attribution will be identified. We will then specify behaviors the child will be encouraged to demonstrate during therapy sessions that will indicate he is employing these cognitive skills. Turning to Box 1–3, we see that talking about attribution is related to the cognitive skill of grouping and regrouping objects according to attribute. This information gives us some direction in creating session goals and procedures. We know that we will be targeting the actions of grouping and regrouping according to some sets of attributes (e. g., size, shape, color, physical properties). We also know that it will be necessary for the clinician to decide *how* best to encourage Jerry to group appropriate materials. Making these decisions will involve reference to principles from learning theory and to background information (which will be discussed below). In addition, the order in which specific attributes will be introduced requires a consideration of factors contributing to the complexity of the learning task. This will be discussed in the section on performance demands.

Collaboration. It is noteworthy that, in the present intervention planning model, behaviors aimed at facilitating development in areas other than language are only specified in session-goal statements. As speech-language pathologists, we usually do not set *long-term* or *short-term* goals in these areas of behavior. Cognitive, sensorimotor, or psychosocial goals are usually determined by allied professionals, such as special educators or physical therapists. We have provided a Collaboration Form for writing such goals in Appendix E.

We recommend that the speech-language clinician collaborate with allied professionals in thinking about short- and long-term achievements in nonlinguistic areas. We also recommend collaboration in setting session goals. If no such colleague is available—or as an adjunct to collaboration—the speech-language clinician may wish to note long-term and short-term goals in areas other than language on the form provided in Appendix E. Collaboration will be discussed in greater depth in Chapter 7.

Learning Theory and Derived Principles. A second major source of information that guides the formulation of session goals and procedures is learning theory. Principles from learning theories provide direction for creating specific activities that will be incorporated in session goals and procedures. Learning principles were first identified in the long-term procedural approach and contributed to the development of linguistic and nonlinguistic contexts at the short-term planning phase.

To recount the application of learning principles at the long- and short-term planning phases we again present data from Seth. The long-term procedural statement for Seth specified that intervention planning would be influenced by principles from social-cognitive and motor-learning theories. Among the principles cited were that learning was facilitated by (a) efforts to match models presented by the clinician and (b) noticing similarities and distinctions among events mediated by adults. The short-term description of a procedural context indicated that the clinician would model target sounds and present comparisons among target and error sounds in minimal pairs.

At the session phase of intervention planning it is necessary to identify the activities in which Seth must engage in order to learn to differentiate a specific sound pair. It is also necessary to describe what Seth and the clinician will *do* during these activities. In other words, we must describe observable behaviors which will be manifested during sessions. Learning principles imply such activities. The information provided in Boxes 1–6 and 1–7 suggests correspondences between learning theories and activities. Returning to Seth, the social-cognitive principle that "matching models" facilitates learning implies imitation. Thus, the clinician may target imitation of a particular articulatory behavior as a session goal (and the clinician's modeling as the complementary session procedure).

Learning principles provide a second category of information related to the formulation of session goals and procedures. However, we are not yet prepared to specify a target behavior or therapeutic context. We need to make decisions about the demands a specific learning task may make on a child's performance. The issue of performance demands will be discussed next.

Performance Demands. A third category of information that affects session goals and procedures involves those factors that add to or lessen performance demands—that is, increase or decrease the complexity of the task of learning a particular behavior. The relative complexity of a particular activity is often reflected in variability in a child's linguistic performance as the child moves from situation to situation.

How performance demands relate to variability in performance. Research in language acquisition and language disorders has demonstrated that aspects of the nonlinguistic and linguistic context influence the amount of speech and language as well as the accuracy of speech and language produced by children. Normally developing children have demonstrated variability in the complexity of productions generally acquired during a single developmental period (see, for example, Bloom, Miller, & Hood, 1975, with reference to sentence constituents, and Klein, 1981a, with reference to phonology). Children with language and speech disorders have been shown to produce a newly acquired structure in some situations but not in others (e.g., Hegde & McCann, 1981; Kent, 1982; Rockman & Elbert, 1984). Kamhi (1988) has referred to contextual and production factors that influence such variability in performance as "performance factors." We shall refer to these factors as "performance demands" or "factors that contribute to the complexity of the learning task."

Using knowledge of performance demands to formulate session goals and procedures. Our knowledge about performance demands comprises important information for the generation of a sequence of session goals and procedures. During a session, we will be asking a child either to produce a new communication form or to generalize one already being produced. In producing a communication form for the first time, we want to provide a linguistic and nonlinguistic context that makes as few demands as possible other than the production of the new form or a related skill. Optimally, the context will actually support production of the form (by being perceptually salient, facilitative of articulatory gestures, or relevant to the content and function of the utterance). In the case of linguistic forms already being produced, we will want to manipulate contextual variables so that the child is challenged to generalize their use to novel linguistic or nonlinguistic environments.

How performance demands relate to generalization. It is important to note that when we talk about increasing the complexity of tasks across sessions, we are talking about transfer of behaviors from one context to another—an aspect of generalization. Issues of generalization have historically been part of the clinical process (e.g., Ainsworth, 1948; Berry & Eisenson, 1956; Van Riper, 1939, 1973, 1978) and continue to be revitalized within new clinical paradigms (e.g., "phonological knowledge", Elbert & Gierut, 1986, discussed below). See also Fey's (1988) introduction to a clinical forum, in which generalization issues are addressed from a variety of theoretical viewpoints.

With reference to the nature of the linguistic target (a new linguistic structure or generalization of a structure already being produced), the clinician will need to envision a sequence of learning tasks that will lead to the achievement of the short-term goal. Sequences derive from the clinician's estimates of the demands made on the learner in performing one particular task relative to another. These estimates of complexity help us to make decisions about which behavior to target and in which contexts—two integral components of the session-goal statement. In the next section of this chapter we will demonstrate how a consideration of performance demands applies across four types of communication disorders: language, phonology, voice, and fluency.

How a Consideration of Performance Demands Affects Session Planning in Four Communication-Disorder Areas

A consideration of performance demands plays a critical role in decision making for session goals and procedures. Consequently, we devote the next section of the chapter to a discussion of performance factors that need to be addressed in four disorder areas: language, articulation-phonology, fluency, and voice.

Language Disorders.   We will first examine sources of variability in the area of language disorders. There is a set of variables that are commonly seen as affecting the child's ability to produce content-form interactions and, therefore, as needing to be manipulated in the formulation of session plans. These variables are (a) perceptual support; (b) the child's sensorimotor action underlying the content of language; (c) pragmatic complexity; (d) phonetic and phonological factors; and (e) conceptual complexity.

Perception and action. The impact of context on language learning and language production was discussed in some depth in Chapter 5. Literature was reviewed that indicates that when children first learn language they talk about objects that they are perceiving, usually in a play context. Only later do they use language to talk about objects and events that they are not presently observing or physically manipulating (e.g., Bloom & Lahey, 1978; Muma, 1978). Children learning language also frequently label and request in familiar game routines with caregivers (e.g., "peek-a-boo" or storytime with a favorite book; Ninio & Bruner, 1978; Ratner & Bruner, 1978).

One implication of these findings is that the provision of *perceptual support* for children learning a new content-form interaction may lessen the performance demands being made on the child. The production of a specific content-form interaction to recollect or anticipate an event that is not observable could be targeted as a more advanced session goal.

A second implication is that *sensorimotor action* supports the production of language. Sensorimotor action involves the physical manipulation of objects and thinking about changes and relationships created by action. In Chapters 1 and 2, in a discussion of constructivist-cognitive learning theory, children's reflection on feedback from their own actions was identified as foundational for the development of cognition and language content (Forman & Hill, 1984;

Moses, 1981; Piaget, 1985). From this point of view, it may be easier for children to represent concepts underlying language while engaged in practical, constructive, problem-solving activities involving the manipulation of concrete objects. Practical, action-oriented, goal-directed activities may also support problem-solving skills such as attending and information retrieval. It may be more difficult for children to learn concepts and problem-solving skills from pictures, verbal explanations, metalinguistic "self-talk," or by being trained behaviorally to perform splinter skills, such as sitting and making eye contact.

It is our position that listening to explanations and observing pictures before engaging in concrete, action-oriented experiences is like putting the cart before the horse (see also Forman & Hill, 1984; Fosnot, 1991; Kamii & DeVries, 1993). This is an especially critical principle to keep in mind for children with language-learning disabilities. Learning concepts through language for a child with a language-learning disability can be disabling. This is a likely consequence of the adult insisting that the child learn by relying on a disabled behavioral system (language) rather than potentially enabled ones (e.g., sensorimotor action, vision; see DeRuiter & Wansart, 1982; Moses, Klein, & Altman, 1990; Reid & Hresko, 1981; Wansart, 1990).

Consider, for example, planning session goals for a six-year-old child with mental retardation. The short-term goal targeted by both the speech-language pathologist and the classroom teacher is "coding attribution." In this case, baseline data revealed deficits in general knowledge of attributes.

Suppose that the clinician decides to focus on "size" as the first attribute for the child to code linguistically. A context should be created that would best facilitate the achievement of this goal. Box 1–3, which lists cognitive correlates of linguistic achievements, is helpful in providing guidance. According to the information in Box 1–3, coding attribution is related to "comparing and ordering objects according to a specific dimension [e.g., size]." Thus, we might engage this child in an activity in which he manipulates objects of various sizes and is encouraged to make size comparisons (e.g., trying to get airplanes of various sizes into small garages, or having to select from a jar of tiny cookies and a jar of large cookies while observing a playmate eating a large cookie). The clinician would initially avoid using pictures of different-sized objects to facilitate the coding of attribution. To "generalize" the use of this linguistic structure, we might introduce pictures in familiar storybooks and, later, more abstract or unfamiliar pictures.

Pragmatic considerations. In a number of sources, perceptual support and sensorimotor action are considered to be pragmatic in nature (e.g., Lahey, 1988; Lund & Duchan, 1988). We have organized these variables as aspects of cognition. We do, however, identify a number of factors belonging to the area of pragmatics that may contribute to task complexity in language cases. These factors are consistent with precepts advanced in MacDonald's ECHO system of language intervention (MacDonald & Carroll, 1992) and in Lund and Duchan's (1988) conceptualization of *fine tuning.* Lund and Duchan describe fine tuning as "how adults alter what they say to children in response to what a child is presumed to be thinking or doing" (p. 64). They note that "the closer the match between the language input and the child's thinking, the better are the conditions for the child to understand and learn about language" (p. 64; see also Barnes, Gutfreund, Satterly, & Wells, 1983; Cross, 1977; Shatz, 1982; Shatz & Gelman, 1973; Snow, 1977).

In a similar vein, Bloom, Miller, and Hood (1975) compared the conditions under which children produced two- and three-constituent utterances. They found that children were more likely to produce three constituents when (a) the lexical items were familiar, (b) the utterance was supported by something in the adult's prior utterance, and (c) there were no new syntactic elements.

As illustrated in the literature reviewed above, certain pragmatic behaviors affect linguistic performance. This research suggests a number of principles which may be applied to intervention planning. For example:

1. Adults' comments that mirror a topic initiated by a child (in play or conversation) are easier to process than comments that shift topics. Lund and Duchan (1988) refer to this close relation between the focus of a child's attention and understanding and the adult's subsequent utterance as *semantic contingency.*

2. Adults' comments that reflect, reiterate, or expand upon a child's utterance are easier to process than comments that do not reflect the child's prior comment. Lund and Duchan (1988) view this relation between the form of the child's utterance and the adult's subsequent statement as another component of semantic contingency.

3. Explicit reference (nominal-nominal) is probably easier to process than anaphoric reference (pronominal-nominal) for children just learning language.

4. Statements by adults to children that do not demand a particular response seem to be, paradoxically, easier to respond to than questions or imperatives. Similarly, *genuine questions,* to which the caretaker really does not know the answer and that are relevant to the child's ongoing actions, are easier to respond to than imperatives or questions that serve no function other than to demand a response. Lund and Duchan (1988) term this relation between the intent of the adult's statement and its demand on the child as *intentional contingency.*

5. Lexical novelty and syntactic complexity increase performance demands.

In sum, the clinician can "fine tune" the linguistic context of the therapeutic session by (a) increasing the alignment between the clinician's utterances and the child's actions, (b) avoiding imperatives and questions meant only to provoke a response, and (c) minimizing lexical novelty and syntactic complexity. Introducing topic shifts and directives using novel linguistic forms would be a means of increasing performance demands. One might wonder why a clinician would increase performance demands this way. One possible reason would be to increase the child's tolerance for demands made in school, where activities are often far from being "child centered."

Phonological factors. There is a body of research that indicates that phonological factors may have an impact upon language learning, particularly at early stages of language development (Klein, 1982; Stoel-Gammon & Cooper, 1984). A number of researchers (e.g., Locke, 1983; Menn,1978; Stoel-Gammon & Cooper, 1984; Vihman, 1976) have found that the first words of normally achieving children are influenced by a child's idiosyncratic "favorite sounds," most frequently produced categories of sounds (stops, glides, nasals produced in anterior positions) and syllabic forms (CV) carried over from babbling. The implication is that careful consideration should be given to the phonetic characteristics of words that a child with a language delay is expected to learn. An early vocabulary constituting stops, glides, and nasals produced in anterior positions; CV syllable forms; and the child's personally preferred sounds should be relatively easy to produce. Words containing fricatives, liquids, blends, and complex multisyllabic forms might pose a greater challenge.

Conceptual complexity. Conceptual complexity is another factor that affects linguistic performance and should be considered in session planning. Developmental hierarchies presented in the literature on normal child development are often useful resources for determining conceptual complexity. Take, for example, the plan to work toward the coding of attribution with the child with mental retardation discussed above. The short-term goal did not specify the attribute to be coded by the child. The complexity of the attribute targeted could have an impact upon the complexity of the learning task. Selecting an attribute to target would be facilitated if we could reference a published developmental hierarchy. Appendix D presents a list of published material on speech and language development in children that provide useful developmental hierarchies.

Some hierarchies, however, are not available. The taxonomy that we referenced to target attribution in the short-term goal (Bloom & Lahey, 1978) does not present a developmental sequence for specific attributes. We must look elsewhere to determine if such a sequence exists. If it does not, we will have to devise a basis for hypothesizing a sequence, ourselves. In this case, a hierarchy was constructed based on information in the literature on young children's understanding of attributes (Smith, 1984) and observations of the child's behavior during play (i.e., the child appeared to make size comparisons rather than those based on shape or color).

Let us consider another example of a planning problem involving conceptual complexity. A short-term goal statement indicates that the child will code a particular linguistic structure while telling a story. Different story grammars (e.g., additive, temporal, causal) involve different levels of conceptual complexity. Planning a session could be facilitated by information about the development of language in the context of narrative story-telling. In this instance, there is a developmental schedule to reference: Lahey (1988). This schedule would serve as a guide for devising a sequence of session goals and procedures of increasing complexity.

Articulation and Phonology. Disorders of articulation and phonology constitute the second area that we will consider with reference to factors that contribute to performance demands. We identify traditional and phonological approaches to this issue. Traditionally, speech-language pathologists have organized the approach to speech-sound production treatment objectives with reference to length of unit (i.e., sound in isolation, syllable, monosyllabic word, multisyllabic word, phrase, sentence, continuous speech) and position in word (initial, final, and medial). These sequences have become very popular because they represent an apparent hierarchy of production complexity (Bernthal & Bankson, 1988). For detailed descriptions of such an approach, see seminal works by Van Riper (1978) and Winitz (1969, 1975) as well as more recent updates (Creaghead, Newman, & Secord, 1989; Bernthal & Bankson, 1988).

More recently, hierarchies with an emphasis on rule development, elimination of phonological processes, and "phonological knowledge" have been formulated on the basis of children's own production patterns. It has been argued that children will demonstrate what they know (or do not know) about the sound system by how they pronounce words. This approach has directed the speech-language pathologist to examine the child's production pattern for information about which factors contribute to complexity (ability to produce a particular sound). Some factors that have been isolated are prosody (stress and serial position of syllable containing the phoneme; Klein, 1981a, 1981b; Klein & Spector, 1985), phonetic environment (e.g., Camarata & Gandour, 1984; Leonard, Devescove, & Ossela, 1987; Wolfe & Blocker, 1990), and underlying phonological representation or "phonological knowledge" (e.g., Elbert, Dinnsen, & Powell, 1984; Elbert, Dinnsen, Swartzlander, & Chin, 1990; Gierut, 1989, 1990; Gierut, Elbert, & Dinnsen, 1987; Powell, 1991). These factors, as the more traditional, provide direction for the planning of a sequence of session goals. In the following section we will discuss the way in which some of these factors may affect session planning.

Word position. Let us consider the child who is fronting as we apply our knowledge of these factors related to performance demands. As is typical in intervention planning, a number of questions comes to mind: (a) Which sound should we start with first, /k/, /g/, /ŋ/, or all? (b) In which word position should the sound be introduced? (c) In which phonetic context should it be embedded? (d) How many syllables should the word contain? (e) How may exemplars are sufficient for generalization to occur?

If we decide to start with /k/, research on phonological development informs us that the final position would be most facilitative, while for /g/ it would be the initial. This is because young children have been reported to produce voiced plosives more readily in the initial position and voiceless more readily in the final (e.g., Ingram, 1989). Difficulties in the acquisition of voicing have been attributed to the complexity of mastering voice onset time adjustments

(Bernthal & Bankson, 1988). It has also been suggested, however, that children only produce voiceless unaspirated stops in both positions (Macken, 1980), which are perceived by adults as voiced in the initial position and voiceless in the final position (Bernthal & Bankson, 1988). Word-position variables, therefore, must be considered in planning a sequence of session goals. If we are targeting place (to eliminate fronting) we would aim to facilitate the production by considering the most facilitating voicing environment. Edwards (1992) proposes similar hierarchical considerations involving place and voicing in her discussion of "process ordering."

Prosody. A second factor that should be considered and is related to position is prosody. If we are interested in generalizing the production of a consonant to medial position we must be careful about the stress and serial position of the syllable in which it is embedded. Klein (1981a, 1981b) demonstrated that children generally maintain consonants from stressed syllables occurring at the end of a sequence. These syllables, therefore, were hypothesized to be less demanding on the child's processing capacities than unstressed syllables beginning a sequence (i.e., giving rise to unstressed syllable deletion). More recent attention to nonlinear aspects of phonology underscores the importance of considering the relationship between segments and syllable structure and segments and stress (see Schwartz, 1992, for a discussion of the relationship of nonlinear phonology to the clinical situation). Thus, stress and serial position of syllable are additional factors to consider in formulating a series of session goals.

Phonetic environment. A third factor that will help us to design a series of session objectives is the phonetic environment of the sound. It is well known that the phonetic environment of the sound will influence its production (e.g., Hodson & Paden, 1991; Kent, 1982). Some neighboring sounds may encourage target sound production, while other sounds may support the error production. For example, a child who is producing /t/ for /k/ will more likely produce a target /k/ in *cake* than in *kite*. The second /k/ in *cake* supports the initial /k/ while the final /t/ in *kite* encourages the production of the error segment in initial position. Both are cases of assimilation, in which one sound becomes more like another; the first case is one of facilitating assimilation, the second is nonfacilitating. It is important for the clinician to be aware of both types of assimilative contexts.

Examples of assimilative tendencies come from the literature on normally developing children and those with delayed speech development. Observation of normally developing children reveals that one sound (1) is more likely to come under the control of another (2) when (1) is not as firmly established in the child's repertoire as (2) (alveolars generally before velars; Macken, 1979; Stoel-Gammon, 1985) or when (2) is in a more favored position than (1) (Smith, 1973). Though these assimilative tendencies are somewhat universal, they need to be assessed for individual children. For example, Camarata and Gandour (1984), Leonard, Devescove, and Ossela (1987), and

Wolfe and Blocker (1990) provide samples of unusual assimilative tendencies exhibited by speech-delayed children.

Assimilation tendencies have been described extensively with reference to clusters. It has been shown that certain clusters facilitate the production of singleton /s/ and /r/ targets (e.g., Swisher's study, cited by Kent, 1982). Also see a comprehensive articulatory classification of clusters by Grunwell (1985) This classification system suggests the articulatory mechanisms underlying the sequencing of consonants, resulting in possible assimilation tendencies. It also provides a very useful framework in which to organize children's cluster errors and plan a sequence of goals based on the complexity of the required articulatory gestures involved.

In summary, knowing about which sounds in words affect the target sound will help the clinician to develop a hierarchy of complexity within phonetic contexts. (For a comprehensive discussion of the impact of aspects of the context on correct sound production—syllable stress, word or syllable position and adjacent sounds—see Kent, 1982.)

Phonological knowledge. A more recent concern in determining what to do first with a speech-disordered client is the client's "phonological knowledge" (for an introduction to and clinical application of this model, see Elbert & Gierut, 1986). This model suggests that target sounds should be selected on the basis of the child's phonological knowledge. This knowledge refers to the way in which "the idiosyncratic properties of morphemes are learned and stored in a speaker's lexicon or mental dictionary" (Elbert & Gierut, 1986, p. 49). Hierarchies of target achievement are developed with reference to *most to least* phonological knowledge or *least to most* phonological knowledge (i.e., Gierut, Elbert, & Dinnsen, 1987). See also Powell's (1991) and Elbert's (1992) rationales for using the principle of "least phonological knowledge" in planning a sequence of goals.

Within the phonological knowledge approach, there has been increased systematic study of the phenomenon of generalization by Elbert and her colleagues (e.g., Elbert, Dinnsen, & Powell, 1984; Elbert, Dinnsen, Swartzlander, & Chin, 1990; Elbert, Powell, & Swartzlander, 1991). These clinical phonologists have studied primarily the way in which a child's phonological knowledge and conditions of the environment influence the type and extent, and kind of generalization that occurs in intervention.

Perceptual support. We can talk about perceptual support in the area of phonology in a number of ways. The first is stimulability. *Stimulability* signifies the ability to produce an utterance following a model. Here the model serves as perceptual support (auditory and visual). Some sounds may be perceived both visually and auditorally (e.g., /f/ and /p/). For this reason such sounds may be more stimulable—that is, more likely to be imitated. The stimulability of a sound is one of the factors that would be considered in determining which sound among a group of sounds (vulnerable to a particular process) would be targeted first.

A second issue related to perceptual support in the area of phonology concerns the linguistic-pragmatic context in which a child is expected to achieve a production. Should the production be imitative or spontaneous? Imitation of model utterances has traditionally been targeted as a goal before the child's spontaneous production, during the establishment phase (Bernthal & Bankson, 1988). Imitation may be seen as utilizing auditory and visual perceptual support for sound production.

Still another form of perceptual support is the printed orthographic symbol. There is no research or clinical data directly regarding the use of printed material to facilitate sound production within a complexity hierarchy of other tasks. It does appear, however, that the printed symbol would serve as perceptual support for the reading child. Consequently, it may be reasonable to expect a child to have greater success in transferring the correct production of a sound to the reading of a word list before he or she will produce these sounds in words spontaneously (i.e., responses to questions or statements).

Summary. In summary, we can see that there are a number of different ways to proceed in making decisions about which sounds (or sound groups) to target first and in which phonetic and prosodic contexts. According to leading clinical phonologists, it is best that one's guiding principles for the development of session goals (or "goal attack strategies"; Fey, 1992a) be consistent with one's particular phonological theory. Various approaches to phonological intervention based on different phonological theories are presented as contributions to a clinical forum (Edwards, 1992; Elbert, 1992; Fey, 1992a, 1992b; Hodson, 1992; Hoffman, 1992; Kamhi, 1992; Schwartz, 1992).

Voice. As with syntax and phonology, this area of treatment requires careful consideration of what may be expected of a child during various points in the treatment process (i.e., a series of session goals). Clinical approaches to voice disorders in children have isolated two primary treatment phases: the awareness phase and the production phase (Andrews, 1986; Wilson, 1987). Within these phases, a number of factors influencing a child's performance have been suggested (e.g., Andrews, 1986; Van Riper, 1978; Wilson, 1987).

The awareness phase. This phase generally initiates the treatment process and targets the child's ability to identify the inadequate vocal behavior and contrast it with the target behavior. The efficacy of listening activities in voice-therapy programs for children is supported by a current investigation (Deal & Belcher, 1990). These authors found that first-, third-, and fifth-grade children were "highly reliable for rating vowel productions as normal or abnormal" (p. 70). Such an awareness or listening component is exemplified cogently in Andrews's (1986), Andrews & Summers's (1993), and Wilson's (1987) therapy approaches for children with voice disorders.

Wilson suggests a four-stage sequence of listening training: (a) awareness of differences in others, (b) gross discrimination of differences in others, (c) fine discrimination of differences in others, and (d) listening to one's own voice. Similarly, Andrews includes two preliminary "awareness" phases in which objectives for the child are primarily metalinguistic. The sequence of these objectives is guided by assumptions about the challenges involved in tasks of identification, differentiation, description, and explanation of appropriate and inappropriate vocal behaviors in others and, then, in oneself. Behaviors of others in each area are targeted before one's own behaviors. Awareness of another's behaviors includes the identification of negative and positive behaviors, the description of the characteristics of these behaviors, discrimination between appropriate and inappropriate behaviors, and suggestion of ways of changing these behaviors. Awareness of one's own behaviors includes identification of the behaviors; explanation of characteristics of the behaviors; explanation of the correct or incorrect physiology associated with the symptoms; identification of symptoms of negative behaviors to change; explanation of how, why, and when inappropriate behaviors are used, and some ways inappropriate behaviors may be avoided or changed.

Beginning with awareness or listening activities suggests that there is less of a performance burden on the client in listening than in producing voice. It also suggests that being able to identify and understand the basis for inappropriate patterns is precursory to the production of adequate vocal characteristics.

The production phase. This phase targets a child's consistent production and use of desired vocal characteristics in spontaneous interpersonal situations. The production phase may also be approached as a progressive sequence of objectives, generally ordered with reference to a number of variables affecting performance demand. Several often-cited variables are (a) perceptual support, (b) physiological aspects, (c) phonetic context, (d) linguistic complexity.

1. Perceptual support. Perceptual support in the area of voice may be visual or auditory. The most common form of perceptual support is auditory and comes in the form of the clinician's model of an appropriate vocal attribute. Visual support is also commonly given in the form of the clinician's demonstration of relaxed muscles (generally around the mouth or throat) as compared with tense muscles (e.g., Wilson, 1987). Visual support may also come in the form of visual imaging—seeing in one's mind an image related to a particular voice type portrayed (Andrews, 1986). Another type of visual support is suggested by Wilson. He creates pictures for the child's notebook that illustrate contrasting voice types (i.e., "hard" represented by waves hitting a rock with force, "easy" by waves hitting a rock smoothly).

One of the most objective types of support comes from instrumentation that provides visual feedback to a child about a target production and his or her own attempt to match it. The Visipitch is one such instrument. It allows for frequency and intensity information to be displayed on an oscilloscope screen. The screen is designed in such a way that the child can compare his or her own production with the target (Andrews, 1986).

The presence of perceptual support (visual or auditory) is an aspect of variability in that it theoretically reduces performance demand. During early treatment sessions it may be difficult to rely entirely on one's mental representation of the target behavior. For this reason, perceptual support in any of its possible forms is generally systematically reduced within a sequence of session-goal objectives.

2. *Physiological aspects.* Andrews (1986) proposes that the physiological process of voice production, itself, suggests a sequence of session goals. She states: "one begins at the beginning of the physiological process (i.e., with respiration) and proceeds in an orderly fashion to link respiration with the onset of phonation, with sustained phonation, then with resonance and articulation. . . the order is predicated on the sequence of events occurring during normal vocalization" (p. 149). Andrews delineates a sequence of tasks that systematically addresses an integration among these basic physiological processes.

3. *Phonetic context.* Andrews (1986) considers the use of selected phonemes for different facets of voice treatment. For example, she suggests that a choice of phonemes is important when attempting to prolong and control airflow during the exhalation phase of respiration. Preferred sounds would be those that are voiced and continuants, such as /z/, /m/, and /v/. (Voiced sounds are preferred because the emission of the airstream is somewhat restricted with vocal fold adduction; continuants may be prolonged as long as the breath lasts.)

Phonetic context is also a consideration in planning a sequence of objectives for phonation training. Andrews describes the utilization of /h/ before a vowel and voiceless consonants before voiced consonants to initiate phonation. Andrews also suggests that back vowels may be more facilitative of easy onset of phonation than front vowels, and lax vowels easier than tense vowels. Wilson (1987) also uses /h/ to initiate phonation. His exercises for "easy" sound initiation increase in performance demand as they move from /h/ preceding a vowel to /h/ preceding monosyllabic words, then to /h/ preceding words in sentences.

4. *Linguistic complexity.* Andrews's "production phase" of treatment includes a sequence of targets (objectives) for the child that are based on increasing communication demands: Some of these are length of utterance (isolated sounds, syllables, words, phrases, sentences) and complexity of utterance (automatic responses, limited repertoire of self-initiated responses, simple self-generated response, complex self-generated response). Issues of linguistic complexity, discussed above with reference to form-content-use interactions, may also be applicable to voice. That is to say, increasing linguistic demands may affect voice production as well as the expression of language. This knowledge will influence identification of linguistic contexts in which the targeted voice quality is expected.

5. *Pragmatic context.* Andrews's final phase of treatment, the "carryover phase," stresses the impact of the communicative context and its participants. Some of the objectives for the child are ordered with reference to (a)

situations in which it is easiest and hardest to maintain target behaviors and (b) individuals who are supportive of the target vocal behaviors. Other pragmatic issues cited above for language disorders will also be applicable to identifying the context in which voice targets are planned.

Fluency. In cases of dysfluency in children, intervention is usually three-pronged in nature: It involves (a) modifying factors in the child's environment that may be contributing to (i.e., maintaining) the fluency problem, (b) helping children distinguish fluent speech patterns from nonfluent patterns, and (c) teaching children new strategies for producing fluent speech. In terms of the first aspect of intervention, the focus is not on working directly with the child to modify his or her language behavior. Instead, the aim of this aspect is a permanent change in the environment that might have a lasting impact on fluency. This first aspect of intervention represents an effort to change a maintaining factor. Usually, in fluency cases, that factor is the family's interpersonal communication patterns, which are often seen as contributing to fluency problems. Thus, *parents'* communication patterns may be targeted for intervention (e.g., Starkweather, Gottwald, & Halfond, 1990). The modification of communication patterns in others represents an effort to address linguistic and psychosocial *maintaining factors,* which were discussed above.

We move beyond a consideration of what maintaining factors to address and focus on the influence of performance demands on fluency when the latter two aspects of intervention become a concern—that is, teaching children discrimination skills and production strategies. We ask ourselves what can be done to reduce the amount of information the child has to process and the number of factors that require the child's attention when he or she is trying to learn the targeted skill.

Information load. One factor that appears to influence the degree of fluency in individuals who stutter, according to Starkweather (1984), is *information load.* This term refers to the "degree of uncertainty associated with a transition from one location to another in a sentence"(p. 34). Uncertainty is related to the speaker's familiarity with the theme of an utterance, the meaning of vocabulary, and a speaker's ability to anticipate the constituent parts of a syntactic structure when speaking (e.g., that the production of an article implies a subsequent noun, which implies a verb). According to Starkweather, fluctuations in information load lead to shifts in speaking effort, which in turn have an impact upon rate and continuity of the speech flow (i.e., fluency).

The implication for intervention planning at the session phase is that familiarity of topic and vocabulary and the child's ability to anticipate the constituents of a syntactic unit should be controlled. Another implication is that techniques that enhance the predictability and control of rhythmicity may be useful in reducing production demand and increasing fluency in children (e.g., the use of poetry or singing).

Phase boundaries and complex content-form interactions. Related to information load, Starkweather (1984) and Colburn and Mysak (1982a, 1982b) identified a covariance between the production of complex linguistic forms and dysfluency (see also Hall, Wray, & Conti, 1986). Starkweather has emphasized that individuals who stutter are not necessarily developmentally less advanced in language skills (i.e., in the ability to generate complex content-form interactions) than individuals who do not stutter. Rather, shifts in performance demands involved in the production of such forms may interfere with the rate and continuity of speech (see also Ratner & Shi, 1987). In line with this assessment Colburn and Mysak (1982a, 1982b) reported that children who do not stutter seem to be most dysfluent when trying to produce emerging syntactic forms.

In an extensive review of the literature on covariation between the structure of language and dysfluencies in stutterers, Starkweather and Gordon (1983) concluded that (a) dysfluencies of the earlier stutterer are likely to occur at the beginning of sentences and at phrase boundaries and (b) stuttering occurs more on function words (prepositions, pronouns, conjunctions) than on content words. These findings suggest that the clinician attend to sentence boundaries and sentence structure (e.g., number of function words, syllabic complexity of individual words, and novelty of syntax) in modulating production demands on the child in session.

Pragmatic factors. We can assume that the pragmatic performance factors identified in the section above on language disorders also contribute to information load in cases of fluency. As with language cases, we may assume that fluency will be enhanced the closer the match between the language of the adult and the child's interest and attention, and the more the child perceives he or she is in control of a dialogue. Some conditions that appear to enhance fluency are as follows:

1. statements by adults to children that do not demand a particular response, as opposed to questions or imperatives;
2. "genuine questions," to which the caretaker really does not know the answer and that are relevant to the child's ongoing actions, as opposed to questions that serve no real function for the child other than responding to the adult (Lund and Duchan, 1988, term this functional relation between question and response *intentional contingency*);
3. adults' comments that mirror a topic initiated by the child (in play or conversation) as opposed to comments that shift topics;
4. adults' comments that reflect, reiterate, or expand upon a child's utterance, as opposed to comments that do not match in any way the child's prior comment.

We can conclude that performance demands in fluency intervention can be modulated by varying the degree of cohesion between the language of the adult, the child's interest and attention, and the child's ability to regulate interactions with others.

Perceptual support. Another factor which may bear upon the relation between information load and fluency is of perceptual support, also discussed above in the sections on language, phonological disorders, and voice. Colburn and Mysak's (1982a, 1982b) work suggests that it is easier for children to talk fluently about events that are observable and objects that are being manipulated than about past or future events. Based on Starkweather's (1984) conclusions about predictability and our comments on pragmatic factors, we infer that a linguistic form modeled by an adult may serve as perceptual support for a fluent production; the form should be modeled relevant to a child's ongoing actions or train of thought and the adult's modeling should not be perceived by the child as critical or unduly directive.

Additional factors. One might view the presentation of words in written form as a type of perceptual support for individuals who are dysfluent. It is not clear from the literature, however, whether the act of reading has any systematic effect on fluency (Conture, 1990). It would appear that the same linguistic factors that may affect fluency in spontaneous speaking do so in reading (Conture, 1990; Wall & Myers, 1984). Any decision to use reading material as a support for fluency should be monitored carefully.

The impact of phonology on dysfluency is another undetermined issue. Wall and Myers (1984) have indicated that words that begin with vowels and words with CV syllable structure may be less likely to exacerbate dysfluencies than words beginning with obstruents and consonant blends. The latter phonetic forms require more complex and rapid coarticulation and greater tension to produce. Starkweather and Gordon (1983) have indicated that individuals who stutter are more likely to be dysfluent on monosyllabic than polysyllabic words. This finding seems somewhat at odds with common sense expectations based on hierarchies of phonological complexity (e.g., Ingram, 1976). The implication for intervention is that the clinician should control for the phonetic structure at the beginning of words that the child will be expected to produce. The clinician should also monitor the child's speech production for evidence of phonetic or phonologic contributions to dysfluent patterns.

Background Information

The final source of reference for writing session goals and procedures is background reference on the child. Some of the information from the case history has already informed us about factors possibly maintaining the child's communication disorder. It is also necessary to review background data to get information about the child's interests, which may be influenced by cultural (Anderson, 1992; Hanson, Lynch, & Wayman, 1990; Terrell & Hale, 1992) and experiential factors (Van Riper & Emerick, 1990). Our knowledge about these factors will assist us in selecting specific activities and materials. This final information source will allow us to complete our description of context in formulating the session goals and procedures.

Additional Issues

Before turning to the four children we have been following, we wish to touch upon three issues that should be considered in session planning: (a) determination of a reward system, (b) criterion for achievement of goals, and (c) modification of plans in the course of a session.

Selecting a Reward System. At the session phase, we must now decide how to respond to a child's successes and failures. This issue was addressed initially at the first phase of intervention planning. Behavioral theory indicates that contingencies following a child's behavior can have powerful effects on strengthening or weakening the behavior (see Chapters 2 and 4). It is well known in clinical practice that a wide range of reinforcement types and schedules exist (Hegde & Davis, 1992). For example, rewards may be tangible (food, stars), social (praise), or intrinsic to activity (appropriate communicative response, such as getting a desired object or action, or resolution of a problem involving concrete objects, such as fitting objects of differing sizes into appropriate containers).

A reward system was specified at the long-term intervention planning phase. The choice of rewards for each child was based on (a) impressions from background information, current testing, and observation about what would be motivating for a particular child and (b) implications of the learning theory referenced to explain language learning (see the discussion in Chapter 4). There is no hard-and-fast rule for specifying rewards in session-goal or procedure statements. If the clinician has decided that the reward will emanate naturally from the child's goal-oriented activity, then no separate description of the provision of a reward is necessary. Instead, the description of the linguistic and nonlinguistic contexts will be an adequate account of reinforcement. If, however, the clinician envisions the award as tangible or social, then the session procedures should make reference to the clinician's provision of such reinforcements.

Criteria for Achievement of Goals. PL 94–142 requires that criteria be specified on IEP forms for the achievement of goals. PL 94–142 mandates that criteria include a description of the targeted behavior, the context in which it will be measured, and a numerical indication of its achievement. Criteria for achievement of all goals (long-term, short-term, and session) are specified at the session phase of planning.

As discussed above, descriptions of context and observable performance are components of session-goal statements. These descriptions are part of the formulation of criteria for the achievement of a goal. It is also necessary to set numerical criteria for determining goal achievement. There are two approaches to setting numerical criteria: frequency count (i.e., how often a target behavior would have to be demonstrated in a delimited period of time for it to be judged as accomplished—five times in one-half hour, for example) or percentage (i.e., how often the child succeeds at demonstrating the target behavior, e.g., eight out of ten or 80% of attempted utterances). All session-goal statements include a specification of a numerical criterion for achievement of the session goal.

Criterion Short-Term Goals For IEPs. As speech-language clinicians who work in special education programs are aware, short-term goals for IEP purposes must be written in the same format as we have presented for writing session goals: in terms of observable behavior in a specified context, with a description of a criterion for accomplishment of the goal. We term such short-term goals written for IEPs "criterion goals." At the session phase, it is possible to formulate a "criterion" goal and procedure for each short-term goal addressed. A "criterion" goal is a short-term goal written in terms of an observable behavior in a specified context that represents the achievement of a short-term goal. The "criterion" procedure is a statement of the clinician's actions to facilitate the expression of this behavior. As noted in Chapter 5, criterion goals are equivalent to short-term goals for IEPs. We will illustrate the formulation of criterion goals and procedures in the portion of this chapter in which session goals and procedures are derived for the four children.

THE DERIVATION OF SESSION GOALS AND PROCEDURES

In this second half of Chapter 6, we will illustrate and elaborate upon the decision-making process at the session phase of intervention planning. We will derive session goals and procedures for the four children we have followed throughout this book: Darryl, Patty, Seth, and Alice. In developing session goals and procedures for each child, we will need to consider maintaining factors, principles from learning theories, and performance demands. The discussion of maintaining factors and learning principles will address the impact of these factors on session planning for all short-term targets. This is because a child's maintaining factors and learning processes will affect the child's acquisition of skills underlying the achievement of all short-term goals. Performance demands will be different for the different short-term goals. Thus, performance demands will be considered separately for each short-term goal.

For each child we will present sample session goals and procedures leading to specified short-term goals. These will comprise "early" session goals and procedures, which would be targeted during the first group of sessions in a given time period, and "later" session goals, which would be targeted as the term progressed. We will also summarize those sources of information that were referenced in the development of each goal (i.e., maintaining factors, learning principles, performance demands). In each goal statement, key words are underlined that refer to the particular aspects of the child's performance targeted as a result of consulting these sources of information. For each short-term goal, we have also included a criterion session goal and procedure, required for completing the short-term portion of IEP forms. A form for recording these criterion goals for IEPs is presented in Appendix B (Form B–4).

Darryl

The first child who will be considered for session planning is Darryl, the five-year-old boy with a developmental language disability. At this phase of intervention planning, our concern is with acts of learning that will lead to the acquisition of the prioritized short-term goals and the context in which they will occur. The complementary session procedure will represent the clinician's actions in session to provoke these acts of learning. In a departure from previous chapters, derived goals and procedures will not be listed prior to the explication of their derivation. Instead, we will begin by deciding in what order to address short-term goals. Questions and sources of information listed in Box 6–1 will guide this set of decisions. Then the derivation of session goals and procedures will be considered with reference to three areas of knowledge that facilitate this derivation: (a) factors suspected of maintaining the child's language problem, (b) learning theory, and (c) factors bearing upon the complexity of the learning task (i.e., performance demands).

Selecting Short-Term Goals to Target First.   Four short-term goals were prioritized at the short-term phase of intervention planning for Darryl (see Chapter 5). Two questions from Box 6–1 provided direction for deciding which of these short-term goals to address first: (a) Can the short-term goals be ordered according to a natural developmental hierarchy? (b) Is the client already producing the target structure in some contexts?

With reference to the first question, there is a developmental sequence implicit in Darryl's short-term goals. All the content-form interactions targeted as short-term goals emerge in normally achieving children at Lahey Phase 5 except existence + copula, which normally is acquired during Phase 4. This developmental information would suggest that existence + copula be targeted before the three Phase-5 structures; these might be targeted, later in the treatment period. With reference to the second question, baseline data indicate that Darryl is already producing two of the structures in some situations (locative action + prepositions and modal + verb phrase). He has not yet begun to produce locative action + possession or existence + copula. Perhaps we should target, first, those structures Darryl is already producing. This might provide a more immediately successful experience for Darryl.

There is an additional factor that can be considered. All short-term goals can be facilitated in a play context (see the sections on maintaining factors, learning theory, and complexity, below). Since all short-term goals could be targeted during the same time frame, a tentative decision is made to do so. This decision, however, raises the third question in Box 6–1: Does Darryl's cognitive status allow for working on multiple targets? It was noted during the second phase of intervention planning that baseline data indicate essentially normal intellectual functioning—with some weakness in inference making about language. An effort was made to avoid subtle inference making in prioritizing the four short-term goals. This information supports the tentative decision to work toward achieving the four short-term goals from the outset. We will suspend a final decision on this matter, however, until we have had an opportunity to think further about how to address maintaining factors, learning principles, and performance demands in individual sessions.

Factors Influencing Goal Construction

Maintaining factors. It was established at the long-term planning phase that cognitive, linguistic, and sensorimotor maintaining factors would be addressed in the design of the clinical context. A review of baseline data concerning Darryl's cognitive functioning indicates that, in nonverbal assessments, Darryl has demonstrated knowledge about objects, locations, possession, and internal states. At this point we are asking Darryl to *coordinate* his ability to talk about these aspects of knowledge—that is, to be able to refer to these content categories in one utterance.

Also relevant to the understanding of Darryl's present cognitive status is baseline data indicating that Darryl produces his most complex utterances in context of play with concrete objects. Hopefully, in the future, Darryl will be able to code complex utterances in other, less perceptually supported contexts, such as in narrative story-telling.

With reference to cognition, it will also be helpful to know what aspects of cognitive functioning are supportive of, foundational to, or interactive with our linguistic goals. Box 1–3 (Chapter 1) provides such information. Corresponding with the acquisition and coordination of complex content-form interactions are two developmentally ordered sets of skills. The first is the ability to engage in multischeme pretend and script play, make part-whole relations, and order objects according to specific attributes. The second is the ability to make part-whole relations, seriations, and classifications in which various combinations of parts and wholes can be envisioned without concrete objects present. We will need to create activities that exercise these cognitive skills. At the previous phase of intervention planning (short-term), we began to think about such activities: for example, building structures and containers for toy cars and trucks.

In addition to cognition, linguistic and sensorimotor factors were identified at the first and second phases of intervention planning as possibly maintaining Darryl's language delay. Baseline data in the area of language indicate that Darryl may have problems perceiving morphemes of low phonetic substance. Therefore, the clinician will stress such structures when modeling. The clinician will also create pragmatic contexts that require Darryl to produce such morphemes with stress.

The influence of Darryl's sensorimotor functioning (mildly high tonicity and mild problems with body stability and segmentation) on linguistic performance will also be addressed in session. As noted at the short-term planning phase, play with concrete objects will provide Darryl with needed sensory feedback, as will a focus on language *production*. Darryl's overall problems with tonicity and body segmentation will be addressed by an occupational therapist (OT). The speech-language clinician will collaborate with the OT and may work with reference to goals set by the OT under the OT's supervision.

Learning theory. At the long- and short-term phases of procedural planning, a therapeutic context was planned for Darryl based on selected principles derived from learning theory, particularly constructivist-cognitive theory. The principles suggested how *the clinician* would interact with Darryl. At this session-planning phase, each principle will suggest behavior that we will expect *Darryl* to demonstrate as a session goal and which we would expect the clinician to encourage in the session procedure. Correspondences between learning principles and behaviors expected of the child are illustrated in Box 6–2.

In sum, at this session phase of intervention planning the behaviors associated with learning principles will be incorporated into session-goal statements. Furthermore, these principles and behaviors will guide us in

---

BOX 6–2. CORRESPONDENCES BETWEEN LEARNING PRINCIPLES AND BEHAVIORS EXPECTED OF DARRYL IN THE SESSION

Principle	*Behavior*
Learning is facilitated by:	Child will:
6. efforts to convey meaning and overcome the miscommunication of meaning successfully	successfully convey meaning and repair communication breakdowns
7. varying actions during problem solving (including the production of erroneous behavior)	engage in problem solving
8. reflection upon personal behavior and the environment, inference making, inductive and deductive reasoning	compare, contrast, distinguish
9. sensory stimulation (i.e., sensory feedback) from movement involved in manipulation of objects	produce language and engage in action oriented tasks

the creation of specific activities. We will need to keep these principles in mind for the time being. We will not be prepared to specify activities until we have considered factors that may have an impact on the complexity of the learning task.

Controlling Performance Demands.   An additional consideration at the session phase of goal and procedure planning concerns the complexity of the learning task and the related issue of generalization. We want to be sure that clinician-child interactions and the activities designed for Darryl are as supportive as possible for learning. In designing activities and interactions, it is important to be aware that subtle changes in the linguistic and nonlinguistic context can affect linguistic performance. With this knowledge in mind, we wish to create a context that, on one hand, will facilitate the child's expression of his current level of communicative competence and, on the other hand, will challenge the child to learn a new behavior or generalize an established behavior to a new context.

A number of decisions were made at the long- and short-term planning phases that bear upon the issue of task complexity. Materials and games were envisioned that were commensurate with Darryl's interests and developmental level in the area of cognition and language. Furthermore, short-term goals were set commensurate with Darryl's current level of linguistic performance. The setting of goals and designing of therapeutic context with reference to the child's developmental level is an important control on task complexity. At this point, let us consider factors that may have an impact upon task complexity and generalization with reference to the individual short-term goals that will be addressed during each session.

Goals 1, 2, and 3: Code locative action + prepositions in *and* on, *locative action + possession, and modal +* to+ *verb phrase.* As noted above, baseline data indicate that Darryl is already producing locative action + prepositions *in* and *on* and modal + to + verb phrase, albeit infrequently and in a limited range of contexts. It appears that Darryl uses these structures to comment on his actions during play. Consequently, learning will involve increasing the frequency of production of these content-form interactions and generalizing their use to new contexts. Darryl does not yet coordinate locative action and possession. This will be a novel acquisition for Darryl. Envisioning a hierarchy of learning tasks to extend frequency and range of use of these structures is based on the following assumptions derived from the literature on normal child language acquisition:

> It is easier for children to use a linguistic structure while manipulating concrete objects than it is for them to discuss a picture or to talk without referential objects present (Lahey, 1988; Tomasello & Farrar, 1984).
>
> Children use more complex language when talking spontaneously about personal action than when answering questions (Bloom & Lahey, 1978).

Using a linguistic structure in a single, noncohesive utterance is easier than using an utterance in a cohesive conversation or in a narrative (Lahey, 1988).

Based on these assumptions, it is possible to envision the following sequence of activities in which use of the targeted structures changes over time:

in familiar play contexts to describe personal action,

in play to respond to requests of the clinician,

in planning an activity without objects present or in reflecting on a just-completed activity,

in a narrative about a past or imagined sequence of events, using pictures or objects for support,

in a narrative describing past or imagined sequences of events, without pictures or objects available.

The idea of Darryl producing targeted structures in narratives requires further consideration. Although the term *narrative story-telling* is relatively specific, it is possible to delimit further the type of narrative Darryl will be expected to produce. Research on normal child development indicates that there is a hierarchy of complexity of story grammars—the complex content-form interactions that account for the cohesiveness of a story (Lahey, 1988). For instance, Lahey (1988) indicates that stories comprising additive chains are less complex than stories comprising causal chains.

A hierarchy of complexity linked to the child's familiarity with a story can also be identified. Telling stories about familiar, real events or stories from books frequently read to the child would be less complex than creating novel stories about unfamiliar or entirely imagined events. Based on hypothesized relations between perceptual support for utterances and task complexity, we expect that telling a story with props is a less complex task than retelling a story from memory alone.

There are two additional issues to consider in determining task complexity for the coordination of modal + verb phrase. The first consideration concerns which modal verb should be targeted first and the order in which modals should be targeted over time: volition (e.g., "want to"), intent (e.g., "gonna"), need (e.g., "have to"), or possibility (e.g., "can"). Baseline data do not help us here. Although these data reveal that Darryl is producing mood + infinitival complement infrequently, they do not indicate which modal form. Bloom and Lahey (1978) indicate that "desire," "need," and "intent" precede "possibility" in the course of development. This is consistent with a developmental principle found in the cognitive literature that indicates that the envisioning of multiple possibilities is a relatively advanced cognitive achievement (Gallagher & Reid, 1984; Piaget, 1987). Thus, we will target volition and intent before need and possibility.

The second consideration concerns the specification of a verb phrase to coordinate with the modal. A verb phrase can belong to a variety of content categories, such as action (e.g., "I want to *eat*") or state (e.g., "I'm gonna *cry*"). Neither Bloom and Lahey (1978) nor Lahey (1988) presents a developmental sequence of content categories that are coordinated with modals. Such a sequence would be indicative of increasing task complexity. However, it is possible to hypothesize about a complexity hierarchy with reference to baseline data and the set of short-term goals that will be addressed during the first group of sessions.

Baseline data indicate that Darryl is producing mood + *to* + infinitival complement infrequently. Unfortunately, baseline data do not indicate which content category Darryl is coordinating with mood. It is important to keep in mind, however, that action and locative action are being targeted during the first group of sessions. As such, targeting the coordination of action and locative action with mood should make the initial learning tasks less complex.

Goal 4: Code the copula in existence and possessive state utterances. Recall that in Chapter 5 we described learning principles that guided procedure planning. It was noted that creating a context in which the use of the copula served an identifiable pragmatic function might increase the linguistic saliency of the copula for Darryl. Given the linguistic and sensorimotor difficulties that have been identified as maintaining factors for Darryl, he should be expected to produce the copula in a context in which this verb serves a pragmatic function and is perceptually salient (i.e., stressed). Such a context would minimize performance demands.

Summary. After considering maintaining factors and learning theories, we have envisioned sequences of activities for each short-term goal that we planned to address with Darryl. These activity sequences were based on inferences we made about factors that contribute to the complexity of the tasks we plan to present to Darryl. With this information in mind, we are now prepared to formulate a set of session goals and procedures.

Sample Session Goals and Procedures and Their Derivation. At this point, we will present sample session-goals and session procedures according to the following format. We will identify the short-term goal that we are seeking to facilitate and then present a sample of an early session goal and corresponding session procedure. Next, we will present a sample of a later session goal and procedure related to achieving that short-term goal. Finally, we will present a criterion goal and procedure, which is a restatement of the short-term goal in observable, measurable terms for use in an IEP. The child's achievement of the criterion goal will represent the accomplishment of the short-term goal. The key terms in each session-goal statement will be italicized. Each session-goal statement will be followed with a list of factors that were referenced in the derivation of the key terms included in the statement. Similarly, any key term in the corresponding procedure statement that was not accounted for in the goal statement and its subsequent derivation will be underlined and derived. Sample session goals and procedures appear in Tables 6–1A through 6–1C.

TABLE 6–1A. Session Goals and Procedures

Client: Darryl	**Clinician:**
Supervisor:	**Semester:**

Short-Term Goal Addressed: (1) Darryl will code locative action + prepositions *in* and *on.*

Early Session Goal:

Darryl will code locative action + in and on to *direct the actions* of the clinician *in a game involving toy vehicles,* five times in a half-hour session.

Derivation:

Maintaining factor(s) addressed: cognition, sensorimotor

Principles from learning theories: 5, 8, 9 (Box 1–7)

Performance demands controlled:

> Linguistic context: use the target utterance in familiar play contexts to describe personal action before responding to requests or narrative story-telling

> Perceptual support: use the target utterance with objects present before recalling objects that are not present

Session Procedure:

Clinician will:

- engage Darryl in play involving the building of block and tunnel structures and the enclosing, supporting, and hiding of toy vehicles;

- comment on where in the room the child is playing;

- ask Darryl to comment on these locations;

- create turn taking and toy vehicle-hiding *problems* involving the location of cars *in* and *on* (losing the objects, getting the objects stuck in tunnels, on top of hard to reach locations);

- provoke Darryl to *provide directives for solving these problems* (e.g., take the truck out of the tunnel);

- model and expand on Darryl's productions of target content-form interactions, stressing target morphemes of low phonetic substance.

Additional Derivation Factors:

Principles from learning theories: 6, 7 (Box 1–7)

Later Session Goal:

Darryl will code locative action + prepositions in and on *while retelling the "Billy Goats Gruff" story using props* after the clinician tells the story five times in a half-hour session.

(continued)

TABLE 6–1A *(continued)*

Derivation:

Maintaining factor(s) addressed: cognition, sensorimotor

Principles from learning theories: 5, 6, 9 (Box 1–7)

Performance demands controlled:

> Context and pragmatics: use of the linguistic structure in narrative story-telling after accomplishing use in familiar play contexts

> Linguistic complexity: use in stories with additive story grammar before temporal before causal

> Perceptual support: use of the structure with objects present before recalling objects that are not present

Session Procedure:

Clinician will:

> tell the "Billy Goats Gruff" story (modified to include many locative action + "in" and "on" utterances) demonstrating the use of props.

Criterion Goal:

Darryl will code locative action + preposition *in* and *on* to recall known locations of familiar objects to initiate a session, five times in fifteen minutes.

Criterion procedure:

The clinician will:

* provide sets of matching objects for self and Darryl to play with;

* identify objects belonging to self and Darryl, stressing possession (the possessive pronoun);

* store objects at the end of session, stressing their location, while modeling locative action statements;

* ask Darryl to direct the storage of objects at the end of sessions and to recall the location of objects belonging to self and the clinician at the beginning of sessions.

TABLE 6–1B.   Session Goals and Procedures

Client: Darryl	Clinician:
Supervisor:	Semester:

Short-Term Goal Addressed: (2)   Darryl will code locative action + possession

Early Session Goal:

Darryl will code locative action + possession to *describe* his actions and the actions of the clinician in context of *play* five times in a half-hour session.

Derivation:

Maintaining factors: cognition, sensorimotor

Principles from learning theories: 5, 9 (Box 1–7)

(continued)

TABLE 6–1B *(continued)*

Performance demands controlled:

Context and use: spontaneous use of the linguistic structure in familiar play contexts to describe personal action before responding to requests or narrative story-telling

Perceptual support: use of the structure with objects present before recalling objects that are not present

Session Procedure:

Clinician will:

- engage Darryl in a game of building structures and hiding toys cars and *create disputes* concerning possession and location of toy cars and trucks;
- model locative action + possession comments, emphasizing target structures during conversational interactions.

Additional Derivation Factors:

Principles from learning theories: 6, 7 (Box 1–7)

Later Goal:

Darryl will code locative action + possession to *recall locations* of personal objects in *constructions built* during a previous session, ten times in a half-hour session.

Derivation:

Maintaining factor(s) addressed: cognition, sensorimotor

Principles from learning theories: 6, 8 (Box 1–7)

Performance demands controlled:

Perceptual support: recall objects not present after achieving use of the structure with objects present

Session Procedure:

Clinician will:

- engage Darryl in a building activity in which furniture and other toy objects are positioned and photographed;
- ask Darryl at the beginning of the following session to recall positions of "your" objects and "my" objects from prior sessions; utilize photographs to check on Darryl's predictions and *encourage Darryl to self-correct if errors* are observed;
- model locative action + possession statements through narration and expansion of Darryl's actions in conversational interactions.

Performance demands controlled:

- Perceptual support: utilize photographs to facilitate recall after the use of concrete objects

(continued)

TABLE 6–1B *(continued)*

Additional Derivation:

Principles from learning theories: 7 (Box 1–7)

Criterion Goal:

Darryl will code locative action + possession to recall known locations of familiar objects to initiate a session five times in fifteen minutes.

Criterion Procedure:

Darryl will code locative action + possession to recall the location of familiar objects.

The clinician will:

- provide sets of matching objects for self and Darryl to play with; identify objects belonging to self and Darryl, stressing possession (the possessive pronoun);
- store these objects at the end of session, stressing their location, while modeling locative action + possession statements;
- ask Darryl to direct the storage of objects used at the end of sessions and to recall the location of objects belonging to self and the clinician at the beginning of sessions.

TABLE 6–1C.   Session Goals and Procedures

Client: Darryl	Clinician:
Supervisor:	Semester:

Short-Term Goal Addressed: (3)   Darryl will code state (modal form) + *to* + verb phrase.

Early Session Goal:

Darryl will code volition + to + locative action to *resolve a turn-taking conflict* with the clinician in context of *play* with toy vehicles five times in a half-hour session.

Derivation:

Maintaining factors: cognition and sensorimotor

Principles from learning theories: 5, 6, 7, 8, 9 (Box 1–7)

Performance demands controlled:

Context and use: spontaneous use of the linguistic structure in familiar play contexts to describe personal action before use in responses to requests or in story-telling

Perceptual support: use of the structure with objects present before recalling objects that are not present

Session Procedure:

Clinician will:

- engage in play with Darryl involving the building of block and tunnel structures and the enclosing, supporting, and hiding of cars;

(continued)

TABLE 6–1C *(continued)*

- create turn-taking problems involving the desire to place blocks on the construction or hide vehicles, anticipate actions by stressing personal intent and by expanding on Darryl's expressions of intent;
- stress target morphemes of low phonetic substance.

Criterion Goal:

Darryl will code intention + *to* + action or locative action to plan four activities prior to a session.

Criterion Procedure:

The clinician will:

- prior to a session, ask Darryl to state four activities that he "is gonna" or "wants to" engage in;
- model intent or volition + verb phrase;
- stress target morphemes of low phonetic substance.

Patty

The following is a detailed derivation of session goals and procedures for Patty, the six-year-old child with a fluency disorder. Recall that session goals represent the child's acts of learning aimed at the achievement of short-term goals. Session procedures describe the clinician's role in facilitating these acts of learning. As with Darryl, we will first prioritize short-term goals to address during individual sessions. We will then determine session goals and procedures that would best facilitate acquisition of these short-term goals. The formulation of session-goal and procedure statements will be influenced by our knowledge of (a) factors suspected of maintaining Patty's communication problem, (b) learning theory, and (c) performance demands. In demonstrating how we arrived at these decisions, we will again refer to questions and sources of information listed in Box 6–1. At the end of the discussion of how we derived session goals, we will present samples of session goals derived for each short-term goal targeted and summarize factors that contributed to the derivation.

Deciding Which Short-Term Goals to Target First. Four goals were targeted for Patty at the short-term phase of intervention planning:

1. To respond to questions with 3+ constituent utterances that function to provide information.
2. To integrate respiration, phonation, and articulation ("easy speech") in words beginning 3+ constituent responses to questions.
3. To integrate respiration, phonation, and articulation ("easy speech") in coding the complex-sentence categories additive, causal, and epistemic.
4. To interact with parents in nonpropositional as well as conversational situations that increase fluent experiences.

Derivation of Session Goals and Procedures.   The first job in session planning is to decide which short-term goals to address first and which to target later in the semester. As was the case in planning for Darryl, above, we will refer to questions in Box 6–1 to guide this aspect of decision making.

Questions from Box 6–1. Question (a) asks: Can the short-term goals be ordered according to a natural developmental hierarchy? Two of the four short-term goals set for Patty (2 and 3) suggest a developmental sequence. Three + constituent structures are acquired before complex content-form interactions in the normal course of development (Bloom & Lahey, 1978). Patty however, has already achieved these linguistic structures. Furthermore, baseline data indicate that she produces 3+ constituent structures fluently most except when responding to questions. This would suggest that Patty is ready to work on fluency in producing complex sentences and responses to questions.

Let us turn to question (b): Is the client already producing the target structure in some contexts? Baseline data indicate, first, that dysfluencies occur on approximately 10% of all Patty's utterances; that is, she is fluent 90% of the time. Patty manifests a 40% to 67% rate of dysfluency in context of questions and complex sentence forms targeted in the short-term goals. Although this represents a significant degree of dysfluency, Patty is still fluent on 33% to 60% of all such utterances. Baseline data indicate, second, that most of Patty's dysfluencies are syllable or word repetitions. Only 2.7 % are sound prolongations, characterized by undue tension. The skill targeted in short-term goals 2 and 3 is "easy speech"—that is, initiating words with reduced tension. Patty appears to be utilizing such a speech pattern in most of her speech. The implication is that our task during sessions will be to *increase* Patty's rate of fluency and intentional control of speech patterns in the linguistic contexts specified in the short-term goals. Since goals 2 and 3 do not represent entirely novel competencies there is no intrinsic reason for prioritizing them in session planning.

Question (c) asks if there are individual skills that could be addressed in ·initial sessions that are foundational to the achievement of multiple short-term goals. The answer is "yes." Every step taken toward teaching Patty to distinguish between "hard" (dysfluent) and "easy" (fluent) speech-production patterns and to intentionally use fluent speech patterns is foundational to the achievement of all the short-term goals. Furthermore, increasing Patty's fluent experiences in interactions with parents (goal 4) should ameliorate a psychosocial factor that is also foundational to the achievement of all short-term goals.

At this point, we are prepared to address short-term goals 2, 3 and 4 in the first set of sessions. What about short-term goal 1: "To respond appropriately to questions with 3+ constituent utterances that function to provide information"? Baseline data indicate that Patty usually answers a question with a question, perhaps as a strategy to avoid stuttering. Facilitating fluency in addressing short-term goal 2 (responding directly to questions) will probably have an impact on this first goal. In addition, addressing this first goal will, in turn, influence the second.

As noted above, Patty's tendency to answer a question with a question may be a secondary symptom of stuttering. As such, this symptom must be reduced (i.e., Patty has to be able to respond directly to a question) to work on "easy speech" (short-term goal 2). Thus, there are many reasons to address short-term goal 1 along with goals 2 through 4 at the outset of clinical intervention with Patty.

The final question in Box 6–1 asks us to consider whether Patty would be able to work on the multiple skills under consideration during individual sessions. Baseline data indicate age-appropriate cognitive, sensorimotor, and psychosocial functions. At this point in the decision-making process, there does not seem to be any compelling reason to begin working on any particular short-term goal before another.

Maintaining factors. The second consideration in session planning concerns maintaining factors that may have to be addressed in the course of therapy. As noted above, baseline data indicate age-appropriate cognitive, sensorimotor, and psychosocial functions. There is a psychosocial factor that is generally discernible in cases of fluency: caretaker-child communication patterns. It is often the case that parents and friends focus their attention on the child's dysfluencies instead of on his or her fluent behavior (Gregory & Hill, 1980; Van Riper, 1973; Wall & Myers, 1984). This attention pattern tends to reinforce and thereby increase dysfluency while punishing the act of speaking. It is generally desirable, therefore, to address parent-child communication patterns at the outset of stuttering therapy (Conture, 1990; Gregory & Hill, 1980; Shine, 1980; Van Riper, 1973; Wall & Myers, 1984). This approach is also consistent with a psychosocial achievement depicted in Box 1–5, which identifies psychosocial correlates of speech-language acquisition. That achievement is the child's ability to be comforted and to develop a sense of security and self-esteem from interactions with caregivers and parental-family stability.

Shapiro (personal communication, September 11, 1992) has emphasized that self-esteem issues bear upon the outcome of fluency treatment with children. Shapiro has created techniques for protecting the child's self-esteem and garnering additional information about the child's awareness and sensitivity to the dysfluency. These techniques include the use of materials such as puppets, to model fluent and dysfluent speech patterns, thereby deflecting potentially critical communications away from the child. Another procedure involves disclosure by the clinician of personal experiences and feelings associated with dysfluency. With reference to the latter suggestion, Shapiro has recommended probes, such as the following conversation he had with a five-year-old: "When I'm tired it's sometimes hard for me to talk." The child responded, "Yes, me too." When Shapiro asked, "How does that make you feel?" the child responded, "It makes me feel embarrassed."

Although baseline data indicate age-appropriate social-emotional functioning, it will be important to address the tendency of caretakers to focus on dysfluency. Session goals and procedures will be developed that target Patty's interactions with her family.

Learning theories. At the long-term phase of procedure planning for Patty, principles from operant, motor, and social learning theories were identified. These principles will be useful in formulating session-goal and procedure statements. They will direct us in the identification of behaviors that are indicative of the learning that is relevant to the achievement of short-term goals. The principles (derived from Box 1–7) and corresponding behaviors expected of Patty during a session appear in Box 6–3.

The behaviors implied by the principles will be incorporated into session goals and will provide direction for the creation of session activities. We will refer back to these principles as we consider each short-term goal and identify factors that we will need to control in formulating session goals and procedures.

Controlling performance demands. In planning session goals and procedures, it is necessary to consider factors that may tax the child's ability to learn or express a particular skill or linguistic structure. The more systematically these factors can be controlled in session planning, the more systematically learning and generalization will be effected.

In the discussion of performance demands in the first part of this chapter, a number of factors were identified that can impinge upon the child's production of fluent speech: (a) length and complexity of linguistic structure and (b) the child's perception of control in interpersonal interactions (e.g., Colburn & Mysak, 1982a, 1982b; Hall, Wray, & Conti, 1986; Starkweather & Gordon, 1983; Stocker & Parker, 1977; Wall & Myers, 1984). With these factors in mind, we now consider each short-term goal that will be addressed during sessions with Patty.

Short-term goal 1: To respond appropriately to questions or requests for information with 3+ constituent utterances that function to provide information. Although this first short-term goal appears to be pragmatic in nature, it is essentially fluency related. As noted earlier, Patty's tendency to answer a question with a question is suspected to be an avoidance behavior in anticipation of dysfluency (see Chapter 5). Answering a question with a question is more stereotyped and devoid of content than is a direct answer to the question. As noted above, children tend to stutter less when producing familiar, stereotypic utterances (Starkweather & Gordon, 1983).

It would be helpful to envision a hierarchy of behaviors that would reduce Patty's fear of dysfluency when responding to requests for information. One factor that might affect Patty's willingness to respond to questions directly is the length and syntactic complexity of the response obligated by the question. Based on the literature reviewed above, we would expect that one-word utterances are more likely to be produced fluently than multiword or multiphrase utterances (Wall & Myers, 1984). Consequently, we will begin by asking questions that obligate single-word responses and work up to questions requiring 3+ constituent responses.

A second variable that could have an impact on Patty's willingness and ability to respond to questions is the content of the response obligated by the

---

BOX 6–3.   CORRESPONDENCES BETWEEN LEARNING PRINCIPLES AND BEHAVIORS EXPECTED OF PATTY IN THE SESSION

Principle	*Behavior*
Learning is facilitated by:	Child will:
1. events following a behavior, which can reinforce (strengthen) or extinguish (weaken) the behavior	produce a target
2. efforts to match models presented by the clinician	imitate models
3. noticing similarities and distinctions among actions and events mediated by adults	indicate awareness of fluent and dysfluent productions
9. sensory stimulation (i.e., sensory feedback) from movement involved in articulation	produce articulatory, phonatory, prosodic gestures of reduced tension ("easy speech")

---

question. Bloom & Lahey (1978) and Brown (1968) provide useful developmental hierarchies for types of questions children ask and can respond to and responses children typically give to questions (see Appendix C). The ability to code existence or action in response to a *what* question about an object or action tends to develop before the coding of causality in response to a *why* question (Bloom, 1991). This suggests that the content of the question (the nature of the subject being asked about), and the content of the response expected of Patty be modulated over time. We should consider first asking Patty questions relevant to identifying objects or actions. We would later work on responses to questions requiring causal reasoning.

A third factor that may be controlled in sessions is the degree of novelty in Patty's responses to questions; the more familiar, stereotyped, and content-free the expected response, the easier it should be to produce fluently (Shine, 1980; Starkweather, 1984). Thus, encouraging Patty to produce familiar names of objects and actions should reduce performance demand. Perhaps, in addition, Patty could initially respond to a question about a familiar object or action with a simple "yes" or "no."

Another aspect of the session plan that may contribute to Patty's ability to respond to requests directly and fluently is the nature of the activity Patty is questioned about. As noted above, Wall and Myers (1984) have indicated that talking about a self-directed play activity involving concrete objects may be a less stressful task than talking about an abstract event in an activity structured by the clinician. In terms of answering questions, however, adult-structured activities may be beneficial; they are more likely to evoke a target response, thus, giving Patty more opportunities to work on the target skill. With reference to these considerations, it may be best during early sessions to create goal-directed concrete play activities, such as constructing Play-Doh animals. Shortly thereafter, we may wish to impose more structure and demand more cooperation, for example, in cooking or game activities involving rules and directions. Still later, we can query Patty about events without the support of concrete objects or ongoing activities.

A final consideration in planning sessions aimed at answering questions is phonological in nature. As discussed above, the relation between phonology and stuttering is not entirely clear. Words beginning with vowels and containing fewer phonemes may make fewer production demands on the individual who stutters than longer words beginning with consonants. There is, however, evidence that individuals who stutter do so less frequently on polysyllabic than on single-syllable words (Starkweather & Gordon, 1983). Baseline data do not provide information about the relation between phonology and dysfluency in Patty's speech. In the absence of such baseline data, the issue of phonology is not expected to be a significant one in Patty's case. Thus, we will control for Patty's knowledge of answers to questions (i.e., with names of objects and actions) when asking Patty questions. We will monitor Patty's responses to discern if she is sensitive to the phonetic structure of words.

Short-term goals 2 and 3: To integrate respiration, phonation, and articulation ("easy speech") in words beginning 3+ constituent responses to questions and to integrate respiration, phonation, and articulation ("easy speech") in coding the complex-sentence categories additive, causal, and epistemic. We have chosen to consider, under one heading, production demands for short-term goals 2 and 3 because there may be a common set of skills related to the achievement of these two goals. Moreover, there is a sequence that has been identified in the achievement of these skills in a number of fluency programs,. These skills, arranged in order of recommended acquisitions, are: (a) distinguishing fluent from nonfluent speech productions in self and others, (b) *intentionally* shaping a fluent response, and (c) applying skills in *a* and *b* to spontaneous speech (e.g., Conture, 1990; Shine, 1980; Wall & Myers, 1984).

Let us consider the first two skills. Although Patty seems to be somewhat sensitive to her dysfluency, as a six-year-old she has probably never formally tried to distinguish fluent from dysfluent speech. Similarly, although Patty is for the most part fluent, she has never *intentionally* tried to produce a particular "easy" speech pattern. Thus, both skills are novel, and an effort should be made to simplify learning them. Based on the literature, the way the concepts *fluency, dysfluency,* and *easy speech* are presented to the child by the clinician and the context (linguistic and nonlinguistic) can have an impact upon the complexity of the learning task.

With children of Patty's age and developmental status, Wall and Myers (1984) suggest describing fluency and dysfluency as "easy to say" and "hard to say." Thus, in a discrimination task, Patty could be asked to tell us when she hears the clinician trying to say a word that is "hard to say."

Shine (1980), Wall and Myers (1984), and others (e.g., Starkweather & Gordon, 1983; Starkweather, 1984) have pointed out that certain phonetic variables surrounding a child's attempt at fluency may interfere with that attempt. Wall and Myers (1984) focus especially on the sounds at the beginning of a word. Words beginning with vowels facilitate the learning of fluent speech patterns, whereas obstruent consonants and consonant blends could interfere. This information suggests that Patty should identify and practice easy speech productions on words of increasingly complex phonetic structure.

We determined above that single words and sentences with one predicate clause are easier to process and produce than complex sentences. Consequently, Patty will first identify or produce easy speech to initiate single words, then 3+ constituent sentences, and finally complex sentences.

The next two issues that require resolution involve the design of the nonlinguistic context. We concluded in an earlier discussion that "low-structure" (i.e., spontaneous, child-structured) concrete play activities tend to promote fluency, whereas highly adult-structured, linguistic activities tend to tax fluency. This hierarchy seems to indicate that speech training should begin in context of play. There is, however, a mitigating factor: the earlier decision that Patty should imitate an adult's model and that she needs to experience much feedback from her own speech acts. Play that is entirely child directed would likely provide minimal opportunities for modeling and imitation—especially in a controlled phonetic and syntactic context. Thus, although spontaneous play may be the most facilitative context for fluent speech, it may not be the ideal context for discrimination and imitation. The adult needs to impose some structure (e.g., see programs such as Conture, 1990; Shames & Florance, 1980; Shine, 1980). Patty's developmental status in the social-emotional and cognitive domains suggests that she could handle that structure. In terms of production exercises, a decision is made initially to utilize an adult-structured activity involving imitation and labeling of objects and pictures in order to control the phonetic and syntactic context of Patty's utterances. After the skill is established in such a context, more play-like activities will be created in which to practice and apply skills acquired.

With reference to psychosocial maintaining factors considered above, the adult-structured activities will be designed to incorporate play. In line with Shapiro's recommendations (personal communication, September 11, 1992), we will incorporate puppetry in exercises on discrimination and fluency techniques. In initial discrimination exercises, we will talk through a turtle (slow, easy-to-say speech) and a rabbit (hard-to-say speech). Patty will talk through these puppets (especially the turtle) in exercises on easy speech patterns.

There are a number of factors that can be considered in simplifying Patty's task of learning fluency techniques. Highly familiar utterances are simpler to produce than novel structures. Consequently, we can first provide Patty with over-learned complex sentences. We can then advance toward the production of novel utterances. Also, it would be easier for Patty to talk about an ongoing, familiar play activity rather than an abstract, temporally distant experience. One kind of activity that would support the modulation of such factors is narrative story-telling. Initially, Patty could be asked to produce simple, over-learned statements in familiar children's stories, such as the wolf's "huff and puff" chant in the tale of the three little pigs.

Over a number of sessions, Patty could begin retelling familiar stories in their entirety, and then begin recalling prior real events. As noted in an earlier discussion, the order of complex sentences targeted in session would follow Lahey's (1988) developmental sequences. The initial production of familiar sections of stories could incorporate songs and other forms of rhythmicity; such exercises have been shown to facilitate fluency (Starkweather, 1980).

4. Short-term goal 4: To interact with parents in nonpropositional as well as conversational situations that increase fluent experiences. In addition to targeted changes in Patty's behavior, we must also work to modify the behavior of Patty's parents. (The inclusion of caretakers in therapy is addressed in some depth in Chapter 8, which deals with collaboration.) In doing so, we need to control the complexity of performance demands for Patty's parents as well as for Patty. Many of the same considerations that influenced our approach to the three prior short-term goals will guide our efforts.

Our primary concern with Patty's parents is modifying their focus of attention—moving it off their child's dysfluencies and onto fluent speech. One way to reduce performance demands is to ask the parents to encourage and reward one type of fluent experience at a time. Furthermore, we need to keep in mind that if Patty's parents are typical, they are quite busy and have many responsibilities. The clinician needs to determine with Patty's parents a reasonable amount of daily time to spend on speech-related activities. Hopefully, giving the family the opportunity to practice a limited range of new behaviors will lead to generalization across communicative interactions that involve Patty. Furthermore, in planning activities for the entire family, it would simplify learning for Patty if these activities were consistent with events that occurred in session.

Summary. We have now decided to work toward achieving four short-term goals during each session. We have identified maintaining factors, principles from learning theories, and performance demands that underlie the achievement of each short-term goal targeted. We are ready to formulate the session-goal and procedure statements. We are also prepared to define criterion goals—that is, a reformulation of the short-term goal statements in terms of observable behaviors that will signal the achievement of each short-term goal targeted. This criterion goal may also be utilized in an IEP. Below, a set of early and later session goals and procedures are presented; each includes a summary of information that was referenced in the derivation of the key components of the goal statements (which are italicized). These session goals, procedures, and derivation summaries are organized according to the short-term goals being addressed (see Table 6–2, A through C).

TABLE 6–2A.   Session Goals and Procedures

Client: Patty	Clinician:
Supervisor:	Semester:

Short-Term Goal Addressed: (1)   Patty will respond to questions with 3 + constituent utterances that function to provide information.

Early Session Goal:

Patty will *label* the pretend-behavior of *a Play-Doh zoo animal using a single word* in response to the examiner's query,"What is the animal doing?", ten times in a half-hour session.

Derivation:

Maintaining factor(s) addressed: psychosocial

Principles from learning theories: 5 (Box 1–7)

Performance demands controlled:

   Lexicon: familiar vocabulary before low frequency vocabulary

   Syntax: single words before 3 + constituent utterances

   Psychosocial context: contingent, fluent responses to questions in context of parallel play before cooperative play

   Perceptual support: responses to questions about ongoing, perceptually supported activity before activities that are not perceptually salient

Session Procedure:

Clinician will:

- engage Patty in the *parallel-play* activity of constructing Play-Doh zoo animals and engaging the animals in pretend actions;

- ask "What is your animal doing?" while Patty is manipulating the animal;

- create, move, and name his own animals to encourage Patty to respond; reiterate the question and *model* a one-constituent response if Patty does not respond to questions.

Additional Derivation Factors:

Principles from learning theories: 9 (Box 1–7)

Later Session Goal:

Patty will code locative action, *using the carrier phrase,*"You hid or you put the (object) in, on, under the (object)," in response to the clinician's question, "Where did I hide the _____," to describe the location of a hidden object in a *hide-and-seek* game, ten times in a half-hour.

Derivation:

Maintaining factor(s) addressed: sensorimotor

(continued)

TABLE 6–2A *(continued)*

Principles from learning theories: 1, 2 (Box 1–7)

Performance demands controlled:

Novelty of utterance: familiar, stereotypic utterances before novel statements

Syntax: 3 + constituent responses after achieving single-word responses to questions

Perceptual support: respond to questions about perceptually supported activity before activities that are not ongoing and perceptually salient

Session Procedure:

Clinician will:

- explain and demonstrate a hide-and-seek game in which Patty and the clinician take turns hiding objects and guessing the location of the hidden objects;

- model the following question-response sequence as part of the explanation of the game: "Where did I hide the object?", "You hid the (object) in, on, under the (object)";

- encourage Patty to use the locative action response by modeling it during the clinician's turn; if Patty does not use the expected question form, the clinician will model it after her nonresponse ("I hid it in the bathtub—right?").

Additional Derivation Factors:

Performance Demands Controlled:

Social context: encourage direct responses to questions in context of cooperative play after parallel play

Criterion Goal:

Patty will use two 3 + constituent utterance to identify session activities in response to the clinician's request for ideas for session activities.

Corresponding Criterion Procedure:

The clinician will:

- initiate the session by asking Patty "What do you want to do?" or "What do you want to play with?";

- encourage Patty to respond spontaneously.

TABLE 6–2B.   Session Goals and Procedures

Client: Patty	**Clinician:**
Supervisor:	**Semester:**

Short-Term Goal Addressed: (2)   To integrate and coordinate respiration, phonation, and articulation (use "easy speech") in words beginning 3 + constituent responses to questions.

(continued)

TABLE 6–2B *(continued)*

(3)	To integrate and coordinate respiration, phonation, and articulation (use "easy speech") when expressing the complex-sentence categories additive, causal, and epistemic.

Early Session Goals (each addresses both short-term goals 2 and 3):

Patty will state *"easy speech"* to describe a *turtle-puppet's* (manipulated by the clinician) pronunciation of a *single word.*

Patty will state *"hard speech"* to describe a *rabbit-puppet's* (manipulated by the clinician) dysfluent pronunciation of a single word.

Derivation:

Maintaining factor(s) addressed:

Sensorimotor: production patterns

Psychosocial: support Patty's self-esteem; mediate initial critiques of dysfluent speech by directing comments to self and others (e.g., puppets) before focusing attention directly on Patty

Principles from learning theories: 3, 4 (Box 1–7)

Performance demands controlled:

Syntax: identify fluent and dysfluent speech patterns in single-word utterances before multiword utterances

Perceptual support: comment about perceptually salient events before nonperceivable events

Session Procedure:

Clinician will:

- introduce a turtle puppet and a rabbit puppet;
- explain that the turtle uses "slow, easy to say speech" and the rabbit sometimes uses "hard to say speech";
- use the turtle to model "easy speech" (slow rate, soft contact) on word-initial sounds or syllables and on phrase-initial words;
- use the rabbit to model "hard to say speech" (repetitions and tense prolongations) in single words on word-initial sounds or syllables;
- ask Patty to say "easy to say" in response to the turtle's fluent speech and "hard to say" in response to the rabbit's dysfluency; if Patty does not respond, model the response by talking to the puppet (e.g., "That was easy to say" or "That was hard to say").

Later Session Goal (addressing short-term goal 2):

Patty will utilize *"easy speech"* to initiate the *responses,* *"You* use it to _____ " and *"It's* (attribute)," in answering clinician's request for information about the attribute or function of an object in a "guessing" game.

(continued)

TABLE 6–2B *(continued)*

Derivation:

Maintaining factor(s) addressed:

Sensorimotor: production patterns

Psychosocial: direct attention to Patty's use of a fluent speech pattern after achieving fluency through the use of a puppet

Principles from learning theories: 4, 9 (Box 1–7)

Performance demands controlled:

Novelty of utterance: familiar, stereotypic utterances before novel statements

Syntax: fluent productions of complex sentences and narratives after achieving fluency on single words and 3 + constituent utterances

Predictability of prosody: fluent productions of complex sentences with predictable, repetitive rhythmic and prosodic patterns before unpredictable rhythmic and prosodic patterns

Content-form interactions: additive complex constructions before temporal, temporal before causal

Session Procedure:

Clinician will:

- describe and demonstrate a game in which a familiar object is partially hidden (behind a screen or in a pail raised to the ceiling on a pulley);

- *model* guessing functions and attributes of the object in response to the phrase "Can you use it to _____?" or "Is it _____?";

- *model* the use of easy speech to initiate the carrier phrase response "You can use it to _____," and "Its _____," to encourage Patty to respond to this request using "easy speech" during a subsequent turn;

- take a turn *modeling* the stereotypic request and response form and the "easy speech" production if Patty does not respond.

Additional Derivation Factors:

Principles from learning theories: 2 (Box 1–7)

Criterion Goal (for short-term goal 2):

Patty will use "easy to say speech" to initiate ten 3 + constituent responses to questions about the names and functions of objects and pictures posed by the clinician.

Corresponding Criterion Procedure:

The clinician will:

- present familiar household objects and pictures of objects to Patty, ask Patty for the names or functions, and encourage Patty to respond using easy speech.

Later Session Goal (addressing short-term goal 3):

Patty will utilize "easy speech" to initiate the *additive chant*, "I'm gonna huff, and I'm gonna puff, and I'm gonna blow your house down," in a Three-Little-Pigs *narrative read* by the clinician.

(continued)

TABLE 6–2B *(continued)*

Derivation:

Maintaining factor(s) addressed:

Sensorimotor: production patterns

Psychosocial: direct attention to Patty's use of a fluent speech pattern through the use of a puppet

Principles from learning theories: 4, 9 (Box 1–7)

Performance demands controlled:

Novelty of utterance: increase novelty in Patty's fluent utterances after achieving fluency on familiar, stereotypic utterances

Syntax: work on fluency in 3 + constituent utterances after achieving fluency on single words

Perceptual support (linguistic): spontaneous expected after imitation

Perceptual support (nonlinguistic): produce fluent speech pattern with perceptual support (objects in a game) before fluent production without perceptual support

Session Procedure:

Clinician will:

- tell the story of the Three Little Pigs using puppets and other props;

- model the additive chant "I'm gonna huff, and I'm gonna puff, and I'm gonna blow your house down," using "easy speech";

- encourage Patty to imitate his production of the chant using "easy speech";

- encourage Patty to recite the chant utilizing "easy speech," each time the wolf comes to blow the house down in the course of the story;

- the clinician will encourage Patty to recite the chant in unison with him if Patty does not respond on her own.

Additional Derivation Factors:

Learning principles: 1, 2 (Box 1–7)

Criterion Goal (for short-term goal 3):

Patty will, when retelling familiar stories using puppets and other objects as props, use "easy to say speech" to initiate 3 additive, 3 causal, and 3 epistemic sentences following the clinician's signal.

Corresponding Criterion Procedure:

The clinician will:

- encourage Patty to retell a familiar story, explaining that he will signal the use of "easy to say speech";

- signal the use of "easy to say speech."

TABLE 6–2C.   Session Goals and Procedures

Client: Patty	Clinician:
Supervisor:	Semester:

Short-Term Goal Addressed:	(4)	Patty will interact with parents in nonpropositional as well as conversational situations that increase fluent experiences.

Early Session Goal:

Patty will *sing* and tape-record a familiar, favorite song *with her mother and father* present, one time each evening for a week.

Derivation:

Maintaining factor(s) addressed:

Psychosocial: support Patty's self-esteem; work with parents to modify punishing reactions to dysfluency and to increase opportunities for fluency

Principles from learning theories: 1, 9 (Box 1–7)

Performance demands controlled:

Novelty of utterance: familiar, stereotypic utterances before novel, content-rich statements.

Predictability of prosody: singing with predictable, repetitive rhythmic and prosodic patterns before unpredictable, variable rhythmic and prosodic patterns.

Session Procedure:

Clinician will:

• meet with parents privately and identify activities in which Patty is reliably fluent;

• ask parents how they respond to dysfluencies;

• stress that a technique of therapy is to focus on experiences that *increase fluent speech.*

Parents will:

• attend therapy session;

• encourage Patty to sing and record a favorite song;

• praise Patty for her singing;

• state, *"Maybe another time. You tell us when you're ready,"* if Patty does not cooperate.

Additional Derivation Factors:

Principles from learning theory: 1 (Box 1–7)

(continued)

TABLE 6–2C *(continued)*

Later Session Goal:

Patty will utilize "easy speech" to initiate "*yes-no*" responses to her *parent's questions* about where objects are hidden in context of a "hide-the-objects" game.

Derivation:

Maintaining factor(s) addressed:

Sensorimotor: production patterns

Psychosocial: support Patty's self-esteem; work with parents to modify punishing reactions to dysfluency and to increase opportunities for fluency

Principles from learning theories: 9 (Box 1–7)

Performance demands controlled:

Language content: familiar, stereotypic utterances before novel, content-rich statements

Session Procedure:

Parents will:

- attend session;

- observe clinician playing a "hide-the-object" game with Patty;

- *ask Patty to explain and model* "easy speech" and to explain the game played with the clinician;

- play the game, using "easy speech" on their turn, *responding excitedly* to Patty's use of "easy say" speech on "yes-no" responses to questions;

- play the game with Patty at home.

Additional Derivation Factors:

Principles from learning theories: 1, 2, 8 (Box 1–7)

Criterion Goal:

Patty will use easy speech to initiate one 3 + constituent utterance, "Let's _____," to identify an after-dinner activity in response to her parents' request for ideas for an activity.

Corresponding Criterion Procedure:

The parents will:

- ask Patty to suggest a family activity after dinner;

- respond affirmatively to Patty's request;

- ignore any dysfluency.

Seth

The first step in the derivation of session goals is to make a decision about whether to target all the short-term goals simultaneously (during the same session) or to prioritize these goals. Let us look at the short-term goals we have decided to address.

Short-term goals:

1. Seth will reduce the phonological processes of fronting and backing in conversational speech.
2. Seth will reduce the stopping of /f/ and /v/ in conversational speech and /ʃ/ in single words.
3. Seth will begin the suppression of the process of gliding (i.e., the production of /l/ in initial position of words).
4. Seth will produce final /z/, and /s/, /z/ clusters coding plural, copula, third person singular, and possessive.

Deciding on a Goal-Approach Strategy. By examining the goals listed, we can see that in goals 1, 2 (part 1), and 4 we are attempting to stabilize sounds already in Seth's repertoire (see Chapter 3 for baseline data). In goals 3 and 2 (part 2), we are attempting to establish a new sound. Working to stabilize sounds, the process of "generalization" to other phonetic and situational contexts, is a gradual process that may take longer with older clients (Hodson & Paden, 1991; see also Bernthal & Bankson, 1988, for a summary of approaches to sound generalization). Generalization may be especially problematic for someone like Seth, who has difficulties in all three behavioral systems associated with speech development (especially sensorimotor). It would not be efficient to wait until Seth has eliminated the processes of fronting, backing, and stopping before we move to gliding. He may never eliminate these processes. Because of his need to remain with constant and consistent attention to these three processes, it would be most efficient to continue to work on reducing these processes as we initiate dissolution of gliding. This decision is in keeping with the "cycles" approach espoused by Hodson and Paden (1991). These clinical phonologists recommend working on a number of processes at once during the same period of time (i.e., two to six hours on each process). Because Seth is an older child and has been working on most of these sounds for some time, we may even plan to address the various short-term targets within a single session.

Factors Influencing Goal Construction. Now that we have decided to target each of the short-term goals from the outset of therapy, we need to consider those factors that will help us formulate a sequence of session goals to reach each short-term target. We need to consider maintaining factors, principles from learning theories, and performance demands. The first two factors will inform us about approaches we need to take across all of the processes. This is because a child's associated behavioral systems will affect the development of any group of sounds. Performance demands (facilitating versus nonfacilitating contexts) will be different for the different processes. The sounds targeted across processes and within each process may be at different levels of production skill (generally measured by percentage of target achievement in obligatory contexts).

Maintaining factors. As we noted earlier, Seth is viewed as having difficulties with cognitive, sensorimotor, and psychosocial maintaining factors. In designing a sequence of session goals, we must keep in mind the modification of or compensation for these factors in order to facilitate the dissolution of the given processes. We turn next to Boxes 1-3 to 1-5 (Chapter 1) to review those sensorimotor, cognitive, and psychosocial accomplishments associated with the elimination of phonological processes. In examining Box 1-4, we can see that the elimination of phonological processes occurs between the ages of four and seven. This is associated with the tongue's complete descent in the oral cavity. Related to tongue descent is increased precision of motor control. At this point in Seth's development there is still some difficulty in directing tongue movements on command and differentiating tongue position (demonstrated in the PSM exam). Seth's maintenance of phonological processes until now further corroborates this finding. In fact, specific articulatory difficulties are suggested by the processes in operation: differentiating and executing contrasting tongue positions (i.e., front and back movements) and release patterns (continuing, stopping). According to the occupational therapist, difficulty with tongue movements is related to low overall body muscle tone, incoordination, and weakness, which is compounded by tactile defensiveness. With this knowledge in mind, our session goals will need to address some aspect of sensorimotor control. Our sequence of sensorimotor accomplishments will be directed by the occupational therapist.

Next we need to look at the cognitive achievements which may be utilized to facilitate the dissolution of phonological processes (see Box 1-3). The skill that appears most appropriate to target for Seth is the last: awareness of language as an entity, distinct from events signified. This skill is believed to underlie the development of metalinguistic knowledge. It has been demonstrated that by the age of seven children can talk about syllable and phoneme segmentation (e.g., Kamhi et al., 1985; Nesdale, Herriman, & Tunmer, 1984) and articulatory-auditory correspondences (Klein et al., 1991). It has not yet been demonstrated that there is a relationship between understanding how sounds are made and the normal development of articulation proficiency (Klein et al., 1991). For a child like Seth, however, who has developmental problems, the knowledge of this relationship may help to stabilize phonological contrasts (e.g., signaled by placement and manner). Also, within the cognitive-metalinguistic domain, it will be necessary for Seth to talk about semantic distinctions signaled by contrasting phonemes (minimal pairs; for an explanation of this concept, see the seminal article by Weiner, 1981). Knowledge about meaningful minimal contrasts has been found to be most expedient in furthering the dissolution of a process once a child has already established the sounds governed by the process (e.g., Hodson & Paden, 1991; Saben & Ingham, 1991).

Box 1–5 presents a listing of the psychosocial achievements related to linguistic performance. Two of the items within later language development appear to be appropriate target skills for Seth: to utilize caregiver directives to mediate problem-solving activity and to be comforted and gain security from parental-family stability. Both these skills are believed to relate to the problem-solving functions of language (i.e., metalinguistic problems) as well as all other aspects of language learning. Baseline data on Seth indicate that there are constraints on his ability to benefit from environmental input. The occupational therapist's report indicates that he is "highly reactive to being touched or handled." The psychologist states that some of his responses reveal, "anxiety, sadness, vulnerability, and low self-esteem." This psychosocial picture of Seth suggests that the above psychosocial skills need to be addressed in formulating session goals.

Summary. At this point in our approach to session-goal planning we know that our session goals will be shaped by efforts to (a) improve tongue movement, (b) increase metalinguistic awareness of sound position and meaning contrasts, and (c) reduce constraints on the utilization of environmental input (e.g., touch, directions).

Principles from learning theories. As discussed at the beginning of this chapter, information about how children learn shapes our thinking about therapy procedures. The way that procedures are derived on the basis of learning principles is demonstrated by the procedural statements at the long-term and short-term phases for Seth. For example, let us look at the part of the long-term procedural approach bearing upon how learning is facilitated (Table 4–6). The following learning principles stated for Seth are derived primarily from social-cognitive learning theory and motor-learning theory (see Boxes 1–6 and 1–7). These principles now influence our session-goal planning. They direct us in deciding what behavior we want Seth to demonstrate during a session (what Seth will do) with reference to a sound target we may have in mind. Each principle suggests one behavior we will expect Seth to demonstrate as a session goal. The relationship between each principle and expected session behaviors is illustrated in Box 6–4.

Summary. At this point in planning our approach to session goals we also know that one of the above behaviors implied by learning principles will be demonstrated as part of a session goal.

Controlling performance demands. As is our practice in planning session goals and procedures, we consider conditions under which the child is expected to perform. The purpose is systematically to design contexts that facilitate learning or promote generalization.

Although we have decided to target all short-term goals simultaneously for Seth, we now need to think about each goal separately. In the case of Seth,

---

BOX 6–4. CORRESPONDENCES BETWEEN LEARNING PRINCIPLES
AND BEHAVIORS EXPECTED OF SETH IN THE SESSION

Principle	*Behavior*
Learning is facilitated by:	
2. efforts to match models presented by the clinician	imitate models
3. noticing similarities and distinctions among actions and events mediated by adults	indicate awareness of similarities and differences
6. efforts to convey meaning and overcome miscommunication successfully	repair error productions
8. reflection upon personal behavior	talk about his productions (how they feel, sound, look)
9. sensory stimulation (i.e., sensory feedback) from movement	produce sounds

---

each process is at a different stage of dissolution and applies to different phonemes. In addition, phonemes within a process are differentially affected by the process (as measured by percentage of correct production) and are vulnerable to different contexts. Sounds that cannot be produced at all may need to be approached with a focus on establishing articulatory and coarticulatory gestures (i.e., production of the sounds in simple contexts—nonsense syllables, words); other phonemes that may already be in the repertoire will require an approach that focuses on appropriate use in meaningful contexts. (These two approaches, in essence, describe the two main facets of phonological learning, cogently summarized by Fey, 1992a, and implemented most clearly in the clinical approach by Hodson & Paden, 1991.)

Short-term goal 1: Seth will reduce the phonological processes of fronting and backing in conversational speech. The elimination of backing has been targeted since Seth was approximately three years of age. At this point we know that he does not have a problem articulating front sounds. He now frequently interchanges the front and back sounds. For this reason we need to make decisions about the environments most facilitating and least facilitating in making these contrasts. This is not a simple matter. For the most part Seth produces each of these sounds appropriately in word lists when each is targeted. It is as though he adopts an articulatory set and proceeds (i.e., everything becomes either a /t/ or a /k/). It is only when he is using these sounds in conversational speech that his productions become variable and not always easily attributable to phonetic surrounds. One lead that we do have is that /k/ sometimes becomes /t/ after a front vowel (week [wit]; make [met]). We can begin to hypothesize that vowels somehow influence the production of consonant placement for Seth, and we can organize early goals in the direction of the most- to least-facilitating vowel contexts in monosyllabic single words. The next step would be to increase the length and complexity of the linguistic unit, gradually introducing a variety of vowel contexts. As noted earlier in this chapter, increases in length and complexity are generally made with reference to syllable number, sentence constituents, syntactic complexity, and prosody (see sources for complexity hierarchies for session goals in Appendix D).

With conversational competence as a goal for Seth, an intervention plan that targets increased phonological complexity within conversational interactions provides a useful framework (Norris & Hoffman, 1990; Hoffman, 1992). Hoffman (1992) describes an intervention approach that is based on a synergistic view of phonological learning and treatment (i.e., phonological knowledge is related to higher levels of language processing). Increased phonological complexity is targeted with increased complexity in other grammatical areas: morphological, semantic, syntactic and pragmatic. This approach aims to give the child "contextually appropriate opportunities to use language" (Hoffman, 1992, p. 257) and incorporates the concept of scaffolding to promote successful performance in the face of increased conversational demands. Contextual support, therefore, is an important ingredient offered in the form of modeling, prompts, questions, storybook print, and story sequences that are organized with reference to the overall conversational demands made on the child.

Short-term goal 2: Seth will reduce the stopping of /f/ and /v/ in conversational speech and /ʃ/ in the initial position of words. We will discuss /f/ and /v/ first because these phonemes are already in Seth's repertoire. (We will look at /ʃ/ with goal 3.) As with goal 1, Seth has established the requisite phonetic gestures. He must learn to use the sounds appropriately and consistently in a variety of contexts. Our focus, therefore, will be guided by the need to organize phonetic contexts from most to least facilitating. We know that in the case of stopping, for example, we want to avoid the common tendency of stopping a fricative when it is in the context of nonfricative sounds (i.e., stops). Presenting an /f/ in *face*, therefore, would be more facilitative of /f/ production than in *fit*, which ends with a stop (Hodson & Paden, 1991; Kent, 1982). Consequently, one framework for organizing a session-goal sequence would be with reference to phonetic context. Also, as in the case of goal 1, further session goals would be designed with reference to increasing phonetic as well as phonological demands.

Short-term goal 3: Seth will begin the suppression of the process of gliding (the production of /l/ in initial position of words). According to most commonly referenced developmental schedules, both liquids, /r/ and /l/, which are vulnerable to gliding, appear about the same time (between thirty-two and thirty-six months) and are mastered after four years of age in normally developing children (Prather, Hedrick, & Kern, 1975). We have chosen to initiate the dissolution of gliding by beginning with /l/ because the required articulatory gestures are more visible and depend on anterior tongue placement, which has been emphasized in the dissolution of backing.

Because Seth is not yet producing liquids, we must assume that the maintenance of gliding is likely the result of articulatory and/or perceptual difficulty. Our approach to remediation will, therefore, include both articulatory-phonetic and phonological components. In terms of production demands, this implies locating the bases for phonetic (articulatory) as well as phonologic (meaning) hierarchies. From an articulatory perspective we want to organize tasks from the most to least facilitative. The traditional approach to the remediation of phonetic errors has been to begin with efforts to insure that the client can identify a given sound (target) and compare that sound with other sounds, specifically the error sound. (For comprehensive treatments of reception approaches see Mysak, 1966; Van Riper, 1978; Winitz, 1975.) While "sound discrimination training" has often been the preferred initial phase of articulation therapy (e.g., Van Riper, 1978; Winitz, 1975), the efficacy of this priority has not yet been established (Bernthal & Bankson, 1988). Although we may begin with identification and discrimination tasks, we rapidly introduce production targets in order to provide a basis for the child to compare his productions with the clinician's productions. A possible early treatment hierarchy for Seth would involve the comparison of error and standard phoneme in the clinician's speech and then in his own speech.

Decisions would need to be made about the contexts in which these discriminations would take place. Since we are targeting initial /l/, complexity hierarchies would be developed through a consideration of the phonetic context (vowels and consonants), syllable number, and canonical form (arrangement of CVs) in which /l/ would occur as the first consonant.

In an effort to target production skill, it is necessary to plan a series of contexts that are predicted to increase in performance demand. A sequence of such contexts may be compiled from popular traditional texts on the remediation of articulation errors (e.g., Van Riper, 1978; Winitz, 1975) as well as from those texts that are more phonologically oriented (Hodson & Paden, 1991). For example, from an articulatory framework we learn that a reasonable sequence of production complexity in initial position may be the following: /l/ + vowel nonsense sequences covering all the available vowels in the language, monosyllabic words beginning with /l/ and followed by a vowel, CVC sequences in which the final consonant is an alveolar consonant, CVC sequences in which the final consonant has a variety of placements (except labial, to avoid the tendency for assimilation to the placement of the error phoneme), CVC sequences including the labials. When Seth has some control over the articulatory gesture and is capable of producing it spontaneously in CV and CVC sequences, it will be time to introduce minimal pair tasks (a phonological emphasis). (While some argue that children will learn to produce sounds because they are confronted by meaning contrasts [Weiner, 1981], others suggest that this demand may be too frustrating for a child with authentic motor difficulties; see Hodson & Paden, 1991; Saben & Ingham, 1991.)

Increase in production demands may next be found by increasing the number of syllables in words. As this is done we must remain cautious about the phonetic context. For example, with an initial increase in syllable number it would be wise to avoid the presence of consonant clusters, which add to overall complexity. Clusters or other agents of complexity (other sounds not in his repertoire) made be added gradually.

Given that /ʃ/ is not within Seth's repertoire, either, our approach to this sound will follow that of /l/, with appropriate modifications for differences in facilitating contexts. It should be noted that the emphasis on continuance versus stopping for the /f/ and /v/ and placement for fronting versus backing is expected to support the acquisition of /ʃ/.

Short-term goal 4: Seth will produce final /z/, and /s/, /z/ clusters coding plural, copula, third person singular, and possessive. This short-term goal is perhaps more complex than the preceding ones because of the interaction of phonologic and morphologic elements. We need to decide which sounds to target and in which morphophonemic contexts. At first glance it seems apparent that we would initially approach singleton targets, then clusters. The selection of *which* singleton is also rather straightforward. Both /s/ and /z/ are within Seth's repertoire, which supports targeting them simultaneously. We then need to decide which of the morphophonemic contexts to target first. To make this decision, we need to consult a hierarchy of morpheme acquisition in normally developing children (e.g., Brown, 1973). According to this hierarchy, the given morphemes appear in the following order: plural, possessive, third person singular, and contractible copula. On the basis of this acquisition order, we reason that this sequence moves from less to more complex and so may guide us in session-goal planning.

Now that we know that our initial goals will target final /s/ and /z/ in plural endings, we need to think about the words in which these will be embedded. We will need to provide lexical contexts that code plural with singleton consonant endings. Our search soon reveals that, in all morphological endings represented by a singleton consonant, that consonant is /z/. A morphophonemic rule realizes all final /s/ morphemes following a vowel as /z/. This is exemplified in plural nouns: *keys* [kiz], *days* [dez]; possessive pronouns: *hers* [hɝz], *his* [hɪz]; possessive nouns: *brother's* [brʌðɚz], *mother's* [mʌðɚz], *boy's* [bɔɪz], *Harry's* [haeriz]; third person singular: *goes* [goz], *sews* [soz]; and contractible copula: *who's* [huz]. Another phonetic realization occurs in bisyllabic renditions. The singleton /z/ also occurs after the vowel /ɪ/ in bisyllabic lexical items coding plural, *witches* [wɪtʃɪz], possessive, *witch's* [wɪtʃɪz], and third person singular, *dances* [daensɪz]. Other phonological realizations for these morphemic endings include clusters formed by the combinations of voiced consonants + /z/: (*eggs* [ɛgz], *man's* [maenz], *hides* [haɪdz]) and voiceless consonants + /s/ (*hats* [haets], *Pat's* [paets], *gets* [gɛts], *what's* [wats]).

In summary, the morphophonemic alternations described above suggest a hierarchy of session goals that will be based on morphological and phonological complexity.

Sample Session Goals and Procedures and Their Derivation.   In this section we would like to present one sample early goal and one later goal with reference to each of the short-term goals above. These sample goals are to be viewed as single behaviors within a series of behaviors designed to achieve the short-term goal. Movement from earlier to later goals within a sequence is based on some scale of complexity referred to above and in Appendix D. For example, targeting the production of sounds in words spontaneously implies the achievement of these sounds as imitations. Targeting the production of sounds in minimal pairs implies the establishment of these sounds within the client's phonetic repertoire. In addition, one criterion goal will be included against which to measure the achievement of each short-term goal. As discussed at the outset of this chapter, criterion goals are necessary for complying with current public laws.

We would also like to demonstrate the derivation of specific elements comprising each goal (i.e., those sources of information that were referenced in the development of each goal). To this end, the underlined words will refer to the particular aspects of the child's performance that were targeted as a result of consulting these sources of information. Sample session goals and procedures for Seth appear in Tables 6–3, A through D, below.

Alice

The first step in the derivation of session goals for Alice is to make a decision about whether to target both short-term goals simultaneously (during the same session) or to prioritize these goals. Let us look at the short-term goals we have decided to address.

Short-term goals:

1. Alice will establish and maintain efficient fundamental frequency and sustained intensity (breath support) to produce 3 and 3+ constituent utterances.
2. Alice will reduce the process of stopping, targeting /z/ in single words and /f/ and /v/ in continuous speech.

Deciding on a Goal-Approach Strategy.   In examining the goals listed, we can see that goals 1 and 2 address different areas of communication impairment. Because these areas of impairment, voice and phonology, often occur in the same child (Ruscello, St. Lewis, & Mason, 1991), they are likely to stem from similar underlying maintaining factors. This may be especially true for Alice, a child viewed as having difficulties in each of the areas of maintaining factors: sensorimotor, cognitive, and psychosocial. Impairments in these areas

TABLE 6–3A. Session Goals and Procedures

Client: Seth	Clinician:
Supervisor:	Semester:

Short-Term Goal Addressed: (1) Seth will reduce the phonological processes of fronting and backing in conversational speech.

Early Session Goal:

Seth will *spontaneously label pictures* representing *monosyllabic* words with final /k, g/ *following back vowels* six out of ten times and *following high front vowels* three out of ten times.

Derivation:

Maintaining factor(s) addressed: sensorimotor-coarticulation

Principles from learning theories: 9 (Box 1–7)

Performance demands controlled:

Phonetic context: back vowels more facilitating than front

Perceptual support: spontaneous expected after imitation achieved (responses to pictures expected after responses to printed stimuli have been achieved)

Number of syllables: monosyllabic more facilitating than polysyllabic

Session Procedure:

Clinician will:

- provide pictures that would elicit words containing final /k, g/ preceded by back vowels and high front vowels;

- model correct productions and request imitations following Seth's error productions;

- provoke Seth to reflect on visual and tactile differences between the use of error and standard sounds.

Additional Derivation Factors:

Learning principles 2, 3, 5 (Box 1–7)

Later Session Goal:

Seth *will produce* /t, d/, /k, g/ contrasts, *without a model,* while asking for objects, *pictured* in cards of a "go fish" game eighteen out of twenty times

Derivation:

Maintaining factor(s) addressed: cognitive-metalinguistic

Principles from learning theories: 1, 6 (Box 1–7)

Performance demands controlled:

Perceptual support: has imitated successfully, ready for spontaneous

Linguistic level: phonetic skill established, phonological contrast requires achievement

(continued)

TABLE 6–3A *(continued)*

Session Procedure:

Clinician will:

- ask Seth what card he wants in order to create a pair;

- reward correct productions by giving Seth the corresponding card;

- demonstrate communication breakdown after incorrect productions by giving Seth the wrong card;

- help Seth reflect on meaning and physical differences between correct and error sound; provide models and request imitation (if spontaneous repair does not result from confrontation).

Additional Derivational Factors:

Principles from learning theories: 3 (Box 1–7)

Criterion Goal:

Seth will produce /t, d/ and /k, g/ appropriately while telling the clinician about what he did in school that day with 75% to 85% accuracy.

Criterion Procedure:

The clinician will engage in conversation about school and ask Seth to relate what he did that morning.

TABLE 6–3B.   Session Goals and Procedures

Client: Seth	Clinician:
Supervisor:	Semester:

Short-Term Goal Addressed:	(2)	Seth will reduce the stopping of /f/ and /v/ in conversational speech and /ʃ/ in single words.

Early Session Goal:

Seth will place *minimal pair picture cards* containing /ʃ/ and /t/ in *initial* and *final* positions in their respective piles after each word is *pronounced* by the *clinician* in eighteen out of twenty trials.

Derivation:

Maintaining factors: sensorimotor

Principles from learning theories: 3 (Box 1–7)

Performance demands controlled:

   Response mode: differentiation before production

   Word position: initial and final positions have already been mastered separately

(continued)

TABLE 6–3B *(continued)*

Session Procedure:

Clinician will:

- produce each word of a set of minimal pair picture cards with the phonemes /ʃ/ and /t/;
- request Seth to place each card on appropriate pile;
- help Seth reflect on his choices when incorrect.

Additional Derivation Factors:

Principles from learning theories: 5 (Box 1–7)

Later Session Goal:

Seth will produce *monosyllabic* words, *without a model*, as he *reads* from a list of words with /ʃ/ in initial and final positions.

Derivation:

Maintaining factor(s) addressed: sensorimotor-establish motor representation

Principles from learning theories: 9 (Box 1–7)

Performance demands controlled:

Perceptual support: spontaneous after imitation (auditory and visual perceptual support), printed stimuli before stimuli without print (written perceptual support)

Syllable number: monosyllabic before polysyllabic

Session Procedure:

Clinician will interact with the client by providing Seth with a list of words that are within his reading level.

Additional Derivation:

Principles from learning theories: 5 (Box 1–7)

Criterion Goal:

Seth will produce /f/ and /v/ with 75% to 85% accuracy as he retells short stories containing a preponderance of /f/ and /v/ words. Seth will produce /ʃ/ in single words while labeling pictures with 75% to 85% accuracy.

Criterion Procedure:

The clinician will tell Seth short stories containing /f/ and /v/ words. He will be asked to retell these stories. The clinician will present pictures represented by words with /ʃ/ in initial position.

TABLE 6–3C.   Session Goals and Procedures

Client: Seth	Clinician:
Supervisor:	Semester:

Short-Term Goal Addressed: (3)   Seth will begin the suppression of the process of gliding (targeting the production of /l/ in initial position of words).

Early Session Goal:

Seth will *produce* alternating *syllables* /ta/, /da/, /na/, and /la/ *after* the clinician.

Derivation:

Maintaining factors: sensorimotor-anterior tongue movement, motor representation

Principles from learning theories: 9 (Box 1–7)

Performance demands controlled:

Linguistic level: syllables before words

Perceptual support: imitation before spontaneous

Session Procedure:

Clinician will

• model syllables /ta/, /da/, /na/, /la/;

• help Seth reflect on his performance.

Additional Derivational Factors:

Principles from learning theories: 2, 8 (Box 1–7)

Later Session Goal:

Seth will *ask* for pictures to complete pairs in a "go fish" game containing *minimal pairs* differentiated by /l/ and /w/.

Derivation:

Maintaining factor(s) addressed:

• sensorimotor-production

• cognitive-metalinguistic

• psychosocial-interacting in game

Principles from learning theories: 6 (Box 1–7)

Performance demands controlled:

Linguistic level: distinguishing minimal pairs after phonetic production is possible

(continued)

TABLE 6–3C *(continued)*

Session Procedure:

Clinician will:

- provide "go fish" game;
- engage in interchange required in game;
- give Seth card he asks for if production is correct;
- give Seth the card he does not expect if the production is wrong;
- encourage Seth to reflect on the wrong-card problem.

Additional Derivation:

Principles from learning theories: 3, 5, 6, 7, 8, 9 (Box 1–7)

Criterion Goal:

Seth will produce /l/ spontaneously in initial position of words with 90% accuracy when identifying an object being described or solving a riddle.

Criterion Procedure:

The clinician will give Seth clues about an object (thing or animal) which begins with /l/. Seth will be asked to guess the correct name.

TABLE 6–3D.   Session Goals and Procedures

Client: Seth	**Clinician:**
Supervisor:	**Semester:**

Short-Term Goal Addressed:	(4)	Seth will produce final /z/, and /s/, /z/ clusters coding plural, copula, third person singular, and possessive.

Early Session Goal:

Seth will *produce* singular and plural *contrasts* (bee-bees) in order to complete minimal pairs in a "go fish" game.

Derivation:

Maintaining factor(s) addressed:	Sensorimotor-production, alveolar placement, coarticulation
	Cognitive-metalinguistic

Principles from learning theories: 3, 9 (Box 1–7)

Performance demands controlled:

Phonetic environment: /z/ before clusters

Linguistic level: minimal-pair contrasts after phonetic ability demonstrated

Linguistic complexity: plural is early developmental morpheme

(continued)

TABLE 6–3D *(continued)*

Session Procedure:

Clinician will:

- provide pictures to represent singular versus plural minimal pairs;
- participate in game turns, asking for cards;
- encourage Seth to reflect on error production.

Additional Derivation Factors:

Principles from learning theories: 5, 6, 7, 8

Later Session Goal:

Seth will, while *following pictures* in a book, *produce* appropriate plural endings (z, Iz, C+s, C+z) as he *retells* a story *told by the clinician* that includes a large proportion of plural items.

Derivation:

Maintaining factor(s) addressed:

   Sensorimotor—coarticulation

   Cognitive—organizing events

   Psychosocial—following adult directives

Principles from learning theories addressed: 3, 5, 6 (Box 1–8)

Performance demands controlled:

   Perceptual support: perceptual support before no perceptual support (clinician's model, pictures)

   Linguistic complexity: continuous speech after word lists and naming pictures

Session Procedure:

Clinician will interact with the client by providing a series of pictures forming a story containing plural lexical items.

Additional Derivation Factors:

Principles from learning theories: 2 (Box 1–7)

Criterion Goal:

Seth will produce final /z/ and /s/, /z/ clusters coding plural, copula, third person singular, and possessive, while retelling a story that necessitates the production of words containing instances of each, with 75% to 85% accuracy.

Corresponding Criterion Procedure:

The clinician will provide Seth with a story that includes instances of /z/, and /s/, /z/ clusters coding a variety of morphemes. Seth will be assisted with pictures and prompts to recall story.

---

have been implicated in cases of phonological disorders (e.g., McDonald, 1964) as well as in voice disorders (Andrews, 1986; Wilson, 1987). It would be reasonable, therefore, to target both of these areas simultaneously, even in the same session. Working through the identified maintaining factors would be beneficial for both disorder types.

Factors Influencing Goal Construction.   Now that we have decided to target both of the short-term goals from the outset of therapy, we need to consider those factors that will help us formulate a sequence of session goals to reach each short-term target. We need to consider maintaining factors, principles from learning theories, and performance demands. The first two factors will inform us about approaches we need to take across both goal targets. This is because a child's associated behavioral systems will affect the development of any aspect of language. Performance demands (facilitating versus nonfacilitating contexts) for voice modification will be different from those for the reduction of phonological processes.

Maintaining factors. As we noted earlier, Alice presents with difficulties in the areas of cognitive, sensorimotor, and psychosocial development. In designing a sequence of session goals, we must keep in mind the modification of or compensation for these factors in order to facilitate the use of appropriate vocal patterns and target speech sounds. We turn to Boxes 1–3 to 1–5 (Chapter 1) to review those sensorimotor, cognitive, and psychosocial accomplishments that are associated with the elimination of phonological processes and the production of appropriate vocal patterns. In examining Box 1–3, we can see that the elimination of phonological processes occurs between four and seven years of age. This is associated with increased precision of motor control. Alice may still be experiencing some difficulty with tongue movement, as evidenced by the operation of gliding and stopping of early developing sounds. She is operating below age expectancy with reference to gliding (/r/ and /l/ are found to emerge in the normal population by thirty-six months of age; Grunwell, 1981; Prather, Hedrick, & Kern, 1975). In addition, the dissolution of stopping should be further advanced. According to Grunwell, stopping no longer applies to /f/ and /s/ by thirty-six months of age; it no longer applies to /v/ and /z/ by approximately forty months of age. (Somewhat later ages are designated by Prather et al., 1975, and Sander, 1972.)

At this point (four years, three months of age), descent of the larynx is not yet complete, which is associated with variability in fundamental frequency, vocal tract posturing, and timing of laryngeal and supralaryngeal adjustments. This immature laryngeal condition may be compounded by sensorimotor problems evidenced in Alice's baseline data. An oral peripheral examination revealed a tense jaw and laryngeal musculature, and raised larynx when vocalizing. Concomitant breathing problems were also noted. These findings suggest that vocal tract posturing and laryngeal and supralaryngeal adjustments are problematic for Alice. It is also likely that the tension exhibited in the laryngeal musculature is related to overall bodily elevated tonicity, inadequate body segmentation, and lack of coordination.

In addition to the possible neuromuscular problems, Alice has a structural laryngeal problem: vocal nodules. With this information from baseline data in mind, our session goals will need to address some aspect of sensorimotor control. Our sequence of sensorimotor accomplishments will be directed by the occupational therapist.

Next we need to look at the cognitive achievements related to the dissolution of phonological processes and modification of vocal parameters (see Box 1–4). The skill that appears most appropriate to target for Alice involves making early part-whole relations, grouping and regrouping objects according to attributes, and ordering objects according to a specific dimension. This skill provides a foundation for making comparisons, distinctions, and inferences. Much of the treatment for the modification of vocal patterns (particularly vocal abuse) during the early stages includes comparisons of adequate and inadequate aspects of voice (pitch, clarity, loudness; Andrews, 1986; Wilson, 1987). For example, children may be asked to describe the differences between making a "hard" sound on /a/ and an "easy" sound on /ha/ (Andrews, p. 151) or to explain basic concepts such as "smooth" versus "rough," "easy" versus "squeezed" (p. 164). The ability to compare one dimension with another is also essential within a phonologic approach. A number of recent articles in clinical phonology have described successful techniques that also involve comparisons of specific dimensions. Here the comparisons are between groups of sounds, generally the target group with the intruder (i.e., continuance versus stopping; frontness versus backness; Howell & Dean, 1987; Tomes & Shelton, 1989). For a child of four years, three months who scores on the low side of the average range cognitively, it is especially important to consider a strong foundation in cognitive skills underlying the understanding of comparisons.

Baseline data in the psychosocial area for Alice reveal that her motivation and attention are variable, that she appears to need approval after performance, and is very competitive with her younger, high-achieving sister, and that her loud volume appears to be associated with the need to engage others and compete with that sister. It is reasonable to believe that Alice's psychosocial difficulties may also be contributing to her voice problem, specifically the development of nodules. A recent survey of children with nodules indicated that these children had higher scores for acting out, distractibility, disturbed peer relations, and immature behaviors than a normal-voice, matched control group (Green, 1989). Although a cause and effect relationship was not definitively made, it was suggested that the speech-language pathologist employ techniques to improve social and communicative skills. These techniques would need to be developed in the formulation of session goals. When necessary, a psychologist should be consulted.

Summary. At this point in our approach to session-goal planning, we know that our session goals will be shaped by efforts to (a) improve tongue movement and decrease tension of laryngeal and surrounding musculature, (b) increase awareness of differences in attributes (features) among sound groups and vocal patterns, and (c) improve interpersonal relationships.

Principles form learning theories. The following learning principles in Alice's case are derived primarily from social-cognitive learning theory and motor-learning theory (see Boxes 1–6 and 1–7). These principles now influence our session-goal planning. They direct us in deciding what behavior we want Alice to demonstrate during a session with reference to a sound target we may have in mind. Each principle suggests one behavior we will expect Alice to demonstrate as a session goal. The relationship between learning principles and session behaviors appears in Box 6–5 below.

Performance demands. Now that we have decided to target voice and phonology in session goals, we are concerned with those factors affecting performance in both areas. Factors that facilitate or impede vocal and articulatory performance were discussed earlier in the chapter. Now these variables will be expanded with reference to the specific goals targeted for Alice.

Short-term goal 1: Alice will establish and maintain efficient fundamental frequency and sustained intensity (breath support) to produce 3 and 3+ constituent utterances. As we indicated in the section on Alice's maintaining factors, we believe that Alice will need to improve her breathing pattern (primarily exhalation phase) and reduce laryngeal tension. In order to plan a sequence of goals incorporating respiration and phonation, we reference Andrews (1986), who states the following: "one begins at the beginning of the physiological process (i.e., with respiration) and proceeds in an orderly fashion to link respiration with the onset of phonation, with sustained phonation, then with resonance and articulation" (p. 149). The integration of respiration and phonation is expanded during Andrews's production phase, in which the child is taught to

---

BOX 6–5. CORRESPONDENCES BETWEEN LEARNING PRINCIPLES AND BEHAVIORS EXPECTED OF ALICE IN THE SESSION

Principle	*Behavior*
Learning is facilitated by:	Child will:
2. efforts to match models presented by the clinician	imitate models
3. noticing similarities and distinctions among actions and events mediated by adults	indicate awareness of similarities and differences among sounds or voice patterns
9. sensory stimulation (i.e., sensory feedback) from movement involved in the performance of articulatory gestures	produce sounds

"produce and monitor target behaviors in a highly structured and controlled situation" (p. 165). Production demands are increased with changes in the complexity of the linguistic context as well as in the cues and monitoring made available to the client. Andrews's production phase of treatment incorporates increases in production demands with reference to (a) interactions of respiration and phonation, (b) phonetic contexts, (c) duration of unit (e.g., word, phrases), (d) complexity of unit, and (e) pragmatic function. As this phase progresses, the responsibility for cueing and monitoring is assumed more and more by the client.

Short-term goal 2: Alice will reduce the process of stopping, targeting /z/ in single words and /ʃ/ and /v/ in continuous speech. Here we have another example of a goal with two parts. It is a single goal in that it addresses an underlying process: stopping. Alice, however, stops the individual fricatives differently. The phonemes /f/ and /v/ are within her phonetic repertoire but are applied variably in continuous speech (stopped 36% to 38% of the time); /z/ is only produced in initial position in isolation after a model. Therefore, we will start with an articulatory phonetic focus for /z/. This will include attempts to establish the articulatory gesture in a number of different contexts (i.e., before a variety of vowels, in different word positions, in monosyllabic words and bisyllabic words, with and without perceptual support). We will expand her knowledge of the use of this sound by introducing minimal-pair contrasts (z, d). For /f/ and /v/ our focus will be use in meaningful contexts. Production challenges will be sequenced with reference to (a) amount of perceptual support (imitation), (b) length of response unit, (c) complexity of response unit, and (d) pragmatic function. Production of /f/, /v/, and /z/ will also be reinforced in conjunction with voice tasks. Samples of session goals addressing each short-term goal appear in Tables 6–4A, 6–4B. These goals exemplify the way in which the categories of information above are applied in the last case presentation.

SUMMARY

The last phase of intervention planning has just been completed. Throughout these first six chapters, we have attempted to articulate a very complex decision-making process. Fortunately, there are two major sources of support available to the clinician. These are (a) allied professionals and the child's family, who can collaborate in the process of intervention planning, and (b) supervisors, who can facilitate mastery of management planning. We address these sources of support in Chapters 7 and 8.

TABLE 6–4A.   Session Goals and Procedures

Client: Alice	**Clinician:**
Supervisor:	**Semester:**

Short-Term Goal Addressed: (1)   Alice will coordinate and sustain airflow and voicing to produce 3 and 3 + constituent utterances.

Early Session Goal:

Alice will *exhale* evenly on /*s*/ for approximately *ten seconds* after a clinician's *model*, ten times during session.

Derivation:

Maintaining factor(s) addressed: Sensorimotor: respiration, laryngeal tension

Principles from learning theories: 2, 5, 9 (Box 1–7)

Performance demands controlled:

Perceptual support: perceptual support before no perceptual support (clinician's model)

Duration of production: ten seconds before a longer duration

Phonetic environment: /s/ focuses on airflow rather than airflow + voice, as cognate /z/

Session Procedure:

Clinician will:

* model controlled emission of air while producing /s/.
* position Alice in a Rifton chair as demonstrated by the occupational therapist.

Later Goal:

Alice will produce *two- and three-word phrases* using easy attack on *vowels* (blending words together) while *pretending to give directions* to doll-house people (e.g., "Sit over here"; "Sit on it"; "Put it here"; "Eat every one") ten times during session.

Derivation:

Maintaining factor(s) addressed:

Sensorimotor: respiration, laryngeal tension, hard glottal attack probably contributing to formation of nodules

Principles from learning theories: 4, 5, 9 (Box 1–7)

Performance demands controlled:

Linguistic complexity: phrases before 3 and 3 + constituent utterances

Phonetic environment: vowels after /h/ and other voiceless continuent consonants; blending words avoids hard attack on initial vowel

(continued)

TABLE 6–4A *(continued)*

Pragmatic functions: pretending to give directions before answering questions

Session Procedure:

Clinician will:

- provide doll-house furniture and dolls, demonstrating the way in which the dolls can be given directions and how they follow;

- have dolls follow directions when voice is produced appropriately and fall or stumble when it is incorrect.

Additional Derivation Factors:

Principles from learning theories: 1 (Box 1–7)

Criterion Goal:

Alice will coordinate and sustain airflow and voicing to produce 3 and 3 + constituent utterances in playing the roles of characters in a children's story with 80% accuracy.

Corresponding Criterion Procedure:

The clinician will tell a familiar story, stopping when a character appears to ask Alice to take the parts of the various characters.

TABLE 6–4B.   Session Goals and Procedures

Client: Alice	**Clinician:**
Supervisor:	**Semester:**

Short-Term Goal Addressed: (2)   Alice will reduce the process of stopping, targeting /z/ in single words and /f/ and /v/ in continuous speech.

Early Session Goal:

Alice will *group pictures* according to the *final sound* of the words, representing them with reference to whether it is a long sound /z/ or a short sound /d/ (i.e., buzz and bud, his and hid) eight out of ten times.

Derivation:

Maintaining factors addressed: Cognitive: grouping according to attributes

Principles from learning theories: 3, 5 (Box 1–7)

Performance demands controlled:

Response mode: awareness of differences in sounds before production

Position in word: final fricatives often acquired before initial; final fricatives easier to prolong

(continued)

TABLE 6–4B *(continued)*

Session Procedure:

Clinician will:

- provide picture cards with /s/ and /z/ in final position;
- acknowledge accuracy of response with "That's good, Alice" or inaccuracy with "Let's try that one again."

Additional Derivation Factors:

Principles from learning theories addressed: 1 (Box 1–7)

Later Session Goal:

Alice will *produce* words representing pictures with /z/ in *each* of three positions after the clinician's *model* eight out of ten times.

Derivation:

Maintaining factor(s) addressed: sensorimotor: articulatory skill

Principles from learning theories referenced: 2, 5, 9 (Box 1–7)

Performance demands controlled:

Response mode: production after awareness

Word position: production in all positions after each introduced separately

Perceptual support: spontaneous productions expected after productions following a model.

Session Procedure:

Clinician will:

- provide models;
- provide pictures representing /z/ in each position.

Criterion Goal (with reference to /z/):

Alice will fill in the missing word containing /z/ in initial-position words ("Animals are found in the *zoo*"); medial-position words ("*Fuzzy wuzzy* was a bear"), and final-position words ("The insects that sting are called *bees*") as part of a guessing game, with accurate productions 80% of the time.

Corresponding Criterion Procedure:

Clinician will:

- create phrases omitting target words;
- read the phrase as prompt, omitting the target word.

7

Collaboration with Allied Professionals and Families

At this juncture, it is evident that a great deal of information needs to be considered in the course of intervention planning. At each phase of management planning, the speech-language pathologist must attend to cognitive, sensorimotor, and psychosocial behaviors and contextual variables that might have an impact upon performance—all in addition to language. In treating relatively uncomplicated communication problems, such as mild articulation disorders, this should not be problematic for the individual speech-language pathologist. In more difficult cases, like the children who have been followed throughout this book, it is *not* likely that any one person would possess expertise in all areas relevant to intervention planning. Thus, when dealing with complex communication disorders in children a collaborative approach is warranted. This chapter is devoted to collaboration in intervention planning.

As we write this chapter, there is currently a movement in the field of speech-language pathology toward collaborative models of assessment and intervention (Creaghead, Estomin, Freilinger, & Peters-Johnson, 1992). Collaboration is not an entirely new idea. The need for communication among disciplines has been widely recognized throughout the history of our field (e.g., Berry & Eisenson, 1956; Johnson, Brown, Curtis, Edney, & Keaster, 1967). It has also been recognized in the field of special education. Communication among disciplines has historically taken place during "rounds" or "interdisciplinary" interactions among allied professionals in hospital, institutional, and school settings (Bricker & Bricker, 1974; Johnson & Mykelbust, 1967). Such interactions have typically involved information sharing following evaluations or treatment sessions conducted by individual staff members. Johnson and Mykelbust (1967) clearly anticipated the present approach to collaboration. In their "clinical" approach to education for individuals with learning disabilities, they did not distinguish between speech-language specialists and classroom teachers in proposing goals, techniques, and setting for treatment.

Like many developments in fields associated with special education, the present movement toward collaboration was stimulated by the passage of

PL 94–142 in 1975. According to PL 94–142 and subsequent legislation, the individualized educational program (IEP) is a legal document that must be developed in collaboration with the child's parents or legal guardians. Within the framework of this legislated mandate, collaboration signifies that the child's family will have *significant* input in the development of intervention goals and procedures and will ultimately have the power of approving or rejecting the IEP (Benner, 1992; Cook, Tessier, & Klein, 1992).

This view of collaboration as involving significant cooperation between professionals and the child's family was revolutionary. Typically, family members were (and still are) included in their child's treatment only as sources of background information in the evaluation process or as recipients of homework assignments (e.g., Larr, 1962). Perhaps only in cases of fluency disorders in children have parents traditionally had the expanded role of carrying through on significant treatment procedures (e.g., Bloodstein, 1969; Van Riper, 1978). PL 94–142 mandated that families join educators and therapists as partners in planning intervention goals and procedures.

A second stimulus to the emergence of collaborative models of service delivery has come from the field of early intervention. In the late 1970s and throughout the 1980s, several books on early intervention described "transdisciplinary" service programs (e.g., Connor, Williamson, & Siepp, 1978; Rossetti, 1986). The term *transdisciplinary* is unique in that it signifies an actual crossover in roles assumed by allied professionals. Transdisciplinary also signifies inclusion of the child's family in the planning and treatment process (Benner, 1992; Cook, Tessier, & Klein, 1992; Rossetti, 1986). In a transdisciplinary interaction, allied professionals, such as speech-language pathologists and occupational therapists, as well as parents work with children with reference to one another's goals and procedures, and learn treatment techniques from one another (Connor, Williamson, & Siepp, 1978).

The recent growth of the "whole language movement" has served as a third catalyst to collaboration. The term "whole language" denotes an underlying linguistic foundation common to the development of oral language, and the achievement of literacy (i.e., reading and writing). Central to both language acquisition and literacy is the child's "construction of meaning" and achievement of personal goals (i.e., the content and use of language; Poplin, 1988). "Naturalistic" intervention techniques, traditionally used by speech-language pathologists to facilitate language development in children (Bloom & Lahey, 1978; Lund & Duchan, 1988), have been applied to the facilitation of literacy in classroom settings (Shapiro, 1992; Schory, 1990). These techniques include the use of concrete, manipulable materials in the classroom; engagement of children in conversations about a variety of subjects; the use of scaffolding techniques, story-telling, and group problem solving (Norris & Damico, 1990; Schory, 1990); and the inclusion of the speech-language pathologist in the planning of classroom programs (Schory, 1990).

A cumulative effect of the developments cited above has been the emergence of collaborative projects in school- and hospital-based programs for children of all ages, types, and degrees of handicapping conditions. For example, Dyer, Williams, & Luce (1991) described a collaborative program for school-age children with autism. Wadle (1991) and Christensen and Luckett (1990) have proposed the integration of related service personnel in regular education classrooms that include children with language-learning disabilities.

In this chapter, we approach collaboration from the perspective of intervention planning. Collaboration may, by necessity, take many forms. That is because speech-language pathologists may be employed in varied settings in which personnel, environment, and possibilities for interactions with allied professionals and children's families may differ considerably. We will leave it to the practicing clinician and practicum supervisor to adapt the ideas concerning collaboration presented below to the culture of a particular setting.

DEFINITIONS

Elaborating on a definition of collaboration presented by Nelson (1993, citing Idol, Paolucci-Whitcomb, & Nevin, 1986; Johnson & Johnson, 1975), we define collaboration for intervention planning as *the shared effort of allied professionals and families to bring diverse perspectives, expertise, and emotional support to the planning and implementation of intervention goals and procedures for children with communication disorders.* A number of key terms in this definition require clarification.

Sharing

The definition refers to collaboration for intervention planning, first, as a shared effort. Sharing indicates that individuals serve as resources for one another. The resources colleagues offer from the perspective of speech-language pathology include (a) information about factors contributing to a child's communication performance, (b) expertise about intervention procedures that could facilitate communication performance, and (c) emotional support for the demanding task of planning and implementing intervention with children and their families. The speech-language pathologist, in a collaborative relationship, would accept information, expertise, and emotional support from relevant others and would endeavor to provide equivalent support to colleagues.

The concept, sharing, varies with different models of collaboration. Sharing was taken to its most extreme position by Creaghead in a teleconference on collaboration in schools (Creaghead et al., 1992). Creaghead depicted collaboration as the abandonment by speech-language pathologists of their traditional role as "the experts" in communication disorders. She advised instead that speech-language clinicians merge roles with others (such as the classroom teacher). A less extreme position is taken by Christensen and Lucket (1990), who described a collaborative program in which the speech-language pathologist delivers speech service in the classroom, while the classroom teacher maintains an academic orientation. Our perspective of collaborative sharing derives from a transdisciplinary model defined by Connor, Williamson and Siepp (1978).

In this model, each member of a team takes primary responsibility for generating goals and procedures in his or her own area. Colleagues from related disciplines, however, bring their points of view to bear on these goals and procedures. Each member of the team observes the same sets of behaviors and baseline data when evaluating a child. This ensures that multiple perspectives will be applied to the identification of factors maintaining a communication disorder and to contextual variables affecting a child's performance. In addition, members of the team treat the child with reference to each other's goals and procedures whenever possible and useful. This ensures consistent treatment of maintaining factors. Thus, although members of the team share professional expertise and responsibilities with one another, each member of the team *retains* a professional identity in his or her respective area of specialized knowledge.

Allied Professionals and Family

The second part of the definition refers to allied professionals and family members as colleagues. The term *allied professionals* refers to regular or consulting participants on a team who hold expertise relevant to communication disorders in children. The expertise that allied professionals bring to the collaborative process is related to maintaining factors. These professionals include physical and occupational therapists, classroom teachers, psychologists, social workers, audiologists, and nurses.

The child's family represents an important component of a collaborative team. We view family as comprising any individual who spends a significant amount of time with the child outside of school. Family may include a child's natural mother and father, siblings, foster parents, grandparents, baby sitters, close friends. It is our clinical experience that family members can play as significant a collaborative role as any professional. Caretakers provide information about a child's communication performance, expertise relevant to the design of intervention procedures that could facilitate communication, and emotional support. Furthermore, the family may be an indispensable resource for the implementation of intervention plans. Families shape children's behavior and can be important catalysts for behavioral change (see also Fey, 1986; Nelson, 1993).

The Planning, Implementation, and Evaluation of Goals and Procedures

The final component of our definition refers to the aim of collaboration: the planning, implementation, and evaluation of intervention goals and procedures. In context of the model of intervention planning that has been outlined in this book, the nature of collaboration changes somewhat as one proceeds across the three phases. At the long- and short-term phases, collaboration focuses on the collection and assessment of baseline data and background information relevant to procedure planning. At the session phase, collaboration becomes a bit more complex. It influences goal setting as well as procedure planning for the client. It may also involve teaching, learning from, supervising, and receiving supervision from colleagues. Let us examine the nature of collaboration across the three phases of intervention planning.

COLLABORATION ACROSS THREE PHASES OF INTERVENTION PLANNING

Long-Term Planning Phase

The long-term phase of intervention planning represents the initial consideration of a management plan. At the long-term planning phase, the speech-language pathologist identifies (a) aspects of a child's speech-language performance to target as long-term goals of intervention, (b) a reasonable time frame in which targeted behaviors may be achieved (i.e., a prognosis), and (c) learning principles and maintaining factors that will guide the derivation of procedures to be followed in the course of therapy. In an ideal situation, a child would have been assessed collaboratively by an appropriate team of professionals. Each member of the team would have participated in the collection and interpretation of baseline data. Consequently, a team familiar with an array of baseline data and knowledgeable about theories of learning, applicable to a broad range of behaviors, would be available for intervention planning.

Unfortunately, this ideal scenario is not always possible as part of service delivery in many hospitals, schools, and private settings. As we remarked in Chapter 4, a child may arrive at a treatment center having been assessed elsewhere, or a particular setting may employ a noncollaborative assessment protocol.

Let us assume such a "least collaborative" scenario. The child arrives at a treatment center, referred by a child-study team for language intervention. The child has been evaluated by a speech-language pathologist and a psychologist. There is minimal information about nonlinguistic factors that may be maintaining the speech-language disorder.

Team Formation. In such a situation, a case in which a child was referred primarily for a speech-language disorder, the speech-language clinician would assume responsibility for organizing and coordinating a collaboration. The clinician would need to coordinate the formation of a collaborative team comprising professionals and the child's parents. The tasks for the professionals on the team would be to (a) identify factors that may be maintaining the speech-language disorder and that may have to be addressed in the course of intervention and (b) to specify principles of learning that could be referenced in designing therapeutic materials and clinician-child interactions. The role of the family on the team would be to contribute to (a) the identification of maintaining factors and (b) the development of long-term goals and procedures, some of which may be focused on the family.

As team coordinator, the speech-language clinician would be responsible for arranging and scheduling team meetings. At these meetings, team members would share and discuss information relevant to an intervention.

Identification of Maintaining Factors. The first task of the collaborative team would be to identify factors that may be maintaining the speech-language disorder. There are two sources of information that will be helpful in this endeavor: case history information and direct observations of child and family.

As team coordinator, the speech-language clinician would be responsible for bringing to the attention of colleagues the case-history information that accompanied the child to the treatment setting. Each professional on the team would review these data and hypothesize about the child's functional status in that professional's area of expertise. For example, in cases of children with severe phonological disorders (like Seth, who was followed in Chapters 3 through 6), a physical or occupational therapist would be consulted concerning the possible contribution of sensorimotor dysfunctions related to body segmentation, stability, and the processing of tactile, kinesthetic, and proprioceptive information. A special educator or psychologist would provide input about the child's cognitive status. These colleagues could also recommend the scheduling of observations of child and family in order to collect additional information. Such observations are generally scheduled if questions arise during the first few therapy sessions. In such cases, long-term goal and procedure statements, formulated initially, would be subject to modification.

Identification of Learning Principles. As discussed in Chapter 4, the identification of maintaining factors that may need to be addressed in the course of intervention provides direction for the development of procedures. Principles of language learning will also provide direction. Allied professionals can alert or instruct the speech-language clinician about those principles of learning that apply to the ameliorization of maintaining factors with reference to their disciplines. Take, for example, the child with multiple phonological deficits. An examination of baseline data in collaboration with a physical therapist may indicate problems with body tonicity and the processing of feedback from oral motor actions. This might alert the speech-language clinician to the significance of motor-learning principles in procedure planning (e.g., learning would be promoted by enhancing sensory stimulation—i.e., sensory feedback—from movement; see Box 1–7). A psychologist or special educator might alert the speech-language clinician to principles of learning relevant to cognitive development, given a child with deficits in the acquisition of content-form interactions.

The Role of Families

Collaboration on goal and procedure planning. Families play an important role in the development of long-term goals and procedures (Nelson, 1993). They are important resources for the identification of maintaining factors. Family members can also help the clinician set feasible long-term goals and procedural parameters. According to Nelson (1993), parents are known to "assume strong advocacy roles to obtain services they feel their children need" (p. 185). Family members can discuss and assess their involvement in terms of available time, energy, and knowledge of recommended intervention targets and approaches.

Collaboration on the prognosis. Perhaps the most challenging aspect of collaboration with families during the long-term planning phase involves the prognostic function of the long-term goal statement. As discussed in Chapter 4, the long-term goal represents a prognosis—that is, a statement of the best performance that can reasonably be expected of the child over a specified time period. In cases governed by the provisions of PL 94–142, parents must approve the long-term goal statement in the IEP.

The task of informing parents of their child's prognosis may be disconcerting in cases of children with severe handicapping conditions. In such situations, the speech-language pathologist may be required to inform parents of possible permanent limitations in their child's potential for development. In these cases, professional colleagues can provide important emotional support for the speech-language clinician and family.

Terminology. It is important to keep in mind that neither family members nor allied professionals are likely to be familiar with linguistic terminology, such as content category, constituents, and pragmatic functions, etc. It will be necessary for the speech-language pathologist to come up with meaningful, conveyable terminology and to educate members of the collaborative team about the linguistic basis of goals—especially at the long- and short-term planning phases. (See Kamhi, 1992, for a discussion of the inappropriate use of technical terminology in the area of phonology.)

Short-Term Planning Phase

During the second phase of intervention planning, attention is directed to the formulation and prioritization of short-term goals and the delineation of a procedural context. When more than one short-term goal is being considered by the speech-language clinician, collaboration can enhance prioritization and procedural decisions. With reference to maintaining factors identified during the long-term planning phase, team members (allied professionals and family) may help us answer the following questions from Boxes 5–1 and 5–2: (a) Does the achievement of any of the goals under consideration have more of an impact than others on the overall communicative success of the child? (b) Is the child capable of working on multiple achievements during one time period? (c) Which among a number of simultaneously occurring achievements (parallel achievements) may be facilitated most readily? For example, the classroom teacher may have suggestions about goals that are most relevant to the child's participation in group interactions (e.g., an emphasis on pragmatics over syntax). The classroom teacher and physical therapist might have insight as to how many goals a child might be able to work on at one time and which could be facilitated most readily. Family members would probably best help us address question (a) with reference to the achievement of communication skills at home.

Allied Professionals.   In considering the role that allied professionals might play in making prioritization and procedural decisions, let us consider a four-year-old child who manifests problems in the area of content-form interactions (coding only existence and action using one to two words) and phonology (using many early processes). The physical therapist has pointed out that this child has sensorimotor involvement affecting tonicity and body segmentation. The psychologist identified a cognitive delay. The speech-language clinician has written long-term goals targeting both phonology and content-form interactions. Recasting the question cited above with reference to the child under consideration, the clinician asks: "Should both phonology and content-form interactions be targeted simultaneously during the first term of treatment?" and "How much emphasis should be placed, initially, on articulation versus content-form interactions?"

The physical therapist, psychologist, and preschool classroom teacher can be helpful in answering these questions, and in fact may wish to plan short-term goals together—which is the ideal approach to collaboration. Working together, the short-term objectives of each member of the team may influence the objectives of the others. For example, in the case of the four-year-old under consideration, the physical therapist intends to work on tonicity, body segmentation, and stability issues. This intervention may have an impact on oral motor functioning, which may be relevant in deciding when to target the suppression of phonologic processes. Perhaps it would be best to do so after the child has spent some time working on sensorimotor objectives. Or perhaps we should work on phonology in tandem with the physical therapist, maybe even incorporating some techniques in our work.

The classroom teacher and psychologist might have some insight as to how many goals the child could work on simultaneously. In addition, the classroom teacher and speech-language clinician may wish to coordinate conceptual and language targets. Suppose, for example, the speech-language clinician wished to target the coding of existence, action, and attribution using three constituents. The classroom teacher may be able to target specific lexicon relevant to those three content categories in classroom contexts such as snack time, play time, circle time. Also, the classroom teacher may have the clearest insight into which goals under consideration may affect the overall communicative success of the child more than others, and which among the achievements under consideration could be facilitated most readily in a preschool setting.

Our professional colleagues can also help us determine the types of materials that should be made available for the child during sessions and the types of elicitations that the clinician should utilize when interacting with the child. Allied professionals such as physical and occupational therapists may have suggestions about adaptive equipment and positioning techniques. The classroom teacher is familiar with toys and other kinds of equipment available throughout the day. In fact, in many preschool, primary, and secondary school settings, speech-language intervention may take place in the classroom—in direct collaboration with the classroom teacher and other team members (e.g., Linder, 1990; MacDonald & Carroll, 1992). We will develop this point further, below, in considering collaboration at the session phase of planning.

Family

Family input into prioritization. The child's family can be an especially important resource at the short-term phase of goal and procedural planning. In terms of making prioritization decisions about short-term goals, family members may be helpful in envisioning which goals under consideration may have more of an impact than others on the overall communicative success of the child, and which among the achievements under consideration could be facilitated most readily at home.

Goals targeting family members. In Chapter 5, we introduced the idea of writing short-term goals that target the parents as well as the children. The idea of writing goals for family members has been addressed by PL 99–457, which extends to preschool age the right of a child with handicaps to a free, appropriate public education (Benner, 1992). According to this law, child-evaluation teams and preschool personnel are to develop Individualized Family Support Plans (IFSPs)—as opposed to Individualized Educational Plans (IEPs), which target children exclusively (Bennett, Lingerfelt, & Nelson, 1990). Although we have not provided examples of goals targeting parents elsewhere in this book, it is possible to develop such goals at the short-term and session planning phases (the *child's* ultimate communicative performance is always the focus of the long-term goal). It might be advisable to do so when the speech-language pathologist determines that modification of the parent-child interaction would be an intermediate step toward the achievement of the long-term goal.

It is important to keep in mind, at the short-term planning phase, that parents and other caretakers are not trained in techniques of speech-language intervention. Caretakers are not typically knowledgeable about or even aware of their own speech patterns, and they may be only vaguely in touch with the specifics of their child's speech-language dysfunction. In such cases, setting short-term goals for parents aimed at facilitating their communication interactions with their children would be indicated.

Furthermore, baseline data concerning the psychosocial history of the child's family in general, and language-relevant caretaker-child interactions specifically, may indicate that difficulties exist. Such difficulties would be a sign that the remediation of a child's speech-language disorder would be facilitated by setting goals for caretakers as well as for children.

It is possible to write short-term goals for caretakers in the same manner that we write them for children. The following are some examples of short-term goals that include family members: "Mother and child will establish joint attention on toys or books during play or book-reading sessions," "Father will narrate the child's actions using three-constituent action and locative action utterances," "Caretaker and child will establish turn-taking routines during play."

If technical terms, such as *three constituent* or *locative action,* are used in the short-term goal statement, time and care must be taken to instruct parents on the meaning of such terms. Otherwise, the goal should be written in lay terms. For example, the term *3-constituent utterances* in the following short-term goal statement was simplified in the second statement in the interest of improving communication with parents: "Mother and father will label objects using *3-constituent utterances* in the presence of the child" was rewritten "Mother and father will label objects using *simple sentences that have a subject, a verb, and an object* in the presence of the child."

Families and short-term procedure planning. As we noted in Chapter 5, decisions concerning the delineation of a procedural approach should also be made with the child's caretakers in mind. Objects used in therapy should be replicated at home. Furthermore, linguistic and nonlinguistic clinician-child interactions should be designed so that their most essential characteristics are replicable by caretakers. The family can instruct the professionals on the team as to the cultural and familial environment of the child and the kinds of objects, play, and communication routines that engage the child.

Session Phase

Perhaps the heart of a collaborative approach to intervention planning lies in the session planning phase. As detailed in Chapter 6, the development of session goals and procedures involves the specification of observable acts of learning that should lead to the acquisition of linguistic competencies specified in short-term objectives. The specification of these acts of learning involves determining actual linguistic and nonlinguistic contexts that will best address maintaining factors and control performance demands. The possibilities for collaboration at this juncture expand from interactions related to goal and procedure planning to interactive intervention. The present "collaborative movement" has envisioned and implemented (a) the development of transdisciplinary (i.e., across discipline) goal statements and procedural techniques, (b) collaborative service delivery in the classroom, (c) the targeting of child-family interactions for modification, and (d) the inclusion of the child's family members in sessions. We will elaborate on the implications of each of these ideas for session planning at the session phase in the remainder of this chapter.

Transdisciplinary Session Goals and Procedures. Session goals and procedures that are transdisciplinary incorporate contextual description affecting child-clinician interactions contributed by allied professionals. An example of a transdisciplinary session goal for a child with a voice problem who manifests sensorimotor involvement is as follows: "Sean will maintain voice for five seconds while stating 'go' to direct a car-racing game while supported in a stable seated position." The caveat, "while supported in a stable seated position," represents the input of the physical therapist.

Connor, Williamson, and Siepp (1978) were among the earliest specialists to propose transdisciplinary goals and procedures. They were influenced by the view of the Bobaths (e.g., Bobath & Bobath, 1981) and others (e.g., Finnie, 1975; Fiorentino, 1972), who demonstrated how addressing the sensorimotor involvement of children with cerebral palsy can affect all aspects of a child's functioning. The concept of transdisciplinary goals and procedures was, perhaps, also influenced by the recognition that cognition and language interact in important ways (e.g., Karmiloff-Smith, 1979, 1986b; Moses, Klein, & Altman, 1990; Rice, 1983). The development of transdisciplinary goals and procedures has gained momentum with the emergence of Individualized Family Support Plans (i.e., Benner, 1992; Linder, 1990). This was foreshadowed in Finnie's (1975) work with families of children with cerebral palsy.

In a transdisciplinary speech-language session goal, the targeted speech-language behavior would be specified as the observable behavior expected of the child (i.e., with reference to the voice goal cited above, "Sean will maintain voice for five seconds while stating 'go' to direct a car-racing game"). The recommendations of allied professionals would be incorporated into the description of the context (i.e., "while supported in a stable seated position," as recommended by the physical therapist). Similarly, the collaborating allied professional(s) could incorporate aspects of the speech-language goal and procedure in their depiction of the context.

The Classroom as the Setting for Intervention. A number of recent articles have proposed that speech-language pathologists intervene in the classroom regardless of grade level or specific disability manifested by children (Christensen

& Luckett, 1990, 1993; Wadle, 1991). This represents an extension of a concept originally developed in the area of early intervention (Linder, 1990; Conner, Williamson, & Siepp, 1978), again foreshadowed in the field of learning disabilities by Johnson and Mykelbust (1967). Some approaches to collaboration are basically *consultative*. In a consultative model, the speech-language pathologist operates as a consultant to the classroom teacher. In this model, the speech-language pathologist makes recommendations about language used by the teacher in conducting lessons and about incorporating language activities into the day's schedule (Cooper, 1991; Creaghead, Estomin, Freilinger, & Peters-Johnson, 1992). There are *whole-language* models of collaboration that advance a still more nontraditional view of the speech-language pathologist in the schools. These whole-language models have the speech-language pathologist sharing or exchanging roles with the classroom teacher (Moses, 1993; Schory, 1990; Wadle, 1991). From this perspective, the achievement of literacy in a variety of subject areas involves communication and language development. Consequently, the speech-language pathologist can contribute to the planning and implementation of classroom activities with reference to linguistic concerns (e.g., the syntax or semantics of math or reading).

It is beyond the scope of this book to discuss in any detail the different roles and approaches to therapy a speech-language pathologist might assume or carry out in classrooms. It is our job, however, to point out that the delivery of speech-language intervention in the classroom requires systematic goal and procedure planning.

The classroom setting—subject area, materials, and interactions—is depicted in session-goal and procedure statements as the *context* in which the target speech-language behavior will be expressed. For example, a session-goal statement for a third grader with a language-learning disability might read, "Sharon will express causality using conjunction in a conversation with science classmates about why sugar and salt disappear in water." The session procedure would indicate that the speech-language pathologist and classroom teacher would encourage children to experiment with dissolving sugar and salt in water and to question and comment on the whereabouts of the sugar and salt after dissolution.

Inclusion of Families In Session.   In many early intervention programs since the 1970s, families of infants and toddlers with developmental disabilities have been included in the treatment of their children (Finnie, 1975; Connor, Williamson, & Siepp, 1978; Linder, 1990). The reason is that parents spend far more time with—and have a potentially far greater impact than therapists—upon their children. Given that developmental disabilities affecting language are extremely serious, and that much consistent attention must be given to their remediation, treating the child's family members as colleagues in any intervention can increase the rate and probability of success (Connor, Williamson, & Siepp, 1978).

The decision to include families in treatment suggests that session goals targeting parent-child interactions be developed. This means, essentially, that the speech-language clinician has a dual focus during any session: the child and the parent. Session goals and procedures need to reflect this dual focus. Session-goal statements that target the child's behavior would refer to the family members' behavior with the child as part of the context statement. A separate session-goal statement targeting the family members' behavior could also be developed in which the child's behavior would constitute the contextual description. For example, "Mother and father will label five doll-house objects using simple sentences that have a subject, a verb, and an object (e.g., 'This is a chair') in the presence of the child."

Additional Considerations.   Collaboration during the session phase of intervention planning itself requires careful planning. If collaborative goals and procedures are to be developed, time must be scheduled for deriving goal and procedure statements for team members and for teaching one another about specific intervention goals and techniques. From our perspective staff development issues are best addressed by scheduling interventions in places where allied professionals and family members may observe one another treating and interacting with children (e.g., in the classroom or in the physical therapy space with family members present). This would be in line with the transdisciplinary or whole-language models of collaboration described above (e.g., Connor, Williamson, & Siepp, 1978).

Successfully instituting a collaborative intervention-planning program requires dealing with additional staff-development matters. These include (a) communication issues (e.g., determining how to convey recommendations and critiques) and (b) issues related to role diffusion (the definition of professional roles and the maintenance of professional and parental self-image in the process of sharing skills and knowledge). These aspects of staff development are potential sources of problems that can have detrimental long-range effects on collaborations (Moses, 1993). We will address staff development issues related to role diffusion, and collaboration in Chapter 8, which deals with supervision relevant to intervention planning.

SUMMARY

In this chapter, we have presented an overview of transdisciplinary collaboration at the three phases of intervention planning. Box 7–1 summarizes the major aspects of collaboration at these phases.

The first three items in Box 7–1 identify contributions of collaborative team members to the development of goals and procedures at each phase of intervention planning. A form designed to facilitate collaborative intervention planning is presented in Appendix E. This form is designed to allow individual members of a collaborative team to write short-term goals and recommended procedures for colleagues to use in developing session goals and procedures (targeting the short-term goal from the perspective of specialists represented on the team).

The last item in the summary identifies four staff development issues that should be considered by supervisors or team leaders working with allied professionals and families. These issues will be addressed in Chapter 8.

BOX 7–1. COLLABORATION AT THE THREE PHASES OF INTERVENTION PLANNING

---

1. *The Long-Term Phase*

   Allied professionals and families provide input for the:

   - identification of maintaining factors
   - identification of learning principles relevant to the modification of maintaining factors
   - communication of prognosis to family

2. *The Short-Term Phase*

   Allied professionals and families provide input for the:

   - prioritization of long-term goals to be addressed at the short-term phase
   - prioritization of possible short-term targets
   - development of goals targeting family-child interactions
   - delineation of a procedural context

3. *The Session Phase*

   Allied professionals and families provide input for the:

   - development of activities that will comprise the context for achievement of session goals
   - development of session goals which involve families

4. *Staff Development Issues*

   Allied professionals and families must address issues related to:

   - role definition
   - role diffusion
   - scheduling
   - communication of recommendations and critiques

8

Clinical Supervision
for Intervention Planning

We began this book by remarking that intervention planning in speech-language pathology is a complex process. We cited the many interacting variables that can affect communication performance and the unpredictability inherent in clinical interactions as contributing to this complexity. Now that we have described intervention planning in some detail, the following issue arises: How do we, as educators, supervisors, and clinicians, facilitate mastery of this complex process?

Clearly, expertise in intervention planning in speech-language pathology is not the product of a cookbook approach to professional training. Attaining expertise requires, first, a strong fundamental base of knowledge in such areas as linguistics; language acquisition and disorders in children; anatomy and physiology; phonetics, phonology, and disorders of articulation; audiology and acoustics; disorders of voice and rhythm; motor-speech disorders; diagnostics and clinical practice. It also requires the acquisition of competencies related specifically to the process of intervention planning, itself (i.e., clinical decision making and problem solving). The achievement of such competencies, characterized by Shapiro and Moses (1989) as a lifelong developmental process, will be our focus in this chapter.

This chapter is addressed to those whose job it is to facilitate professional development. This task is traditionally seen as belonging to the domain of the clinical supervisor and the university professor. More recently, a literature on *self-supervision* has emerged that has endeavored to help higher educators and supervisors share responsibility for professional development with the practicing clinician (Anderson, 1988; Farmer & Farmer, 1989; Shapiro & Anderson, 1988).

Our concern with the teaching of intervention-planning skills is in line with a nationwide movement toward the assessment and improvement of teaching practices in higher education (e.g., Brandt, 1991; Duckworth, 1984; Fosnot, 1991) and in "Title III" projects proliferating at universities across the

United States. This concern is also consistent with the focus of problem solving and decision making in a number of publications in the area of supervision (e.g., Anderson, 1988; Farmer & Farmer, 1989).

In this chapter, a set of clinical challenges will be abstracted from our account of the intervention-planning process. One challenge—the revision of client goals and procedures following a clinical session—will be examined in some detail. A framework will then be proposed for conceptualizing the development of expertise in clinical intervention planning. This framework details the kinds of professional competencies that may underlie resolution of challenges related to intervention planning. The identification of these competencies will guide the supervisor in setting goals and planning procedures for clinician, directed toward the development of expertise in intervention planning.

CHALLENGING CONCEPTS AND DECISIONS
RELATED TO INTERVENTION PLANNING

Overview

The process of effective intervention planning presents a unique set of challenges to the speech-language pathologist. We identify ten challenges that have the greatest potential for being problematic. These challenges, and the aspects of intervention planning to which they relate, are presented in Box 8–1.

The challenges refer to the formation of beliefs and concepts about language and language learning, the envisioning of others' perspectives (the child's in therapy and the theoretic views of researchers), and the development of information-processing capabilities and problem-solving skills. Student clinicians as well as seasoned clinicians have the opportunity to develop such competencies as they make decisions relevant to goal and procedure planning that were discussed throughout this book. The degree of difficulty and stress associated with the meeting of each challenge will vary with individual clinicians and clients. The difficulty of each challenge will change as clinicians successfully solve problems in the course of planning goals and procedures. Furthermore, challenges may assume different degrees of importance as the clinician moves from one phase of intervention planning to another.

Intervention-planning decisions related to the first nine challenges were elaborated in previous chapters. The revision of intervention plans (challenge 10), however, has not yet been discussed. We will consider the developmental nature of all of these challenges, and relevant supervisory goals and procedures. First, however, we will examine the revision of goals and procedures.

BOX 8–1.   INTERVENTION-PLANNING CHALLENGES

Challenge	*Where Encountered in Intervention Planning*
1. Viewing language as comprising three interactive components: content, form, and use	Goal planning, all phases
2. Envisioning language as influenced by nonlinguistic behavioral systems (i.e., maintaining factors)	Procedures planning, all phases Session-goal planning
3. Conceptualizing the nature of linguistic organization	Goal and procedure planning, all phases
4. Contemplating the child's active role in language learning	Procedure planning, all phases
5. Accepting the existence of multiple theories of language learning and the possibility that more than one theory may offer valuable information for intervention planning	Procedure planning, all phases
6. Recognizing one's own beliefs about language and language learning	Goal and procedure planning, all phases
7. Appreciating the context-sensitive nature of linguistic behavior	Session planning
8. Managing the large amount of information that needs to be considered in planning goals and procedures	Goal and procedure planning, all phases
9. Collaborating with parents, allied professionals, and paraprofessionals	Goal and procedure planning, all phases
10. Revising intervention plans	Session planning

Revising Goals and Procedures

There are three points at which intervention plans are typically revised: (a) at regularly scheduled reevaluation periods, usually mandated by city, state or federal regulations tied to IEPs (e.g., presently once a year at the New York City Board of Education); (b) between clinical sessions, when the speech-language pathologist has time to reflect on the success or failure of the last interaction with the client; and (c) during a session.

Revising Plans on a Regular Basis.   Revising plans on a scheduled basis requires, essentially, an "informed" reengagement in the three phases of the intervention-planning process. We refer to this reengagement as "informed" because the clinician will have gained knowledge from hands-on experience with the child. This knowledge will be about long-term, short-term, and session goals that have been achieved; procedures that have worked; and procedures that have failed. This information will inform the clinician's decisions about whether to continue treatment, and about appropriate goals and procedures if continuation is merited.

Revising Plans Between Sessions.   Clinicians usually revise intervention plans between sessions, when planning the next session. Revisions are based on direct experiences with clients (e.g., what worked and what did not work). These experiences should be viewed in light of the three bodies of information that contributed to the formulation of the original set of session goals and procedures: learning principles, maintaining factors, and performance demands (i.e., variables contributing to the complexity of the learning task).

Revising Plans During a Session.   As carefully as we may have planned, therapeutic interactions with children retain a certain degree of unpredictability. As such, clinicians are often challenged to make on-the-spot changes in plans during a session. Decision making *during an actual session* is somewhat different than decision making when planning goals and procedures before the initiation of therapy or between sessions, but it is just as challenging. The clinician has less time to reflect on all of the bodies of information that have been identified as contributing to intervention planning. Instead, personally held beliefs about language, language learning, and problem-solving skills tend to guide decision making.

In the remainder of this chapter, we will present a developmental framework for facilitating expertise in clinical intervention planning. This framework addresses the clinician's active role in learning and problem solving, which is grounded in the clinician's personal beliefs about language and language learning.

A FRAMEWORK FOR SUPERVISION
IN INTERVENTION PLANNING

As noted above, to meet challenges inherent in intervention planning, students need a strong knowledge base, exposure to information about the intervention process (i.e., phases, decisions, expected outcomes, sources of information involved in intervention planning), and supervised practicum experience. In addition to *presenting* information to students and practicing clinicians, supervisors need to consider the clinician's own point of view about language and language intervention (Duckworth, 1984; Fosnot, 1991; Perry, 1970). Supervisors also need to consider the clinician's *developmental level* in a number of specifiable areas relevant to the conceptualization of language, decision making, and problem solving.

Based on a model of professional development proposed by Shapiro and Moses (1989), intervention planning may be seen as comprising a set of novel problem-solving experiences. According to these authors, attaining expertise in intervention planning entails passing through a sequence of developmental phases that are a natural consequence of learning how to plan clinical interventions and solve clinical problems. These developmental phases involve transformations in how clinicians organize and interpret information that they believe to be relevant to intervention planning and problem solving.

With reference to this model of professional development, we identify four competencies that may underlie the clinician's mastery of the challenges identified in Box 8–1. These involve (a) shifting perspective (with reference to the child and theories of language learning); (b) engaging in causal reasoning about linguistic structures and interactions among maintaining factors; (c) envisioning multiple possible solutions to problems; and (d) engaging in role diffusion. We view these competencies as developmental in nature. We will consider each competency, and the way in which the competency applies to the challenges of intervention planning. Later in the chapter we will offer suggestions (goals and procedures) for facilitating these competencies.

Shifting Perspective

At each phase of intervention planning, the clinician is challenged to view significant events and crucial constructs from multiple perspectives. The ability to shift perspective signifies that the clinician understands that single events can be experienced differently by different people. This competency has two dimensions as it applies to intervention planning. The clinician must be able to (a) envision a clinical event from the perspective of the child, and (b) appreciate that a number of theories of language learning have important implications for the development of intervention plans.

Viewing Events from the Child's Perspective. The clinician's ability to envision clinical events from the child's perspective as well as from his or her own is a critical competency at all phases of intervention planning. Choosing materials and designing interactions that are engaging to children involve this competency. This competency is relevant to recognizing the child's active role in language learning, and to the appreciation of (a) constructivist-cognitive learning theory (Chapters 1 and 2), (b) information relevant to the child's developmental status contained in baseline data and developmental taxonomies (Chapters 1 to 6).

According to Moses and Shapiro (1992), learning how to view clinical events from the perspective of the child (as well as from perspective of the adult clinician) is developmental in nature, i.e., achievement of this competency can require a fundamental reorganization or revision of the way a clinician reasons about a clinical event. It is not often observed in novice clinicians.

The inability to shift perspective may be reflected in the clinician's choice of material that is not age or culturally appropriate for a particular child (e.g., using pictures instead of concrete objects with a three-year-old child who has severe developmental disabilities in cognition and language). This inability may be seen in the frequent reprimands directed at children who have trouble engaging in a planned activity. In supervisory interactions, this difficulty is apparent in the clinician's tendency to blame the child for problems (e.g., short attention span, lack of motivation). An entirely different approach to clinical planning and problem solving is seen in the clinician who is able to shift perspective. Clinicians who recognize the child's perspective and demonstrate an intrinsic interest in the child's involvement with material and spontaneous communication are able to adjust on-the-spot to clinical problems with reference to the child's developmental status and session goals.

Viewing Language Learning from Multiple Theoretical Perspectives.   Another important aspect of perspective taking that is relevant to intervention planning is the ability to appreciate the role that theories play in professional endeavors (Perry, 1970). Throughout this book we have emphasized the existence of different points of view about the nature of language and language learning. The ability to identify principles from theories of language and language learning is essential to goal and procedure planning. Thus, clinicians in training need to be acquainted with these different theories. Students also need to learn how to derive principles from theories, and to appreciate the generativity of theoretically grounded principles. (See Chapters 1 and 2 for discussion of theories and principles.) Ultimately, students need to understand that more than one theory can have merit—this will facilitate their ability to base procedures on principles of learning theories. Students also may discover that it is possible to commit oneself professionally to a personal view of language and language learning amid various possible views. Perry (1970) has identified this insight as a crucial stage in professional development.

Causal Reasoning by Clinicians

Clinicians are regularly required to think about causality in the course of intervention planning. Two types of causal reasoning are most relevant to goal setting and procedural planning: (a) the identification of linguistic organization, which involves inferential reasoning about an entity (organization) that is not directly observable, but that is presumed to underlie observable behavior; and (b) the specification of interactions among variables that may have an impact on linguistic performance. Each of these types of causal reasoning has a developmental component that requires attention in supervision.

Beyond the Information Given: Inferring Linguistic Structures.   A hallmark of a child's development is being able to *go beyond the information given* (e.g.,

Bruner, 1964; Piaget, 1954). *Going beyond the information given* signifies the ability to infer the existence of variables that may not be perceivable, but which may cause observable events. Some examples are a child's knowledge that force can be invisibly transmitted across objects, that objects are made of molecules, and that sugar continues to exist even when it dissolves. The ability to infer the existence of objects or events that are not directly observable may be viewed as a central developmental achievement in the acquisition of professional expertise (Gentner & Stevens, 1983).

Throughout this book, we have been referring to causal entities that are not directly observable. These entities are linguistic structures, such as content categories, syntactic rules, and phonologic processes, that are causal in that they account for ways in which the child organizes behavior and the environment (e.g., Bloom & Lahey, 1978; Osherson & Lasnik, 1990).

Linguistic structures must be inferred from observable behavior. This inferential process is a complex cognitive task. It involves the observation and comparison of a variety of different behaviors. The clinician's task is to identify underlying similarities or patterns among seemingly diffuse behaviors. Consider the following utterances: "Cat sit chair"; "Mommy go car"; "Daddy jump bed"; "Doggie go house." When the semantic relations encoded in each of these phrases are compared, an underlying consistency is inferable. These semantic relations may be classified as referring to "locative action" (Lahey, 1988).

We believe that such linguistic structures underlie and generate linguistic behaviors and, as such, are legitimate targets of speech-language intervention. The ability of student clinicians to conceptualize the existence of such linguistic structures is not automatic; it is a developmental achievement. Students may have to pass through a sequence of intermediate developmental phases when learning to identify such structures. Performance at intermediate phases of development may be reflected in specific problems related to goal and procedure planning.

Effects on goal planning. As noted above, causal reasoning by novices often involves an inability to conceive of nonobservable entities as contributing to the cause of an event. The focus in causal explanations, instead, is on self or on things that can be seen directly (Kuhn, 1989; Gentner & Stevens, 1983; Moses, 1990; Moses, Klein, & Altman, 1990). It is possible, therefore, that novice clinicians will encounter difficulties writing goals with reference to linguistic organization, which is not directly observable (e.g., content categories, phonological processes). Instead, novice clinicians may be prone to writing goals in overly general, nonlinguistic terms (e.g., "to improve vocabulary") or with reference to relatively concrete, nonlinguistic categories (e.g., "the child will use kitchen vocabulary [stove, cook, hot, cold, eat, drink, glass, sour, plate, cup, sweet] in complete sentences to talk about snack-related activities"). In these goal statements, there is no reference to linguistic organization (i.e., no reference to semantic categories [objects, actions, attributes] in the selection of vocabulary). There seems to be no consideration of organizational parameters as driving language behavior and no thought given to the developmental status of the child.

Effects on procedure planning. In procedure planning novice clinicians may fail to address principles of learning theories that account for the child's role in the development of linguistic structures. The clinician might overlook the child's problem-solving efforts, reasoning, and inference making. The clinician may fail to consider the child's developmental status in selecting materials for therapy and the possibility that "erroneous behavior" could be acceptable when that behavior represents an intermediate step in the child's construction of linguistic knowledge.

With development of the ability to conceive of nonobservable causes, the targeting of linguistic structures should make more sense to the clinician. Learning theories that endeavor to account for the development of linguistic structures should become more compelling. Our task as supervisors and educators is to convince students that these structures might actually exist and to provide students a means to infer their existence.

Evaluating Causal Interactions. We have identified variables that may contribute to a speech-language disorder, and that need to be addressed across the three phases of intervention planning. These are *maintaining factors* and *performance demands.* They involve cognitive, sensorimotor, psychosocial, and linguistic competencies and contextual issues. Reasoning about the impact of such variables on speech and language performance presents a challenge. It is especially challenging in session, when clinicians have to make on-the-spot decisions about the ongoing flow of information generated by client-clinician interactions. Research on causal reasoning by adults confronted with novel complex problems indicates that adults may pass through a series of developmental stages to attain such expertise (Gentner & Stevens, 1983; Moses, 1990; Moses & Shapiro, 1992).

Adults faced with complex problems in unfamiliar areas often tend to overlook variables at the causal "center" of the event under consideration. Instead, observable attributes of an event are initially seen as causal. In the area of intervention planning, the novice clinician's focus might be on the correctness or incorrectness of a linguistic act, and the practicing of "correct" behavior. Little attention would be paid to less obvious maintaining factors or performance demands.

With development, attention is drawn to overlooked variables that might underlie observable performance. Cognizance of these multiple variables can produce feelings of being overwhelmed and unable to handle such a complex task (Goldberg, 1993). With time, however, clinicians learn to target maintaining factors in planning goals and procedures. Collaborations with allied professionals that are aimed at incorporating targeted maintaining factors into session goals and procedures become important. Attention should be paid to variability in performance relevant to the session goal, and to the systematic control of materials and interactions that might be contributing to that variability. When problems arise during sessions, the advanced clinician modifies tasks or interactions presented to clients, while remaining goal oriented (Moses & Shapiro, 1992).

Envisioning Multiple Possible Solutions to Problems

Moses and Shapiro (1992) identified the ability to envision multiple possible solutions to problems as characteristic of expert clinical practice in speech-language pathology. This competency is central to the revision of intervention plans during and after actual clinical interactions. It is reflected in the ability to revise procedures while keeping the aim of intervention constant. The revision of procedures may involve a reassessment of materials, the demands of a task, or the pragmatic contour of clinical interactions. Envisioning possibilities is developmental in nature (Piaget, 1980). Moses and Shapiro (1992) found that novice clinicians tended to repeat prior procedures in the face of evidence that those procedures were ineffective or otherwise problematic. Novice clinicians also tended to lose track of goals when engaged in problem solving during sessions. Developmentally advanced clinicians were able to modify procedures in the face of clinical problems while remaining goal oriented.

Role Diffusion

In Chapter 7, we suggested that speech-language pathologists need to practice *role diffusion*. We defined *role diffusion* as involving the mutual sharing of expertise and support among allied professionals, paraprofessionals, and families. For the speech-language pathologist working with children, this involves recognizing that parents, allied professionals (e.g., teachers, physical therapists), paraprofessionals, and parents may know something about how to facilitate communication in a particular child. It also involves a willingness to share knowledge with others. As we remarked in Chapter 7, the ability to engage in role diffusion is an important and sometimes challenging professional skill. Engaging in role diffusion requires a measure of self-esteem on the part of the speech-language clinician. One has to feel competent to be willing to share one's expertise with others (who can be potentially critical) and to admit that one can learn from others without being perceived as professionally weak.

The competency we term *role diffusion* is acquired with clinical experience. It also has a developmental component. We will consider how to facilitate this competency in the sections below on goals and procedures for the supervision of intervention planning.

Summary

We have identified four areas of clinician development (i.e., competencies) that are relevant to the attainment of expertise in intervention planning in speech-language pathology: perspective taking, conceiving of possible solutions to problems, causal reasoning, and role diffusion. We related each aspect of clinician development to the resolution of specific challenges that clinicians encounter in the course of intervention planning. Box 8–2 presents a summary of intervention-planning challenges, relevant aspects of clinician development, and developmental patterns reflected in clinician performance during intervention planning.

Knowledge of these challenges and underlying developmental issues can be used by supervisors to assess clinician performance in the process of intervention

---

BOX 8–2. CORRESPONDENCES AMONG CLINICAL COMPETENCIES, INTERVENTION-PLANNING CHALLENGES, AND DEVELOPMENTAL PATTERNS IN CLINICIAN PERFORMANCE

Competencies	Intervention Planning Challenges (and Intervention Phases)	Developmental Patterns in Clinician Performance
Shifting perspective	Goal and procedural planning (all phases) Use of baseline data and developmental taxonomies in planning goals and procedures (all phases)	From: Tendency to reference adult performance in setting goals and designing procedures Tendency to control interactions in a didactic manner To: Use of developmental taxonomies and baseline data about the child's interests in setting goals and designing procedures Application of principles from a variety of learning theories to the design of clinical interactions Relegation to child of some control during the clinical session
Inferring linguistic structures	Setting long- and short-term goals in linguistic terms (phases 1 & 2) Use of principles from learning theories in targeting linguistic structures in procedure planning (all phases)	From: Tendency to set long- and short-term goals with reference to the performance of either overly general or overly specific tasks, such as "improving receptive language" or "sequencing abilities"

BOX 8–2 *(continued)*

Lack of interest in how
and why linguistic
structures are acquired

To: Tendency to set
long- and short-term goals
with reference to linguistic
structures (semantic,
syntactic, or pragmatic)
Interest in learning theories
that explain the child's
role in acquiring linguistic
structures and that deal,
in general, with how and
why linguistic structures
are acquired
Use of principles from
learning theories in
procedural planning

Evaluating functional and causal interactions among multiple variables	Goal planning (phases 2 and 3) Procedural planning (all phases) Revision of intervention plans Attention to maintaining factors, performance demands, and principles from learning theory in setting and sequencing short-term and session goals	From: Tendency to teach behaviors targeted in long- and short-term goal statements directly, without addressing maintaining factors and other variables affecting performance Repetition of procedures in response to clinical problems Little attention to sequencing goals at the short-term and session-planning phases

To: Consideration of
maintaining factors,
performance demands,
and principles from
learning theory in
planning session goals,
sequencing short-term
goals, planning
procedures, and modifying
plans in response to
clinical problems

(continued)

BOX 8–2 *(continued)*

Envisioning possible solutions to problems	Planning session goal and procedures Revision of session plans	From: Conception of one procedural approach and limited creativity in creation of materials Repetition of a single clinical procedure in response to problems experienced in session
		To: Creation of a variety of materials and types of clinical interactions Ability to reference principles from different learning theories in goal and procedure planning Ability to modify goals and procedures in response to problems experienced in session
Role diffusion	Collaboration in goal and procedure planning (all phases)	From: Tendency to plan goals and procedures without collaborating with allied professionals, paraprofessionals, and families
		To: Collaboration with allied professionals, paraprofessionals, and families when setting goals and planning procedures

planning. This knowledge also would be useful in establishing goals for clinicians relevant to the development of expertise in intervention planning.

SETTING GOALS TO FACILITATE EXPERTISE IN INTERVENTION PLANNING

We have identified a set of challenges that confront the speech-language pathologist engaged in intervention planning and five areas of development that underlie the resolution of these challenges. Based on this framework, we have derived the following set of possible long-term goals for practicum students, relevant to the achievement of skill in intervention planning:

When planning goals and procedures for children with communication disorders, the clinician will:

1. reference an adequate fund of knowledge about speech-language development and disorders;
2. identify the perspective of the child and others (e.g., family) with reference to the child's communication disorder and specific therapeutic interactions;
3. envision multiple possible solutions to clinical problems;
4. recognize organization inherent in linguistic behavior (semantic, syntactic, and pragmatic);
5. identify and address interactions among variables that may be maintaining a speech-language disorder;
6. identify variables that may be making demands on the child's performance during a session;
7. practice role diffusion.

In keeping with the basic tenets of intervention planning, it is necessary to establish a hierarchy of short-term goals that can be achieved by student clinicians during the course of a semester, and that represent a step in the achievement of a long-term goal. We have derived a group of short-term goals from the ten intervention planning challenges identified earlier (Box 8–1). These short-term goal(s) and corresponding long-term goals are presented in Box 8–3.

BOX 8–3. CORRESPONDING SHORT- AND LONG-TERM GOALS FOR FACILITATING EXPERTISE IN INTERVENTION PLANNING

Long-Term Goals	*Short-Term Goals*
The clinician will:	The clinician will
1. reference an adequate fund of knowledge about speech-language development and disorders;	A. identify and define concepts and procedures related to content courses and apply knowledge in practica;

2. shift perspective—identify the perspective of others with reference to therapeutic interactions;	A. appreciate the child's active role in language learning by
	   1. identifying and using developmental taxonomies in content courses such as diagnostics, and intervention planning;
	   2. identifying and justifying principles from constructivist-cognitive learning theories in course work and in the formulation and enactment of intervention plans;
	 B. distinguish and apply multiple theories of language learning in course work and in the formulation and enactment of intervention plans;

(continued)

BOX 8–3 *(continued)*

<table>
<tr>
<td></td>
<td>C. specify personal beliefs about the nature of language and language learning in course work, in diagnostics, and intervention planning;</td>
</tr>
<tr>
<td></td>
<td>D. apply principles from various learning theories to intervention planning;</td>
</tr>
<tr>
<td>3. infer linguistic structures;</td>
<td>A. exhibit knowledge of developmental taxonomies and parameters of linguistic organization in the areas of semantics, syntax, phonology, morphology, and pragmatics in course work;</td>
</tr>
<tr>
<td></td>
<td>B. exhibit knowledge of interactions among systems of respiration, phonation, resonation, and articulation in voice and fluency;</td>
</tr>
<tr>
<td></td>
<td>C. conduct naturalistic assessments of linguistic organization;</td>
</tr>
<tr>
<td></td>
<td>D. set long-term and short-term goals with reference to parameters of linguistic organization;</td>
</tr>
<tr>
<td></td>
<td>E. evaluate learning theories as applied to the development of linguistic organization;</td>
</tr>
<tr>
<td>4. envision multiple possible solutions to problems;</td>
<td>A. create procedural approaches at the long- and short-term phases of intervention planning that address learning principles, maintaining factors, and performance demands;</td>
</tr>
<tr>
<td></td>
<td>B. plan a variety of session activities with reference to specified goals;</td>
</tr>
<tr>
<td></td>
<td>C. modify linguistic, cognitive, psychosocial, and sensorimotor aspects of procedures during sessions, keeping goal constant;</td>
</tr>
<tr>
<td>5. identify and address causal interactions among multiple variables;</td>
<td>A. identify nonlinguistic behavioral systems (i.e., maintaining factors that may be influencing linguistic performance);</td>
</tr>
<tr>
<td></td>
<td>B. identify factors accounting for variability in a child's performance during session (performance demands);</td>
</tr>
</table>

BOX 8–3 *(continued)*

	C. identify semantic, syntactic, phonologic, and pragmatic components of language;
	D. create goals and procedures at all phases of intervention planning that address semantic, syntactic, phonologic, and pragmatic components of language, principles of learning theory, maintaining factors, and performance demands;
	E. modify goals and procedures between sessions and at regularly scheduled intervals with reference to semantic, syntactic, phonologic, and pragmatic components of language, principles of learning theories, maintaining factors, and performance demands;
	F. generate hypotheses about causes of problems identified in session with reference to semantic, syntactic, phonologic, and pragmatic components of language and language learning during supervisory clinical and classroom interactions;
6. practice role diffusion.	A. invite allied professionals, paraprofessionals, and parents to participate in goal and procedure planning at all phases of decision making;
	B. enact interventions in classrooms and with allied professionals, paraprofessionals, and parents present whenever appropriate;
	C. modify intervention plans in collaboration with allied professionals, paraprofessionals, and parents present whenever appropriate;
	D. demonstrate communication skills relevant to collaboration with allied professionals, paraprofessionals, and parents;
	E. discuss emotions and other issues related to collaboration with members of the team.

The information in Box 8–3 can be used by supervisors to plan short-term goals for clinician performance relevant to intervention planning. We will leave it to the reader (i.e., the professor, supervisor, or clinician) to devise "session goals" for clinicians to address on a daily basis. Session goals are suggested by the practical nature of the short-term goals listed in Box 8–3. For example, short-term goal B (which relates to long-term goal 4) is "The clinician will plan a variety of session activities with reference to specified short-term goals and corresponding procedures." Derivative session goals might be "The clinician will plan three session activities for (a specified client) that address a (specified short-term goal)," and "The clinician will justify the derivation of each activity with reference to principles of learning theories and maintaining factors identified in the corresponding procedural approach and procedural context plans." The supervisor also may find ideas for session goals in the following discussion of procedures for the supervision of intervention planning.

A PROCEDURAL APPROACH TO THE SUPERVISION OF INTERVENTION PLANNING

Having proposed a framework for deriving goals of supervision relevant to intervention planning, we turn to procedures. We view procedure planning in supervision as we do procedure planning in all areas of speech-language pathology. Procedures need to be oriented toward the achievement of specified goals. They need to be based on principles derived from theories of learning and development. Furthermore, attention needs to be paid to factors that may be maintaining problematic behavior and otherwise influencing performance.

The discussion that follows is based on the assumption that the achievement of the goals listed in Box 8–3 rests on a strong knowledge of language and interacting behavioral systems. As noted above, clinicians need to be exposed to various theories of language and language learning, and to practice deriving principles from theories. They need to understand the contribution of maintaining factors to linguistic performance. The discussion also assumes that, in keeping with ASHA guidelines, students will receive supervised diagnostic and clinical practicum experiences and related coursework. Our focus will be on "hidden," often overlooked issues that may arise in practicum or content courses. These are issues related to the four areas of clinician development: perspective taking, causal reasoning, envisioning multiple possible solutions to problems, and role diffusion. Proposals for facilitating clinician development in these areas derive from literature on supervision, and a newly emerging literature on the teaching of professional skills in speech-language pathology (Michael, Klee, Bransford, & Warren, 1993; Rassi & McElroy, 1992; Shapiro & Moses, 1989), and related fields (Duckworth, 1984; Fosnot, 1991; Perry, 1970). Our primary focus will be the resolution of conflicts related to the tendency of student clinicians and their supervisors to view clinical events from different developmental perspectives. We also will examine conflict resolution with reference to causal reasoning, the conception of multiple problem-solving procedures, and collaboration.

Perspective Taking

The ability to view events from multiple perspectives was identified, above, as a central competency underlying several aspects of intervention planning. These include the use of information from learning theory, baseline data, and developmental taxonomies in goal and procedure planning. In the area of perspective taking, three target achievements were suggested for clinicians: the clinician should understand that (a) a child's behavioral organization and view of the world are necessarily different from an adult's, (b) different theories of language and language learning may have merit, and (c) the clinician always has a *personal* point of view about language and language learning.

With reference to achievement (c), Perry (1970) has found that college students often are not aware that they have a point of view about issues raised by their teachers. Professors, too, often are unaware of this. Nevertheless, students do indeed have points of view that influence their judgments and reactions to information presented in class. Perry demonstrated that conflicts often arise in the university classroom, when information presented by the professor conflicts with students' implicit beliefs and assumptions about the subject. These conflicts may interfere with learning, unless explicitly addressed by the professor. In classes relevant to intervention planning, there are many opportunities for theory-related conflicts to arise. The discussion that follows identifies conflicts related to specific learning theories and conflicts that may arise when students must refer to more than one learning theory. This discussion is followed by a consideration of specific procedures aimed at the facilitation of perspective taking and resolution of conflicts.

Conflicts Related to Specific Learning Theories. Conflicts may arise in the supervision of intervention planning when students, personal beliefs about language learning—often unspecified and unarticulated—conflict with principles from learning theories that are presented by the supervisor. It is worthwhile noting that students just beginning their clinical training can be expected to have deeply entrenched beliefs about language and language learning. Our students probably began to think about language learning at a very early age, perhaps when they were five or six years old pretending to be mommies, daddies, or school teachers.

Evidence of conflicts rooted in theory and belief systems typically emerges during therapy sessions. One type of conflict is seen when the clinician finds that it is difficult to apply theoretical principles about language and language learning that were presented in the classroom or supervisory interaction. The student may have expressed theoretic principles on paper in justifying goals and procedures; nevertheless, principles and related goals and procedures may be forgotten during actual clinical interactions.

For example, one learning principle that was referenced in planning for a child with a language delay involved encouraging the child to reflect on concrete, problem-solving activities (Box 1–7, principle 8). Theoretically, the child's reflection on such activities can provide a basis for the emergence of content categories such as *action* and *attribution*. In carrying through on such an idea in an actual session with a client, the clinician would have to provide opportunities for the child to engage in relevant problem-solving activities. Often, when children are engaged in such activities, they do not talk. In fact, from the perspective of constructivist-cognitive theory, they are not expected to talk continuously. Children need some time to engage in goal-directed problem-solving activities and reflection. Ideas that grow from such activities embody the content of language (Duckworth, 1972; Sinclair, 1970). The following is an anecdotal account of a clinical session involving a student clinician, which further exemplifies a conflict in theoretic viewpoint. The clinician planned a session with reference to the above principle while holding an opposing belief about language learning.

The clinician decided to teach a child about comparatives and the attributes *heavy* and *light* according to the constructivist-cognitive principle cited above. The clinician, however, personally believed that children learn language by following adult directions and by imitation (this was revealed in a subsequent supervisory dialogue).

The clinician provided a scale and objects for the child to balance. The child spontaneously placed dolls on the scale and began to play "see-saw." The child did not talk as she made the dolls go up and down. From the perspective of constructivist-cognitive principles, the clinician should give the child a chance to engage in and reflect on the goal-directed activity she initiated (see-saw) *before* compelling the child to produce a particular behavior (Forman & Hill, 1984). The clinician might use the see-saw activity to model a target utterance or to introduce the idea of balancing. The clinician, however, should not direct the child to behave in a particular way before the child had an opportunity to engage with the problem. Despite this clinician's reference to constructivist principles in intervention planning, the clinician took the dolls off of the scale, and said to the child, "This is heavy, this is light. Now you say it." The clinician subsequently modeled "same" and "different," and demonstrated how to balance the dolls and other objects on the scale. The clinician subsequently revealed in supervision that the child's see-saw activity and silence were unacceptable. These behaviors conflicted with the clinician's belief in the need for direction from an adult.

Conflicts That Arise from Referencing More Than One Learning Theory. A different type of conflict in perspective may arise when the clinician needs to reference principles from more than one learning theory in intervention planning.

The clinician may only be able to reference one model of language learning. Take, for example, a session involving Darryl, the child with a language delay who we have been following throughout the book. Suppose that during transitions between activities, Darryl had a tantrum . The psychologist prescribed using an operant approach to modify this behavior. She recommended that the therapist withdraw attention from the child until he uses "acceptable" communication to gain her attention. The speech-language clinician, who focused on a "child-centered" therapy approach using principles from constructive-cognitive learning theory, reacted to the tantrum by stroking Darryl's head, offering him toys, and asking him "What is the problem?". The observing psychologist reacted with displeasure, because it did not incorporate the recommended withdrawal of attention. The psychologist concluded that the speech-language clinician was not interested in her recommendations. It may be, however, that the clinician was unable to use the psychologist's suggestion because it conflicted, in principle, with her own constructivist orientation, and required a context-specific shift to a different model of learning.

Procedures for Facilitating Perspective Taking.   Shapiro and Moses (1989) proposed several techniques for the facilitation of perspective taking. These techniques involved the explication of students' beliefs about clinical events, and the clarification of differences in the perspectives of supervisors and clinicians. Michael, Klee, Bransford, and Warren (1993) have proposed and validated a teaching method termed "anchored instruction." This method was designed to facilitate the transition from learning about theory in the college classroom to the use of theory to guide clinical intervention. Several of Shapiro and Moses's recommendations for facilitating perspective taking will be examined, followed by a consideration of anchored instruction.

Recommendations of Shapiro and Moses

1. Work to identify situations that hold potential for change and therefore warrant careful attention. Situations that hold potential for change arise with regularity at many points in the course of intervention planning for particular clients. Often these are interactions that cause supervisors discomfort and frustration. The clinician seems to be resisting the supervisor's suggestion about clinical interactions. Such situations also arise in the classroom. Professors lecture with excitement about principles of language and language learning that have special personal significance (e.g., generativity, principles of behavioral organization, behavioral techniques for shaping performance); nevertheless, students' eyes seem to glaze over, and during exams students omit the essence of the professor's explanations.

Although such experiences tend to cause discomfort, these situations may hold the greatest potential for facilitating clinician development. Such situations can be transformed into learning experiences if the supervisor recognizes the developmental basis for clinicians' behavior and employs techniques aimed at provoking development. The following suggestions from Shapiro and Moses (1989) represent techniques for transforming such discouraging interactions into learning experiences.

2. *Evaluate your own point of view about the situation and about learning and change.* Supervisors should keep in mind that *perspective taking* is the objective of clinician development. Consequently, before meeting with clinicians, supervisors should explicate their personal perspectives about the specific aspect of intervention planning under consideration. The supervisor also needs to identify the theory or theories that have contributed to his or her views about language, language learning, and specific intervention procedures.

3. *Evaluate the situation from the perspective of all participants involved or affected.* The supervisor needs to take steps to evaluate the clinician's perspective and underlying developmental status with reference to the specific clinical event under consideration and language in general. According to Shapiro and Moses (1989), the supervisor (or professor) would conduct the assessment of the clinician's perspective as follows:

> Ask questions to uncover the clinician's perspective. These questions should provoke the explication of a point of view about the child's role in learning and language production as well as the nature of language and language learning. This can be done in courses such as "Language Acquisition in Children" and in supervisory sessions related to clinical practicum.
>
> Evaluate the clinician's performance with reference to a developmental framework (e.g., the framework presented in Box 8–2).
>
> Observe the clinician in session or in class to identify specific behaviors indicative of the clinician's perspective. In a recent study on professional competencies of speech-language pathologists in clinical problem solving, Moses and Shapiro (1992) identified developmental profiles of clinician performance in clinical and supervisory interactions relevant to perspective taking. Among the behaviors indicative of a novice clinician were (a) overreliance on the use of questions and commands, (b) excessive attention to the client's problematic behaviors and indications to the client that behavior is unacceptable, (c) establishment of developmentally and/or culturally inappropriate goals, (d) formulation of developmentally and/or culturally inappropriate procedures, (e) consistent shifting of goals in session, and (f) failure to modify goal-directed procedures in session with reference to the child's spontaneous behavior. (Often, the child was reprimanded for not following the clinician's preplanned procedures.)

In contrast to the behavioral profile just presented, performance characteristics indicative of advanced developmental achievements include: (a) the use of conversational interactions in session, (b) a focus on client successes, (c) the setting of developmentally and culturally appropriate goals and procedures, (d) a consistent focus on a delimited set of goals in session, even when problems arise, (e) acknowledgment of the intent of children's spontaneous messages, and (f) modification of goal-directed procedures in session by incorporating aspects of children's spontaneous behavior into procedural plans.

4. Interact with the clinician in ways that provoke conflict resolution and perspective changing. Some suggestions for supervisors and professors aimed at conflict resolution and perspective changing, abstracted from Shapiro and Moses (1989, pp. 328–329), are as follows:

> Ask questions designed to encourage the clinician to explicate a point of view about the child's role in learning and language production, as well as the nature of language, and language learning (as when conducting an assessment of the clinician's developmental status in this area).
>
> Encourage and accept ideas that do not agree with your own point of view. This supports the clinician's thinking and independence in problem solving, and heightens awareness that the clinician's point of view is valuable and is a point of departure.
>
> Present your own point of view as another possibility to consider. This helps the clinician to identify and differentiate perspectives. It also helps identify sources of conflict and disequilibrium.
>
> Encourage the clinician to debate and justify clinical decisions in the course of intervention planning. According to Shapiro and Moses, it is sometimes advisable for the teacher or supervisor to intentionally contradict students to provoke such debates. The purpose is to shed light on conflicts arising from different perspectives and to provoke resolution.

Anchored Instruction. The technique of "anchored instruction" described by Michael et al. (1993) was designed to facilitate the generalization of knowledge about learning theories from the college classroom to clinical practice. It involves the promotion of collaborative problem solving in college classrooms. The supervisor or professor presents videotaped excerpts from actual speech-language intervention sessions and assigns groups of students the task of explaining the dynamics of the videotaped clinical interaction from the perspective of different learning theories. Students first view the clinical interactions applying principles derived from one particular learning theory (e.g., Vygotsky's social-cognitive theory). Then they reexamine the interaction from a different perspective (e.g., operant learning theory). In perhaps the only empirical data-based study of college-teaching techniques to date, Michael et al. compared the efficacy of traditional classroom instruction and anchored instruction on the transfer of knowledge of principles from three learning theories (operant, sociolinguistic, and Vygotsky's cognitive theory) to clinical practice in twenty-two speech-language pathology graduate students. They found that the students who received anchored instruction scored significantly higher on two measures of transfer-analyses of written and videotaped clinician-child interactions. Anchored instruction appears to facilitate the clinician's ability to use principles from various learning theories for planning and revising goals and procedures.

Facilitating Causal Reasoning in Clinicians

As we emphasized in the first part of this chapter, our model of intervention planning rests on the idea that linguistic performance is a product of a number of interacting variables. These include the components of language (form, content, and use), nonlinguistic maintaining factors (cognitive, psychosocial, and sensorimotor), and the nature of the immediate environment in which the child is expected to perform (i.e., context). As such, expertise in intervention planning necessitates the ability to reason about causal relations among this multitude of variables and the child's linguistic performance. It is essential that supervisors design procedures to help students engage in causal reasoning.

Inferring Linguistic Structures.   As discussed above, one of the most challenging aspects of causal reasoning for students is conceptualizing the nature and function of linguistic structures, such as content categories and syntactic rules. Students are similarly challenged to conceptualize the structure and function of other behavioral systems relevant to language, such as the valvular function of the oral musculature. Such structures, which are targeted at all phases of intervention planning, are not directly observable. They are, in reality, organizational or functional parameters of behavior. Their existence must be inferred. The student must observe and compare a variety of behaviors that appear to be different from one another. The task of the clinician is to identify underlying similarities or patterns that are consistent across seemingly disparate behaviors.

Our task as supervisors is twofold: It is to teach students how to identify such structures, and to aid students in developing a feeling for their nature and significance.

Students first encounter information relevant to this task in content courses such as linguistics, language acquisition, language disorders, phonology, and diagnostics. It is in these courses that students become familiar with developmental research and taxonomies, and learn procedures for performing developmental assessments. Referencing linguistic structures in intervention planning is, in part, theory driven. It makes sense if one believes that such structures actually exist in the mind. Nativist and constructivist theorists take such a position (Bloom, 1970; Chomsky, 1982a; Pinker, 1984, 1991). Behavioral and connectionist theorists do not (e.g., Mclelland & Rummelhart, 1986). See Pinker and Mehler (1988) for critiques of connectionism.

Given that the identification of linguistic structures is theory driven, it would be helpful for students to be exposed to supervisors who believed in such theories. It also is important that students' beliefs about language be considered during instruction. Furthermore, specific techniques should be developed to help students learn to evaluate linguistic organization. Some suggestions for supervisors in this area are:

1. Treat student's errors as information about the student's developmental status. Try not to react emotionally—with frustration or anger—at the clinician's behavior. Do not label the clinician's behavior with negative personality characteristics such as "stubbornness" or "laziness."

2. Make sure that the student has had coursework on child development, is familiar with developmental taxonomies, and has received instruction about procedures for conducting developmental assessments.

3. Videotape clinical interactions.

4. Encourage clinicians to describe clinician-child interactions objectively.

5. Have clinicians identify patterns of similarity in behavior described.

6. Encourage clinicians to work with peer groups in these problem-solving assignments.

7. Encourage clinicians to hypothesize about behavioral patterns, even if hypotheses do not agree with yours. Offer your insights as another set of possibilities to consider.

8. Encourage clinicians to consult published taxonomies and developmental research to guide the identification of patterns in children's behavior.

9. Encourage clinicians to discuss theoretical issues relevant to procedure planning, such as:

   —Where do organizational parameters come from (mind, environment, or interaction of the two)?

   —If parameters originate in the mind, how do these parameters develop?

   —If parameters originate in the environment or in an interaction, what conditions contribute to their development?

10. Tie these theoretic discussions to readings about theories of language learning.

Functional and Causal Interactions among Multiple Variables. Another challenging aspect of causal reasoning in intervention planning is the need to consider the interaction of multiple variables (the form, content, and use of language, nonlinguistic maintaining factors, and the nature of the immediate environment in which the child is expected to perform). Trends in clinician development related to this aspect of causal reasoning were discussed earlier and summarized in Box 8–3. The information in Box 8–3 illustrates that novices may naturally try to reduce the amount of information needing attention at any one time. The supervisor's job is to increase the clinician's capacity to consider interactions among multiple variables. Some procedural suggestions are as follows:

1. Make sure the clinician has taken courses that deal with the range of maintaining factors and other variables affecting performance. Often speech-language pathologists have not had background in social-emotional or sensorimotor development and their relations to speech and language (including the development of locomotor and oral motor functions). Sensorimotor information may be found in courses on cerebral palsy or in introductory courses offered by allied professionals.

2. Use videotaped excerpts of clinical interactions to illustrate factors that may be maintaining speech-language disabilities.

3. Engage students in problem-solving activities in which they think about possible interactions among variables that may be contributing to a child's speech-language performance. Be sure to have baseline data available to reference. Reward hypothesis generating and testing and the generation of possibilities, not only correct answers. Such problem-solving activities are particularly helpful after a clinical session. The student (perhaps with peers) should review sessions on videotape, identify problems that arise, and consider possible factors contributing to the problem.

4. Give students the opportunity to interact and engage in problem solving with allied professionals whose expertise lies in the areas of the maintaining factors. This requires coordinating clinical programs with allied fields at the university level. In all areas of speech and language, we find interactions with occupational and physical therapists to be especially useful.

Envisioning Multiple Possible Solutions to Problems

The next developmental competency relevant to intervention planning that will be considered is the ability to envision multiple possible solutions to problems. This competency interacts with perspective taking and the general ability to handle information. As such, this competency is central to planning and revising intervention procedures while keeping goals constant. Novice clinicians often are able to think of one type of clinical procedure per goal (Moses & Shapiro, 1992; in progress). The following are some suggestions for facilitating this developmental skill:

1. Spend time familiarizing students with principles of learning theories. Encourage students to design a number of materials, games, and interactions with reference to specific principles. The objective is to help students discover that theoretical principles are generative, i.e., they lead to many different procedural possibilities.

2. Allow students time to play with children. Ask students to design materials, games, and interactions. The purpose should be to engage children in goal-directed activity (allowing the child to set goals, too) and to have fun. Encourage students to hypothesize what children might learn from specific play activities.

3. Engage students in collaborative problem solving after clinical sessions. Students should identify clinical problems and variables contributing to the problem, and suggest possible alternative solutions with reference to causal factors identified. Again, reward hypothesis generating and testing (i.e., the generation of possibilities). The supervisor should not be concerned solely with the correctness or incorrectness of the clinician's ideas.

4. As suggested above, give students the opportunity to engage in problem solving with allied professionals who are knowledgable about behaviors that may be maintaining a speech-language disorder. Also give students the opportunity to interact with caretakers. Students may discover a wealth of procedural possibilities—and learn about available resources—by collaborating with allied professionals and the child's caretakers.

Role Diffusion

The ability to engage in role diffusion is the final competency we have targeted for supervision in intervention planning. Recall that we defined role diffusion as the sharing of expertise with others and acceptance of professional guidance from others who may not be speech-language pathologists (see Chapter 7). It is our experience that many conflicts arise in the course of collaboration related to role diffusion. These conflicts are tied to issues of self-esteem, funds of knowledge, and ability to evaluate multiple dimensions of behavior from multiple perspectives (Connor, Williamson, & Siepp, 1978; Linder, 1990). Thus, role diffusion comprises a developmental component that needs to be addressed in the course of clinical training and supervision. The following are some procedural suggestions:

1. Give students the opportunity, at all phases of intervention planning, to collaborate with their clients' families, with fellow students, and with allied professionals.
2. Set goals that target communication skills relevant to collaboration. These goals would involve pragmatic skills related to leadership, peer interactions, persuasion, and conflict identification and resolution.
3. Circumscribe professional boundaries that need to be *maintained* during collaboration. Although we believe that the sharing of expertise is important, we also believe that each member of a team brings a special expertise to intervention planning. This expertise is central to the collaborative process, and to the sharing and learning that are central to role diffusion. Each member of a team needs to perceive himself or herself as knowledgable and as the recipient of respect from colleagues.
4. Pay attention to the emotional status of the speech-language clinician. Acknowledge feelings of anxiety and shame, as well as those of confidence, excitement, and professional commitment. The emotional aspect of professional life is easily overlooked. Emotional well-being is, however, most crucial to professional development.

Case Management Forms

A set of case management forms has been provided in the appendices. Appendix B includes the following forms: Areas of Assessment for Intervention Planning (B–1), Summary of Baseline Data for Intervention Planning (B–2), Management Plan (B–3, Long-Term Goals and Procedures, Short-Term Goals and Procedures, Session Goals and Procedures), and IEP Conversion Form (B–4). Collaboration forms may be found in Appendix E. These forms serve several functions.

The management forms have two purposes: First, they may be used for systematic recordkeeping on individual clients enrolled in the university clinic. They also are designed to serve a number of instructional functions. Forms B–1 and B–2 may be referenced by students enrolled in a diagnostic practicum. When these forms are completed they provide a summary of baseline data for intervention planning and illustrate the relationship between diagnostic and intervention processes. Form B–3 provides a framework in which the student may develop goals and procedures across the three phases of intervention planning. The forms have been designed to obligate the student to think through the formulation of goal and procedure statements. The student must include rationales that incorporate information consistent with the model of intervention planning presented in this book (e.g., baseline data, maintaining factors, etc.). By engaging students in problem solving relative to these rationales, the competencies underlying expertise in intervention planning (Chapter 8) may be facilitated. In addition, Form B–3 (comprising three sections) is presented as a single unit to emphasize the continuity necessary across phases of intervention.

References

Adams, R. (1980). The young stutterer: Diagnosis, treatment and assessment of progress. *Seminars in Speech, Language and Hearing, 1,* 289–299.

Ainsworth, S. (1948). *Speech correction methods.* New York: Prentice-Hall.

American Speech-Language-Hearing Association. Committee on Supervision in Speech-Language Pathology and Audiology. (1985). Clinical supervision in speech-language pathology and audiology (Position statement). *ASHA, 27,* 57–60.

American Speech-Language-Hearing Association. Committee on Supervision in Speech-Language Pathology and Audiology. (1989). Preparation models for the supervisory process in speech-language pathology and audiology (A tutorial). *ASHA, 31,* 97–106.

American Speech-Language-Hearing Association. (1991). A model for collaborative service delivery for students with language-learning disorders in the public school. *ASHA, 33* (Suppl. 5), 44–50.

Anderson, J.L. (1988). *The supervisory process in speech-language pathology and audiology.* Boston: Little Brown/College Hill.

Anderson, N.B. (1991). Understanding cultural diversity. *American Journal of Speech Language Pathology, 1,* 9–10.

Andrews, M.L. (1986). *Voice therapy for children.* New York: Longman.

Andrews, M.L., & Summers, A.C. (1993). A voice stimulation program for preschoolers: Theory and practice. *Language, Speech, and Hearing Services, 24,* 140–145.

Aram, D., & Nation, J. (1982). *Child language disorders.* St. Louis: Mosby.

Atkinson, R.C., & Shiffrin, R.M. (1971). The control of short-term memory. *Scientific American, 225,* 82–90.

Barnes, S., Gutfreund, M., Satterly, D., & Wells, G. (1983). Characteristics of adult speech which predict children's language development. *Journal of Child Language, 10,* 65–84.

Bates, E., Benigni, L., Bretherton, I., Camaioni, L., & Volterra, V. (1979). *The emergence of symbols: Communication and cognition in infancy.* New York: Academic Press.

Bateson, G. (1980). *Mind and nature: A necessary unity.* New York: Bantam.

Bellugi, U. (1967). *The acquisition of negation.* Unpublished doctoral dissertation, Harvard University.

Benner, S. (1992). *Assessing young children with special needs.* White Plains, NY: Longman.

Bennett, T., Lingerfelt, B.V., & Nelson, D.E. (1990). *Developing individualized family support plans.* Cambridge, MA: Brookline.

Bernstein-Ratner, N. (1988). Patterns of parental vocabulary selection in speech to very young children. *Journal of Child Language, 15,* 481–492.

Bernthal J.E., & Bankson, N. (1988). *Articulation and phonological disorders* (2nd ed.). Englewood Cliffs, NJ: Prentice-Hall.

Berry, M., & Eisenson, J. (1956). *Speech disorders: Principles and practices of therapy.* New York: Appleton-Century-Crofts.

Bigge, J. (1988). *Curriculum based instruction for special education students.* Mountain View, CA: Mayfield.

Blank, M., Rose, S., & Berlin, L. (1978). *Preschool language assessment instrument: The language of learning in practice.* New York: Grune & Stratton.

Bloodstein, O. (1969). *A handbook on stuttering.* Chicago: National Easter Seal Society.

Bloodstein, O. (1981). *A handbook on stuttering.* Chicago: National Easter Seal Society.

Bloom, K. (1988). Quality of adult vocalizations affects the quality of infant vocalizations. *Journal of Child Language, 15,* 469–480.

Bloom, L. (1970) *Language development: Form and function in emerging grammars.* Cambridge, MA: Massachusetts Institute of Technology Press.

Bloom, L. (1991). *Language development from two to three.* New York: Cambridge University Press.

Bloom, L., Beckwith, R., Capatides, J., & Hafitz, J. (1988). Expression through affect and words in the transition from infancy to language. In P. Baltes, D. Feathernam, & R. Lerner (Eds.), *Life-span development and behavior* (Vol. 8, pp. 99–127). Hillsdale, NJ: Erlbaum.

Bloom L., & Capatides, J. (1987). Expression of affect and the emergence of language. *Child Development, 58,* 1513–1522.

Bloom, L., Hood, L., & Lightbown, P. (1974). Imitation in language development: If, when, and why. *Cognitive Psychology, 6,* 380–420.

Bloom, L., & Lahey, M. (1978). *Language development and language disorders.* New York: Wiley.

Bloom, L., Lahey, M., Hood, L., Lifter, K., & Fiess, K. (1980). Complex sentences: Acquisition of syntactic connectives and the semantic relations they encode. *Journal of Child Language, 7,* 235–261.

Bloom, L., Lightbown, P., & Hood, L. (1975). Structure and variation in child language. *Monographs of the society for research in child development, 40* (2, Serial No. 160).

Bloom, L., Miller, P., & Hood, L. (1975). Variation and reduction as aspects of competence in language development. In A. Pick (Ed.), *Minnesota Symposia on Child Psychology* (Vol. 9, pp. 3–55). Minneapolis: University of Minnesota Press.

Bloom, L., Rispoli, M., Gartner, B., & Hafitz, J. (1989). Acquisition of complementation. *Journal of Child Language, 16,* 101–120.

Bloom, L., Rocissano, L., & Hood, L. (1976). Adult-child discourse: Developmental intervention between information processing and linguistic knowledge. *Cognitive Psychology, 8,* 521–552.

Bloom, L., Tackeff, J., & Lahey, M. (1984). Learning *to* in complement constructions. *Journal of Child Language, 11,* 391–406.

Bobath, B. (1971a). *Abnormal postural reflex activity caused by brain lesions.* London: Heinemann.

Bobath, B. (1971b). Motor development, its effect on general development, and application to the treatment of cerebral palsy. *Physiotherapy, 57,* 1–7.

Bobath, B. & Bobath, K. (1981). *Motor development in the different types of cerebral palsy.* London: Heinemann.

Bornstein, M.H. (1984). Color name versus shape-name learning in young children. *Journal of Child Language, 12,* 387–393.

Bracken, B. (1984). *Bracken basic concept scale.* San Antonio, TX: Psychological Corporation.

Braine, M.D.S. (1963). The ontogeny of English phrase structure: The first phase. *Language, 39,* 1–13.

Braine, M.D.S. (1990). The "natural logic" approach to reasoning. In W.F. Overton (Ed.), *Reasoning, necessity, and logic* (pp. 135–138). Hillsdale, NJ: Erlbaum.

Brandt, R. (Ed.). (1991). The reflective educator. *Educational Leadership, 48,* 10.

Bransford, J., Sherwood, R., Vye, N., & Reiser, J. (1986). Teaching, thinking, and problem-solving. *American Psychologist, 41,* 1078–1089.

Bricker, W.A., & Bricker, D.D. (1974). An early language-training strategy. In R.L. Schiefelbusch, & L.L. Lloyd (Eds.), Language perspectives to Acquistion, retardation, and intervention (pp. 431–468). Baltimore: University Park Press.

Brown, R. (1968). The development of Wh questions in child speech. *Journal of Verbal Learning and Verbal Behavior, 7,* 279–290.

Brown, R. (1973). *A first language: The early stages.* Cambridge, MA: Harvard University Press.

Brown, R., & Belluggi, U. (1964). Three processes in the acquisition of syntax. *Harvard Educational Review, 34,* 133–151.

Bruner, J.S. (1964). The course of cognitive growth. *American Psychologist, 19,* 1–15.

Bruner J.S. (1975). The ontogenesis of speech acts. *Journal of Child Language, 2,* 1–19.

Bruner, J.S. (1983). *Child talk.* New York: Norton.

Byrnes, J.P. (1988). Formal operations: A systematic reformulation. *Developmental Review, 8,* 1–22.

Camarata, S., & Gandour, J. (1984). On describing idiosyncratic phonologic systems. *Journal of Speech and Hearing Disorders, 49,* 262–266.

Campbell, T., & Bain, B. (1991). How long to treat: A multiple outcome approach. *Language, Speech, and Hearing Services in Schools, 22,* 271–276.

Carney, P. (1991). Competence: An ethical decision. *ASHA, 33,* 7–8.

Carrow-Woolfolk, E. (1985). *Test for auditory comprehension of language.* Allen, TX: DLM Teaching Resources.

Carrow-Woolfolk, E. (1988). *Theory, assessment, and intervention in language disorders: an integrative approach.* New York: Grune and Stratton.

Case, R. (1985). *Intellectual development from birth to adulthood.* Orlando, FL: Academic Press.

Casey, P.L., Smith, K.J., & Ulrich, S.R. (1988). *Self-supervision: A career tool for audiologists and speech-language pathologists.* Rockville, MD: National Student Speech-Language-Hearing Association.

Cecconi, C.P., Hood, S.B., & Tucker, R.K. (1977). Influence of reading level difficulty on the disfluencies of normal children. *Journal of Speech and Hearing Research, 20,* 475–494.

Cheng, P., & Holyoake, K. (1985). Pragmatic reasoning schemas. *Cognitive Psychology, 17,* 391–416.

Chiesa, M. (1992). Radical behaviorism and scientific frameworks: From mechanistic to relational accounts. *American Psychologist, 47,* 1287–1299.

Chomsky, N. (1957). *Syntactic structures*. The Hague: Mouton.

Chomsky, N. (1959). Review of "Verbal Behavior" by B.F. Skinner. *Language, 35,* 26–58.

Chomsky, N. (1965). *Aspects of the theory of syntax*. Cambridge, MA: Massachusetts Institute of Technology Press.

Chomsky, N. (1982a). *The generative enterprise: A discussion with Riny Huybregts and Henk van Riemsdijk*. Dordecht, Holland: Foris.

Chomsky, N. (1982b). Some concepts and consequences of the theory of government and binding. *Linguistic Inquiry Monograph, 6*. Cambridge, MA: Massachusetts Institute of Technology Press.

Chomsky, N., & Halle, M. (1968). *The sound pattern of English*. New York: Harper and Row.

Christensen, S.S., & Luckett, C.H. (1990). Getting into the classroom and making it work. *Language, Speech and Hearing Services in Schools, 21,* 110–113.

Colburn, N., & Mysak, E. (1982a). Developmental dysfluency and emerging grammar I: Dysfluency characteristics in early syntactic utterances. *Journal of Speech and Hearing Research, 25,* 414–420.

Colburn, N., & Mysak, E.D. (1982b). Developmental dysfluency and emerging grammar II: Co-occurrence of dysfluency with specified semantic-syntactic structures. *Journal of Speech and Hearing Research, 25,* 421–427.

Cole, K., & Dale, P. (1986). Direct language instruction and interactive language instruction with language delayed preschool children: A comparison study. *Journal of Speech & Hearing Research, 29,* 206–217.

Compton, A.J. (1970). Generative studies of children's phonological disorders. *Journal of Speech and Hearing Disorders, 35,* 315–339.

Connell, P. (1987). An effect of modeling and imitation teaching procedures on children with and without specific language impairment. *Journal of Speech and Hearing Research, 30,* 105–113.

Connor, F.P., Williamson, G.G., & Siepp, J.M. (1978). *Program guide for infants and toddlers with neuromotor and other developmental disabilities*. New York: Teachers College Press.

Conture, E.G. (1990). *Stuttering*. Englewood Cliffs, NJ: Prentice-Hall.

Cook, R.E., Tessier, A., & Klein, M.D. (1992). *Adapting early childhood curricula for children with special needs*. New York: Merill.

Cooper, C.S. (1991). Using collaborative/consultative service delivery models for fluency intervention and carryover. *Language, Speech and Hearing Services in Schools, 22,* 152–153.

Cornett, B., & Chabon, S. (1988). *The clinical practice of speech-language pathology*. Columbus, OH: Merrill.

Courtright, J., & Courtright, I. (1976). Imitative modeling as a theoretical base for instructing language-disordered children. *Journal of Speech and Hearing Research, 19,* 655–663.

Courtright, J., & Courtright, I. (1979). Imitative modeling as a language intervention strategy: The effects of two mediating variables. *Journal of Speech and Hearing Research, 22,* 389–402.

Craik, F.I.M., & Lockhart, R.S. (1972). Levels of processing: A framework for memory research. *Journal of Verbal Learning and Verbal Behavior, 11,* 671–684.

Craik, F.I.M., & Tulving, E. (1975). Depth of processing and the retention of words in episodic memory. *Journal of Experimental Psychology, 104,* 268–294.

Creaghead, N.A., Estomin, E.R., Freilinger, J.J., & Peters-Johnson, C. (1992). *ASHA transcript series: Classroom integration and collaborative consultation as service delivery models*. Rockville Pike, MD: American Speech-Language-Hearing Association.

Creaghead, N.A., Newman, P.W., & Secord, W.A. (1989). *Assessment and remediation of articulatory and phonological disorders*. Columbus, OH: Merrill.

Crelin, E.S. (1973). *Functional anatomy of the newborn*. New Haven, CT: Yale University Press.

Crelin, E.S. (1976). Development of the upper respiratory system. *Ciba Clinical Symposia, 28*, 3–26.

Cross, T. (1977). Mothers' speech adjustments: The contribution of selected child listener variables. In C. Snow & C. Ferguson (Eds.), *Talking to children.* (pp. 151–188). New York: Cambridge University Press.

Cruickshank, W.M. (1967). *The brain-injured child in home, school, and society*. New York: Syracuse University Press.

Culatta, B., Horn, D.G., & Theodore, G. (1992). *Scripted play and story enactments to facilitate language and literacy*. Seminar presented at the 1992 national convention of the American Speech-Language-Hearing Association, San Antonio, TX, October 22.

Culatta, B., Page, L.L., & Ellis, J. (1983). Story retelling as a communicative performance screening tool. *Speech, Language, and Hearing Services in Schools, 14*, 66–74.

Davis, L. (1987). Respiration and phonation in cerebral palsy: A developmental model. *Seminars in Speech and Language, 8*, 101–105.

Deal, R.E., & Belcher, R.A. (1990). Reliability of children's ratings of vocal roughness. *Language, Speech, and Hearing Services in Schools, 21*, 68–71.

DeRuiter, J.A., & Wansart, W.L. (1982). *Psychology of learning disabilities*. Rockville, MD: Aspen.

deVilliers, J., & DeVilliers, P. (1978). *Language acquisition*. Cambridge, MA.: Harvard University Press.

Dickson, S. (Ed.). (1984). *Communication disorders: Remedial principles and practices* (2nd. ed.). Glenview, IL: Scott Foresman.

Dinnsen, D., Chin, S., Elbert, M., & Powell, T. (1990). Some constraints on functionally disordered phonologies: Phonetic inventories and phonotactics. *Journal of Speech and Hearing Research, 33*, 28–37.

Dollaghan, C., & Kaston, N. (1986). A comprehension monitoring program for language impaired children. *Journal of Speech and Hearing Disorders, 51*, 264–271.

Dore, J. (1974). A pragmatic description of early language development. *Journal of Psycholinguistic Research, 3*, 343–348.

Dowling, S. (1992). *Implementing the supervisory process: Theory and practice*. Englewood Cliffs, NJ: Prentice-Hall.

Duchan, J., & Weitzner-Lin, B. (1987). Nurturant-naturalistic intervention for language- impaired children: Implications for planning lessons and tracking progress. *ASHA, 28*, 45–49.

Duckworth, E. (1972). The having of wonderful ideas. *Harvard Educational Review, 42*, 217–231.

Duckworth, E. (1976). And some comments on learning to spell. *The Urban Review, 9*, 121–123.

Duckworth, E. (1984). Symposium on the year of the reports: Responses from the educational community. *Harvard Educational Review, 54*, 297–312.

Dunn, L., & Dunn, L. (1981). *Peabody picture vocabulary test—revised.* Circle Pines, MN: American Guidance Service.

Dyer, K., Williams, L., & Luce, S.C. (1991). Training teachers to use naturalistic communication strategies in classrooms for students with autism and other severe handicaps. *Language, Speech, and Hearing Services in Schools, 22,* 313–321.

Edwards, M.L. (1992). Clinical forum: Phonological assessment and treatment: In support of phonological processes. *Language, Speech, and Hearing Services in Schools, 23,* 233–240.

Edwards, M.L., & Shriberg, L. (1983). *Phonology: Applications in communicative disorders.* San Diego: College Hill Press.

Eiger, D. (1988). Accountability in action: Entry, measurement, exit. *Seminars in Speech and Language, 9,* 299–319.

Eiger, D., Chabon, S., Mient, M., & Cushman, B. (1986). When is enough, enough? Articulation therapy dismissal considerations in the public schools. *ASHA, 28,* 23–25.

Eilers, R.E. (1980). Infant speech perception: History and mystery. In G. Yeni-Komshian, J. Kavanagh, & C.A. Ferguson (Eds.), *Child Phonology: Vol. 2. Perception* (pp. 23–39). New York: Academic Press.

Eimas, P. (1985). The perception of speech in early infancy. *Scientific American, 252,* 46–61.

Elbert, M. (1992). Clinical forum: Phonological assessment and treatment: Consideration of error types: A response to Fey. *Language, Speech, and Hearing Services in Schools, 23,* 241–246.

Elbert, M., Dinnsen, D., & Powell, T. (1984). On the prediction of phonologic generalization learning patterns. *Journal of Speech and Hearing Disorders, 49,* 309–317.

Elbert, M., Dinnsen, D., Swartzlander, P., & Chin, S. (1990). Generalization to conversational speech. *Journal of Speech and Hearing Disorders, 55,* 694–699.

Elbert, M., & Gierut, J. (1986). *Handbook of clinical phonology: Approaches to assessment and treatment.* San Diego: College Hill Press.

Elbert, M., Powell, T., & Swartzlander, P. (1991). Toward a technology of generalization: How many exemplars are sufficient? *Journal of Speech and Hearing Research, 34,* 81–87.

Emslie, C., & Stevenson, J. (1981). Pre-school children's use of the articles in definite and indefinite referring expressions. *Journal of Child Language, 8,* 313–328.

Englemann, S., & Bruner, E.C. (1969). *DISTAR: An instructional system.* Chicago: Science Research Associates.

Englemann, S., & Osborne, J. (1972). *DISTAR: Lnguage levels I and II.* Chicago, IL: Science Research Associates.

Ervin-Tripp, S., & Mitchell-Kernan, C. (Eds.). (1977). *Child discourse.* New York: Academic Press.

Farber, N.G. (1990). Puzzled minds and weird creatures: Spontaneous inquiry and phases in knowledge construction. In I. Harel (Ed.), *Constructionist learning.* (pp. 1–16). Cambridge, MA: Massachusetts Institute of Technology Media Laboratory.

Farmer, S.S., & Farmer, J.L. (1989). *Supervision in communication disorders.* Columbus, OH: Merrill.

Ferguson, C.A. (1978). Learning to pronounce: The earliest stages of phonological development in the child. In F. D. Minifie & L.L. Lloyd (Eds.), *Communicative and cognitive abilities: early behavioral assessment* (pp. 237–297). Baltimore: University Park Press.

Ferguson, C.A., & Macken, M.A. (1980). Phonological development in children: Play and cognition. *Papers and Reports in Child Language Development, 18,* 133–177.

Fey, M.E. (1986). *Language intervention with young children.* San Diego: College Hill Press.

Fey, M.E. (1988). Generalization issues facing language interventionists: An introduction. *Language, Speech, and Hearing Services in Schools, 19,* 272–281.

Fey, M.E. (1992a). Clinical forum: Phonological assessment and treatment: Articulation and phonology: Inextricable constructs in speech pathology. *Language, Speech, and Hearing Services in Schools, 23,* 225–232.

Fey, M.E. (1992b). Clinical forum: Phonological assessment and treatment: Articulation and phonology: An addendum. *Language, Speech, and Hearing Services in Schools, 23,* 277–282.

Finnie, N.R. (1975). *Handling the young cerebral palsy child at home.* New York: Dutton.

Fiorentino, M.R. (1972). *Normal and abnormal development: The influence of primitive reflexes on motor development.* Springfield, IL: Thomas.

Fischer, K.W. (1989). *The failure of competence: How context contributes directly to skill.* Paper presented at the Nineteenth Annual Symposium of the Jean Piaget Society, Philadelphia, PA, June 1.

Fischer, K.W. (1980). A theory of cognitive development: The control and construction of hierarchies of skills. *Psychological Review, 87,* 477–531.

Fischer, K.W., & Pipp, S.L. (1984). Processes of cognitive development: Optimal level and skill acquisition. In R. Sternberg (Ed.), *Mechanisms of cognitive development* (pp. 45–80). New York: Freeman.

Forman, G.E. (Ed.). (1982). *Action and thought: From sensorimotor schemes to symbolic operations.* New York: Academic Press.

Forman, G.E., & Hill, F. (1984). *Constructive play: Applying Piaget in the preschool.* Montvale, CA: Wellesley.

Fosnot, K. (1991). *Enquiring learners, enquiring teachers.* New York: Teachers College Press.

Friedlander, B.Z. (1970). Receptive language development in infancy: Issues and problems. *Merrill-Palmer Quarterly, 16,* 7–51.

Furrow, D., & Nelson, K. (1986). A further look at the motherese hypothesis: a reply to Gleitman, Newport & Gleitman. *Journal of Child Language, 13,* 163–176.

Furrow, D., Nelson, K., & Benedict, H. (1979). Mothers' speech to children and syntactic development: Some simple relationships. *Journal of Child Language, 6,* 423–442.

Galambos, J.A., Abelson, R.P., & Block, J.B. (Eds.). (1986). *Knowledge structures.* Hillsdale, NJ: Erlbaum.

Gallagher, J., & Reid, D.K. (1984). *The learning theory of Piaget and Inhelder.* Austin, TX: Pro Ed.

Gantwerk, B. (1985). Issues to address in criteria development. In American Speech-Language-Hearing Association (Ed.): *Caseload issues in schools: How to make better decisions.* Rockville, MD: American Speech-Language-Hearing Association (pp. 43–45).

Gardner, R. (1983). *One-word expressive vocabulary test.* Novato, CA: Academic Therapy Publications.

Garvey, C. (1975). Requests and responses in children's speech. *Journal of Child Language, 2,* 41–63.

Gelmen, S.A., & Markman, E.M. (1984). Implicit contrast in adjectives vs. nouns: Implications for word-learning in preschoolers. *Journal of Child Language, 11,* 125–143.

Gentner, D., & Stevens, A.L. (1983). *Mental models.* Hillsdale, NJ: Erlbaum.

Geschwind, N. (1984). The brain of a learning disabled child. *Annals of Dyslexia, 34,* 613–620.

Gierut, J. (1989). Maximal opposition approach to phonological treatment. *Journal of Speech and Hearing Disorders, 54,* 9–19.

Gierut, J. (1990). Differential learning of phonological oppositions. *Journal of Speech and Hearing Research, 33,* 540–549.

Gierut, J., Elbert, M., & Dinnsen, D. (1987). A functional analysis of phonological knowledge and generalization learning in misarticulating children. *Journal of Speech and Hearing Research, 30,* 462–479.

Ginsberg, G., & Kilbourne, B. (1988). Emergence of vocal alternation in mother-infant interchanges. *Journal of Child Language, 15,* 221–235.

Gleitman, L.R., Newport, E.L., & Gleitman, H. (1984). The current status of the motherese hypothesis. *Journal of Child Language, 11,* 43–79.

Glenn, S., Ellis, J., & Greenspoon, J. (1992). On the revolutionary nature of the operant as a unit of behavioral selection. *American Psychologist, 47,* 1329–1336.

Goldberg, S.A. (1993). *Clinical intervention: A philosophy and methodology for clinical practice.* New York: Macmillan.

Goldman, R., & Fristoe, M. (1986). *The Goldman-Fristoe test of articulation.* Circle Pines, MN: American Guidance Service.

Goldstein, K. (1948). *Language and language disturbances.* New York: Grune & Stratton.

Gopnik, A. (1984). The acquisition of *gone* and the development of object concept. *Journal of Child Language, 11,* 273–292.

Gopnik, A., & Meltzoff, A. (1984). Semantic and cognitive development in 15–21-month old children. *Journal of Child Language, 11,* 495–514.

Gopnik, A., & Meltzoff, A. (1987). The development of categorization in the second year and its relation to other cognitive and linguistic developments. *Child Development, 58,* 1523–1531.

Green, G. (1989). Psycho-behavioral characteristics of children with vocal nodules: WPBIC ratings. *Journal of Speech and Hearing Disorders, 54,* 306–312.

Greenfield, P.M., & Smith, J.H. (1976). *The structure of communication in early language development.* New York: Academic Press.

Gregory, H., & Hill, D. (1980). Stuttering therapy for children. *Seminars in Speech, Language, and Hearing, 1,* 351–363.

Gropen, J., Pinker, S., Hollander, M., & Goldberg, R. (1991). Syntax and semantics in the acquisition of locative verbs. *Journal of Child Language, 18,* 115–152.

Grunwell, P. (1981). *The nature of phonological disability in children.* New York: Academic Press.

Grunwell, P. (1985). *Phonological assessment of child speech.* San Diego: College Hill Press.

Guess, D., Sailor, W., & Baer, D.M. (1974). To teach language to retarded children. In R.L. Schiefelbusch & L.L. Lloyd (Eds.), *Language perspectives—Acquisition, retardation, intervention* (pp. 529–606). Baltimore: University Park Press.

Hall, D.E., Wray, D.F., & Conti, D.M. (1986). The language-dysfluency relation. *Hearsay, 2,* 110–113.

Halliday, M.A.K. (1975). *Learning how to mean: Explorations in the development of language.* London: Edward Arnold.

Hammill, D.D. (1985). *Detroit tests of learning aptitude.* Austin, TX: Pro Ed.

Hammill, D.D., & Bartel, N.R. (Eds.). (1985). *Teaching children with learning and behavior problems.* Boston: Allyn & Bacon.

Hammill, D., & Newcomer, P.L. (1982). *Test of language development—Intermediate edition.* San Antonio, TX: Psychological Corporation.

Hanson, M. J., Lynch, E.W., & Wayman, K.I. (1990). Honoring the cultural diversity of families when gathering data. *Topics in Early Childhood Special Education, 10,* 112–131.

Hayes, S.C., & Hayes, L.J. (1992). Verbal relations and the evolution of behavior analysis. *American Psychologist, 47,* 1383–1395.

Hegde, M.N. (1985). *Treatment procedures in communicative disorders.* Boston: Little Brown.

Hegde, M.N., & Davis, D. (1992). *Clinical methods and practicum in speech-language pathology.* San Diego: Singular.

Hegde, M., & McCann, J. (1981). Language training: Some data on response classes and generalization to an occupational setting. *Journal of Speech and Hearing Disorders, 46,* 353–358.

Hirano, M., Kurita, S., & Nakashima, T. (1981). The structure of the vocal folds. In N. Stevens & M. Hirano (Eds.), *Vocal fold physiology* (pp. 33–41). Tokyo: University of Tokyo Press.

Hodson, B. (1992). Clinical forum: Phonological assessment and treatment: Applied phonology: Constructs, contributions, and issues. *Language, Speech, and Hearing Services in Schools, 23,* 247–253.

Hodson, B., & Paden, E. (1991). *Targeting intelligible speech.* Austin, TX: Pro Ed.

Hoff-Ginsberg, E. (1985). Some contributions of mothers' speech to their children's syntactic growth. *Journal of Child Language, 12,* 367–386.

Hoff-Ginsberg, E. (1990). Maternal speech and the child's development of syntax: A further look. *Journal of Child Language, 17,* 85–99.

Hoffman, P.R. (1992). Clinical forum: Phonological assessment and treatment: Synergistic development of phonetic skill. *Language, Speech, and Hearing Services in Schools, 23,* 254–260.

Howell, J., & Dean, E. (1987). I think that's a noisy sound: Reflection and learning in the therapeutic situation. *Clinical Language Teaching and Therapy, 3,* 259–266.

Hsu, J.R., Cairns, H.S., Eisenberg, S., & Schlisselberg, G. (1989). Control and coreference in early child language. *Journal of Child Language, 16,* 339–353.

Hsu, J.R., Cairns, H.S., & Fiengo, R. (1985). The development of grammars underlying children's interpretations of complex sentences. *Cognition, 20,* 25–48.

Hsu, J.R., Cairns, H.S., & Schlisselberg, G. (1991). When do children avoid backwards coreference? *Journal of Child Language, 18,* 339–353.

Hubbell, R.D. (1988). *A handbook of English grammar and language sampling.* Englewood Cliffs, NJ: Prentice-Hall.

Hyams, N. (1986). *Language acquisition and the theory of parameters.* Dordecht, Holland: D. Reidel.

Hymes, D. (1971). Compentence and performance in linguistic theory. In R. Huxley & E. Ingram (Eds.), *Language acquisition models and methods* (pp. 3–24). New York: Academic Press.

Idol, L., Paolucci-Whitcomb, P., & Nevin, A. (1986). *Collaborative consultation.* Rockville, MD: Aspen.

Ingram, D. (1974). Phonological rules in young children. *Journal of Child Language, 1,* 49–64.

Ingram, D. (1976). *Phonological disability in children.* New York: Elsevier.

Ingram, D. (1989a). *First language acquisition: Method, description and explanation.* New York: Cambridge University Press.

Ingram, D. (1989b). *Phonological disability in children.* (2nd ed.). San Diego: Singular Publishing Group.

Inhelder, B., & Piaget, J. (1958). *The growth of logical thinking from childhood to adolescence.* New York: Basic Books.

Inhelder, B., Sinclair, H., & Bovet, M. (1974). *Learning and the development of cognition.* Cambridge, MA: Harvard University Press.

Jackson, H. (1915). *Selected writings of J. Hughlings Jackson.* London: Hodder and Stoughton.

James, S., & Seebach, M. (1982). The pragmatic function of children's questions. *Journal of Speech and Hearing Research, 25,* 2–11.

Johnson, C. (1985). The emergence of present perfect verb forms: Semantic influences on selective imitation. *Journal of Child Language, 12,* 325–352.

Johnson, D.J., & Myklebust, H.R. (1967). *Learning disabilities: Educational principles and practices.* New York: Grune & Stratton.

Johnson, D.W., & Johnson, R. (1975). *Learning together and alone.* Englewood Cliffs, NJ: Prentice-Hall.

Johnson, E.G. (1977). The development of color knowledge in preschool children. *Child Development, 48,* 308–311.

Johnson, W., Brown, S.F., Curtis, J.F., Edney, C.W., & Keaster, J. (1967). *Speech handicapped school children.* New York: Harper & Row.

Jones, S.S., & Smith, L.S. (1991). Object properties and knowledge in early lexical learning. *Child Development, 62,* 499–516.

Kagan, J., & Lemkin, J. (1961). Form, color, and size in children's conceptual behavior. *Child Development, 32,* 25–28.

Kahane, J.C. (1983). Postnatal development and aging of the human larynx. *Seminars in Speech and Language, 4,* 189–303.

Kamhi, A., Lee, R., & Nelson, L. (1985). Word, syllable and sound awareness in language disordered children. *Journal of Speech and Hearing Disorders, 50,* 207–212.

Kamhi, A. G. (1982). Overextensions and underextensions: How different are they? *Journal of Child Language, 9,* 243–247.

Kamhi, A.G. (1988). A reconceptualization and generalization problems. *Language, Speech, and Hearing Services in Schools, 19,* 304–313.

Kamhi, A.G. (1989). Nonlinguistic symbolic and conceptual abilities of language-impaired and normally developing children. *Journal of Speech and Hearing Research, 24,* 446–453.

Kamhi, A.G. (1992). Clinical forum: Phonological assessment and treatment: The need for a broad based model of phonological disorders. *Language, Speech, and Hearing Services in Schools, 23,* 261–268.

Kamhi, A.G. (1993). Research into practice: Some problems with the marriage between theory and clinical practice. *Language, Speech, and Hearing Services in Schools, 24,* 57–60.

Kamii, C.K., & DeVries, R. (1993). *Physical knowledge in preschool education: Implications of Piaget's theory.* New York: Teachers College Press.

Kamii, C.K. (1985). *Young children reinvent arithmetic: Implications of Piaget's theory.* New York: Teachers College Press.

Kaplan, E.L. (1970). Intonation and language acquisition. *Child language and development.* Number 1: committee on linguistics, Stanford, CA: Stanford University.

Karmiloff-Smith, A. (1979). *A functional approach to child language.* Cambridge, UK: Cambridge University Press.

Karmiloff-Smith, A. (1986a). From meta-processes to conscious access: Evidence from children's metalinguistic and repair data. *Cognition, 23,* 95–147.

Karmiloff-Smith, A. (1986b). Stage/structure versus phase/process in modelling linguistic and cognitive development. In I. Levin (Ed.), *Stage and Structure* (pp. 192–212). Norwood, NJ: Ablex.

Karmiloff-Smith, A., & Inhelder, B. (1975). If you want to get ahead, get a theory. *Cognition, 3,* 192–212.

Kemp, J. (1983). The timing of language intervention for the pediatric population. In J. Miller, D. Yoder, & R. Schiefelbusch (Eds.), *Contemporary issues in language intervention* (pp. 183–195). ASHA Report No. 12.

Kent, R.D. (1976). Tutorial: Anatomical and neuromuscular maturation of the speech mechanism. *Journal of Speech and Hearing Research, 19,* 421–447.

Kent, R.D. (1980). Articulatory and acoustic perspectives on speech development. In A.P. Reilly (Ed.), *The communication game: perspectives on the development of speech, language, and non-verbal communication skills.* (Johnson & Johnson Pediatric Round Table Series: 4), 38–43.

Kent, R.D. (1982). Contextual facilitation of correct sound production. *Language, Speech, and Hearing Services in Schools, 13,* 66–76.

Kent, R.D. (1992). The biology of phonological development. In C.A. Ferguson, L. Menn, & C. Stoel-Gammon (Eds.), *Phonological development: Models, research implications* (pp. 65–90). Timonium, MD: York Press.

Kent, R.D., & Bauer, H. (1985). Vocalizations of one-year-olds. *Journal of Child Language, 12,* 491–526.

Kent, R.D., & Lybolt, J.T. (1982) Techniques of therapy based on motor learning theory. In W.H. Perkins (Ed.), *General principles of therapy* (pp. 13–25). New York: Thieme-Stratton.

Kent, R.D., & Murray, A.D. (1982). Acoustic features of infant vocalic utterances at 3, 6, and 9 months. *Journal of the Acoustical Society of America, 72,* 353–365.

Kirk, S.A., McCarthy, J., & Kirk, W.D. (1968). *The Illinois test of psycholinguistic abilities.* (rev. ed.) Urbana, IL: University of Illinois Press.

Kirk, U. (1983). *Neuropsychology of language, reading, and spelling.* Orlando, FL: Academic Press.

Klein, H.B. (1981a). Productive strategies for the pronunciation of early polysyllabic lexical items. *Journal of Speech and Hearing Research, 24,* 389–405.

Klein, H.B. (1981b). Perceptual strategies for the replication of consonants from polysyllabic lexical models. *Journal of Speech and Hearing Research, 24,* 535–551.

Klein, H.B. (1982). Hippopotamus is hard to say: The integration of lexical and phonological information. *Seminars in Speech, Language, and Hearing, 3,* 127–137.

Klein, H.B. (1984). Learning to stress: A case study. *Journal of Child Language, 11,* 375–390.

Klein, H.B. (1985). The relationship between early pronunciation processes and later pronunciation skill. *Journal of Speech and Hearing Disorders, 50,* 156–165.

Klein, H.B., Moses, N., & Altman, E. (1990). Communication of adults with learning disabilities: Self and others perceptions. *Journal of Learning Disabilities, 23,* 220–229.

Klein, H.B., Lederer, S.H., & Cortese, E.E. (1991). Children's knowledge of auditory/articulatory correspondences: Phonologic and metaphonologic. *Journal of Speech and Hearing Research, 34,* 559–564.

Klein, H.B., & Spector, C.C. (1985). Effect of syllable stress and serial position on error variability in polysyllabic productions of speech-delayed children. *Journal of Speech and Hearing Disorders, 50,* 391–402.

Kuhn, D. (1989). Children and adults as intuitive scientists. *Psychological Review, 96,* 674–689.

Lahey, M. (1988). *Language disorders and language development.* New York: Macmillan.

Lahey, M. (1990). Who shall be called language disordered: Some reflections and perspective. *Journal of Speech and Hearing Disorders, 55,* 612–620.

Laitman, J.T., & Crelin, E.S. (1976). Postnatal development of the basicranium and vocal tract region in man. In J.F. Bosma (Ed.), *Symposium on development of the basicranium* (pp. 206–220). Washington, DC: Department of Health, Education and Welfare.

Larr, A.F. (1962). *Tongue thrust and speech correction.* San Francisco: Fearon.

Launer, P., & Lahey, M. (1981). Passages: from the 50's to the 80's in language assessment. *Topics in Language Disorders, 1,* 11–29.

Lee, L. (1974). *Developmental sentence analysis.* Evanston, IL.: Northwestern University Press.

Leith, W. (1984). *Handbook of clinical methods in communication disorders.* San Diego: College Hill Press.

Lenneberg, E., & Lenneberg, E. (1975). *Foundations of language development: A multidisciplinary approach.* (Volumes 1 and 2). New York: Academic Press.

Leonard, L.B., Devescove, A., & Ossela, T. (1987). Context sensitive phonological patterns in children with poor intelligibility. *Child Language, Teaching and Therapy, 3,* 125–132.

Leonard, L.B. (1979). Language impairment in children. *Merrill-Palmer Quarterly, 25,* 205–232.

Leonard, L.B. (1989). Language learnability and specific language impairment in children. *Applied Psycholinguistics, 10,* 179–202.

Linder, T.W. (1990). *Transdisciplinary play-based assessment: A functional approach to working with young children.* Baltimore: Brookes.

Locke, J.L. (1980). The inference of speech perception in the phonologically disordered. Part II: Some clinically novel procedures, their use, some findings. *Journal of Speech and Hearing Disorders, 45,* 444–468.

Locke, J.L. (1983). *Phonological acquisition and change.* New York: Academic Press.

Loftus, G.R., & Loftus, E.F. (1976). *Human memory: The processing of information.* Hillsdale, NJ: Erlbaum.

Lund, N., & Duchan, J. (1988). *Assessing children's language in naturalistic contexts* (2nd ed.). Englewood Cliffs, NJ: Prentice-Hall.

Luper, H.L., & Mulder, R.L. (1964). *Stuttering: Therapy for children.* Englewood Cliffs, NJ: Prentice-Hall.

MacDonald, J.D., & Carroll, J.Y. (1992). Communicating with young children: An ecological model for clinicians, parents, and collaborative professionals. *American Journal of Speech-Language Pathology: A Journal of Clinical Practice, 1,* 39–48.

Macken, M.A. (1979). Developmental reorganization of phonology: A hierarchy of basic units of acquisition. *Lingua, 49,* 11–49.

Macken, M.A. (1980). Aspects of the acquisition of stop systems: A cross-linguistic perspective. In G. Yeni-Komshian, J.F. Kaabanagh, & C.A. Ferguson (Eds.), *Child Phonology* (Vol 1; pp. 143–168). New York: Academic Press.

Magnusson, E. (1991). Metalinguistic awareness in phonologically disordered children. In M.S. Yavis (Ed.), *Phonological disorders in children* (pp. 87–120). New York: Routledge.

McCarthy, D. (1974). *McCarthy Scales of children's abilities.* New York: Psychological Corporation.

McCune-Nicolich, L. (1981). The cognitive bases of relational words in the single word period. *Journal of Child Language, 8,* 15–34.

McCune, L. (1987). The complementary roles of differentiation and integration in the transition to symbolization. In J. Montangero, A. Tryphon, & S. Sionnet (Eds.). *Symbolism and knowledge* (pp. 119–128). Geneva: Fondation Archives Jean Piaget.

McDonald, E.T. (1964). *Articulation testing and treatment: A sensorimotor approach.* Pittsburgh: Stanwix House.

McLean, J., & Snyder-McLean, L. (1978). *A transactional approach to early language training.* Columbus, OH: Merrill.

Mclelland, J.L., Rummelhart, D.E., & the PDP Research Group (Eds.). (1986). *Parallel distributed processing: Explorations in the microstructure of cognition. Volume 1: Foundations.* Cambridge, MA: Massachusetts Institute of Technology Press.

McReynolds, L.V., & Elbert, M. (1981). Generalization of correct articulation in clusters. *Applied Psycholinguistics, 2,* 119–132.

Meitus, I.J., & Weinberg, B. (Eds.). (1983). *Diagnosis in speech-language pathology.* Baltimore: University Park Press.

Menn, L. (1978). Phonological units in beginning speech. In A. Bell & J.B. Hooper (Eds.). *Syllables and Segments* (pp. 157–171). New York: North Holland.

Menyuk, P. (1964). Comparison of grammar in children with functionally deviant and normal speech. *Journal of Speech and Hearing Reserch, 7,* 109–121.

Menyuk, P. (1969). *Sentences that children use.* Cambridge, MA: Massachusetts Institute of Technology Press.

Menyuk, P. (1990). Metalinguistic abilities and language disorder. In J. Miller (Ed.), *Research in child language disorders: A decade of progress* (pp. 387–398). Austin, TX: Pro Ed.

Menyuk, P., Menn, L., & Silber, R. (1986). Early strategies for the perception and production of words and sounds. In P. Fletcher & M. Garman (Eds.), *Language acquisition* (2nd ed., pp. 192–222). New York: Cambridge University Press.

Michael, A., Klee, T., Bransford, J.D., & Warren, S.F. (1993). The transition from theory to therapy: Test of two instructional methods. *Applied Cognitive Psychology, 7,* 139–154.

Miller, J.F., & Chapman, R. (1981). The relation between age and mean length of utterance in morphemes. *Journal of Speech and Hearing Research, 24,* 154–161.

Miller, J.F., & Yoder, D.E. (1973). A syntax teaching program. In J.E. McClean, D.E. Yoder, & R.L. Schiefelusch (Eds.). *Language intervention with the retarded* (pp. 89–110). Baltimore: University Park Press.

Miller, L. (1984). Problem solving and language disorders. In G. Wallach & K. Butler (Eds.), *Language learning disabilities in school-age children* (pp. 199–229). Baltimore: Williams and Wilkins.

Moses, N. (1981). Applying Piagetian principles to the education of children with learning disabilities. *Topics in Learning and Learning Disabilities, 1,* 11–20.

Moses, N. (1990). *The relation between causal and procedural knowledge in adults engaged in a tractor-trailer task.* Paper presented at the Twentieth Annual Symposium of the Jean Piaget Society, Philadelphia, PA, June.

Moses, N. (1993). *TYCL: A collaborative preschool classroom language program.* Unpublished manuscript.

Moses, N., Klein, H., & Altman, E. (1990). An approach to assessing and facilitating causal language in learning disabled adults based on Piagetian theory. *Journal of Learning Disabilities, 23,* 220–229.

Moses, N., & Papish, M. (1984). Mainstreaming from a cognitive perspective. *Learning Disabilities Quarterly, 7,* 212–220.

Moses, N., & Shapiro, D.A. (1992). Assessing and facilitating clinical problem solving in the supervisory process. In S. Dowling (Ed.), *Total Quality Supervision: Effecting Optimal Performance. Proceedings of the 1992 National Conference of Supervision.* (pp. 70–77). Houston: University of Houston.

Moses, N., & Siskin-Spector, L. (1991). *A transdisciplinary classroom language program for children with autism and other developmental disabilities.* Paper presented at the annual conference of the New York State Speech, Language, and Hearing Association, Kiamesha Lake, NY.

Mounoud, P., & Hauert, C.A. (1982). Development of sensorimotor organization in young children: Grasping and lifting objects. In G. Forman (Ed.), *Action and thought: From sensorimotor schemes to symbolic operations* (pp. 3–35). New York: Academic Press.

Mowrer, D. (1977). *Methods of modifying speech behaviors* (2nd ed.). Columbus, OH: Merrill.

Muma, J. (1978). *Language handbook: Concepts, assessment, intervention.* Englewood Cliffs, NJ: Prentice-Hall.

Murray, L., & Trevarthen, C. (1986). The infant's role in mother-infant communications. *Journal of Child Language, 13,* 15–29.

Musslewhite, C.M. (1986). *Adaptive play for special needs children.* San Diego: College Hill Press.

Myklebust, H.R. (1954). *Auditory disorders in children.* New York: Grune & Stratton.

Mysak, E.D. (1966). *Speech pathology and feedback theory.* Springfield, IL.: Charles C. Thomas.

Mysak, E.D. (1980). *Neurospeech therapy for the cerebral palsied: A neuroevolutional approach.* New York: Teachers College Press.

Nation, J., & Aram, D. (1984). *Diagnosis of speech and language disorders* (2nd ed.). San Diego: College Hill Press.

Nelson, K. (1986). *Event knowledge: Structure and function in development.* Hillsdale, NJ: Erlbaum.

Nelson, N.W. (1993). *Childhood language disorders in context: Infancy through adolescence.* New York Macmillan.

Nesdale, A.R., Herriman, M.L., & Tunmer, W.E. (1984). Phonological awareness in children. In W.E. Tunmer, C. Pratt, & M.L. Herriman (Eds.), *Metalinguistic awareness in children* (pp. 56–72). New York: Springer-Verlag.

Netsell, R. (1980). Speech motor control development. In A.P. Reilly (Ed.), *The communication game: perspectives on the development of speech, language, and non-verbal communication skills.* (Johnson & Johnson Pediatric Round Table Series: 4), 33–38.

Netsell, R., & Daniel, B. (1979). Dysarthria in adults: Physiologic approach to rehabilitation. *Archives of Physical Medicine and Rehabilitation, 60,* 502–508.

Newcomer, P.L., & Hammill, D.D. (1982). *The test of language development—primary edition.* San Antonio, TX: Psychological Corporation.

Newell, A. (1981). Reasoning, problem solving, and decision processes: The problem space as a fundamental category (pp. 150–195). In. R.S. Nickerson (Ed.), *Attention and performance VIII.* Hillsdale, NJ: Erlbaum.

Newell, A., & Simon, H.A. (1972). *Human problem solving.* Englewood Cliffs, NJ: Prentice-Hall.

Newhoff, M., & Leonard, L. (1983). Diagnosis of developmental language disorders. In I. Meitus & B. Weinberg (Eds.), *Diagnosis in speech-language pathology* (pp. 71–112). Baltimore: University Park Press.

Newport, E.L., Gleitman, H., & Gleitman, L.R. (1977). Mother I'd rather do it myself: Some effects and non-effects of maternal speech style. In C. Snow & C. Ferguson (Eds.), *Talking to children: Language input and acquisition* (pp. 109–149). New York: Cambridge University Press.

Nicolich, L. (1977). Beyond sensorimotor intelligence: Assessment of symbolic maturity through analysis of pretend play. *Merrill-Palmer Quarterly, 23,* 89–99.

Ninio, A., & Bruner, J. (1978). The achievement of antecedents of labelling. *Journal of Child Language, 5,* 1–5.

Nippold, M. (1985). Comprehension of figurative language in youth. *Topics in Language Disorders, 5,* 1–20.

Nittrouer, S., & Cheney, C. (1984). Operant techniques used in stuttering therapy: A review. *Journal of Fluency Disorders, 9,* 169–190.

Norris, J.A., & Damico, J.S. (1990). Whole language in theory and practice: Implications for language intervention. *Language, Speech, and Hearing Services in Schools, 21,* 212–220.

Norris, J.A., & Hoffman, P. (1990). Language intervention within natural environments. *Language, Speech, and Hearing Services in Schools, 21,* 72–84.

Oller, D.K. (1980). The emergence of the sounds of speech in infancy. In G.H. Yeni-Komshian, J.F. Kavanagh, & C.A. Ferguson (Eds.), *Child phonology: Production* (Vol. 1, pp. 93–112). New York: Academic Press.

Olswang, L.B. (1990). Treatment efficacy: The breadth of research. In L.B. Olswang, C.K. Thompson, S.F. Warren, & N.J. Minghetti (Eds.). *Treatment Efficacy Research in Communication Disorders* (pp. 99–103) Rockville, MD: The American Speech-Language-Hearing Foundation.

Olswang, L.B., & Carpenter, R.L. (1982a). The ontogenesis of agent: Cognitive notion. *Journal of Speech and Hearing Research, 25,* 297–305.

Olswang, L.B., & Carpenter, R.L. (1982b). The ontogenesis of agent: Linguistic notion. *Journal of Speech and Hearing Research, 25,* 306–314.

Orton, S.T. (1937). *Reading, writing, and speech problems in children: A presentation of certain types of disorders in the development of the language faculty.* New York: Norton.

Osgood, C.E., & Miron, M.S. (1963). *Approaches to the study of aphasia.* Urbana, IL: University of Illinois Press.

Osherson, D.N., & Lasnik, H. (1990). *An invitation to cognitive science: Language* (Vol. 1–4). Cambridge, MA: Massachusetts Institute of Technology Press.

Owens, R.E., Jr. (1992). *Language development* (3rd ed.). Columbus, OH: Merrill.

Ozer, M.N. (Ed.) (1979). *A cybernetic approach to the assessment of children: Toward a more humane use of human beings.* Boulder, CO: Westview Press.

Parnell, M., Patterson, S., & Harding, M. (1984). Answers to Wh questions: A developmental study. *Journal of Speech and Hearing Research, 27,* 297–305.

Paul, R., & Shriberg, L. (1982). Associations between phonology and syntax in speech delayed children. *Journal of Speech and Hearing Research, 25,* 536–546.

Pendergast, K., Dickey, S., Selmer, T., & Soder, A. (1969). *The photo articulation test,* (2nd. ed.). Danville, IL: Interstate Press.

Penfield, W., & Rasmussen, T. (1968). *The cerebral cortex of man.* New York: Haffner.

Penfield, W., & Roberts, L. (1959). *Speech and brain mechanisms.* Princeton, NJ: Princeton University Press.

Perkins, W.H. (Ed.). (1983). *Phonologic-articulatory disorders.* New York: Thieme-Stratton.

Perkins, W.H. (Ed.). (1982). *General principles of therapy.* New York: Thieme-Stratton.

Perry, W.G. (1970). *Forms of intellectual and ethical development in the college years: A scheme.* New York: Holt, Rinehart, & Winston.

Piaget, J. (1954). *The construction of reality in the child.* New York: Basic Books.

Piaget, J. (1962). *Play, dreams, & imitation.* New York: Norton.

Piaget, J. (1971). *Biology and knowledge.* Chicago: University of Chicago Press.

Piaget, J. (1976). The gaps in empiricism. In B. Inhelder, H.H. Chipman, & C. Zwingman (Eds.), *Piaget and his school* (pp. 24–35). New York: Springer-Verlag.

Piaget, J. (1977). The role of action in the development of thinking. In W.F. Overton & J.M. Gallagher (Eds.), *Knowledge & development.* New York: Plenum.

Piaget, J. (1985). *The equilibration of cognitive structures.* Chicago: University of Chicago Press.

Piaget, J. (1987). *Possibility and necessity* (Vols. 1 and 2). Minneapolis: University of Minnesota Press.

Piaget, J., & Garcia, A. (1991). *Toward a logic of meaning.* Hillsdale, NJ: Erlbaum.

Piaget, J., & Inhelder, B. (1969). *The developmental psychology of Jean Piaget.* New York: Basic.

Piatelli-Palmarini, M. (Ed.). (1980). *Language and learning: The debate between Jean Piaget and Noam Chomsky.* Cambridge, MA: Harvard University Press.

Pickering, M. (1987). Interpersonal communication and the supervisory process: A search for Ariadne's thread. In M.B. Crago & M. Pickering (Eds.), *Supervision in human communication disorders: Perspectives on a process* (pp. 203–225). San Diego: Singular.

Pinker, S. (1984). *Language learnability.* Cambridge, MA: Massachusetts Institute of Technology Press.

Pinker, S. (1989). *Learnability and cognition: The acquisition of argument structure.* Cambridge, MA: Massachusetts Institute of Technology Press.

Pinker, S. (1990). Language acquisition. In D.N. Osherson & H. Lasnik (Eds.), *An invitation to cognitive science* (pp. 197–241). Cambridge, MA: Massachusetts Institute of Technology Press.

Pinker, S. (1991). *Learnability and cognition.* Cambridge, MA: Massachusetts Institute of Technology Press.

Pinker, S., & Mehler, J. (Eds.). (1988). *Connections and symbols.* Cambridge, MA: Massachusetts Institute of Technology Press.

Platt, J., & Coggins, T. (1990). Comprehension of social-action games in prelinguistic children: Levels of participation and effect of adult structure. *Journal of Speech and Hearing Disorders, 55,* 315–326.

Poplin, M.S. (1988). Holistic/constructivist principles of the teaching/learning process: Implications for the field of learning disabilities. *Journal of Learning Disabilities, 21,* 401–416.

Potter, M.C. (1990). Remembering. In D.N. Osherson & E.E. Smith (Eds.), *An invitation to cognitive science: Thinking* (Vol. 1, pp. 3–32). Cambridge, MA: Massachusetts Institute of Technology Press.

Powell, T.W. (1991). Planning for phonological generalization: An approach to treatment target selection. *American Journal of Speech-Language Pathology: A Journal of Clinical Practice, 1,* 21–27.

Powell, T.W., Elbert, M., & Dinnsen, D.A. (1991). Stimulability as a factor in the phonological generalization of misarticulating preschool children. *Journal of Speech and Hearing Research, 34,* 1318–1328.

Prather, E., Hedrick, D., & Kern, C. (1975). Articulation development in children ages two to four years. *Journal of Speech and Hearing Research, 40,* 179–191.

Pressley, M., Forrest-Pressley, D.L., Elliot-Faust, D., & Miller, G. (1985). Children's use of cognitive strategies, how to teach strategies, and what to do if they can't be taught. In M. Pressley & C.J. Brainerd (Eds.), *Cognitive learning and memory research: Progress in cognitive developmental research* (pp. 1–48). New York: Springer-Verlag.

Prinz, W., & Saunders, A.F. (Eds.). (1984). *Cognition and motor processes.* New York: Springer-Verlag.

Proctor, A. (1989). Stages of normal noncry vocal development in infancy, *Topics in Language Development, 10,* 26–42.

Rassi, J.A., & McElroy, J.A. (1992). *The education of audiologists and speech-language pathologist.* Timonium, MD: York Press.

Ratner, M.B., & Shi, C.C. (1987). Effects of gradual increases in sentence length and complexity on children's dysfluency. *Journal of Speech and Hearing Disorders, 52,* 278–287.

Ratner, N., & Bruner, J. (1978). Games, social exchange and the acquisition of language. *Journal of Child Language, 5,* 391–402.

Rees, N.S. (1978). Pragmatics of language. In R.L. Schiefelbusch (Ed.), *Bases of language intervention* (pp. 191–268). Baltimore: University Park Press.

Reid, D.K. (1988). *Teaching the learning disabled: A cognitive developmental approach.* Needham, MA: Allyn & Bacon.

Reid, D.K., & Hresko, W.P. (1981). *A cognitive approach to learning disabilities.* New York: McGraw-Hill.

Reiser, B.J. (1986). The encoding and retrieval of memories of real-world experiences. In J.A. Galambos, R.P. Abelson, & J.B. Black (Eds.), *Knowledge structures,* (pp. 71–100). Hillsdale, NJ: Erlbaum.

Rescorla, L. (1980). Overextension in early language development. *Journal of Child Language, 7,* 321–337.

Rice, M.L. (1983). Contemporary accounts of the cognition/language relationship: Implications for speech-language clinicians. *Journal of Speech and Hearing Disorders, 48,* 347–359.

Rice, M.L., & Kemper, S. (1984). *Child language and cognition.* Baltimore: University Park Press.

Rockman, B.K., & Elbert, M. (1984). Untrained acquisition of /s/ in a phonologically disordered child. *Journal of Speech and Hearing Disorders, 49,* 246–254.

Rondal, J. (1980). Father's and mother's speech in early language development. *Journal of Child Language, 7,* 353–370.

Rosen, A., & Proctor, E. (1981). Distinctions between treatment outcomes and their implications for treatment evaluation. *Journal of Consulting and Clinical Psychology*, *49*, 418–425.

Rossetti, L. (1986). *High-risk infants: Identification, assessment, and intervention.* San Diego: College Hill Press.

Roth, F., & Spekman, N. (1984a). Assessing the pragmatic abilities of children: Part I: Organizational framework and assessment parameters. *Journal of Speech and Hearing Disorders*, *49*, 2–11.

Roth, F., & Spekman, N. (1984b). Assessing the pragmatic abilities of children: Part II: Guidelines, considerations and specific education procedures. *Journal of Speech and Hearing Disorders*, *49*, 12–17.

Ruscello, D.M., St. Louis, K.O., & Mason, N. (1991). School-aged children with phonological disorders: Coexistence with other speech/language disorders. *Journal of Speech and Hearing Research*, *34*, 236–242.

Saben, C.B., & Ingham, J.C. (1991). The effects of minimal pairs treatment on two children with phonologic disorders. *Journal of Speech and Hearing Disorders*, *34*, 1023–1040.

Sander, E. (1972). When are speech sounds learned? *Journal of Speech and Hearing Disorders*, *37*, 55–63.

Scarborough, H., & Wyckoff, J. (1986). Mother, I'd still rather do it myself: Some further non-effects of 'motherese.' *Journal of Child Language*, *13*, 431–437.

Scherer, N., & Olswang, L. (1989). Using structured discourse as a language intervention technique with autistic children. *Journal of Speech and Hearing Disorders*, *54*, 383–394.

Schiefelbusch, R.L., & LLoyd, L.L. (Eds.). *Language perspectives—acquisition, retardation, and intervention* (pp. 431–468). Baltimore: University Park Press.

Schiff, N. (1979). The influence of deviant maternal imput on the development of language during the preschool years. *Journal of Speech and Hearing Research*, *22*, 581–603.

Schiff-Myers, N. (1983). From pronoun reversals to correct pronoun usage: A case study of a normally developing child. *Journal of Speech and Hearing Disorders*, *48*, 394–402.

Schiff-Myers, N., & Klein, H. (1985). The effect of deaf parents' speech on hearing children's phonological development. *Journal of Speech and Hearing Research*, *28*, 466–474.

Schory, M.E. (1990). Whole language and the speech-language pathologist. *Language, Speech, and Hearing Services in Schools*, *21*, 206–211.

Schwabe, A., Olswang, L., & Kriegsmann, E. (1986). Requests for information: Linguistic, cognitive, pragmatic, and environmental variables. *Language, Speech, and Hearing Services in Schools*, *17*, 38–55.

Schwartz, R.G. (1992). Clinical forum: Phonological assessment and treatment: Clinical application of recent advances in phonology theory. *Language, Speech, and Hearing Services in Schools*, *23*, 269–276.

Schwartz, R.G., Leonard, L., Folger, L., & Wilcox, M. (1980). Evidence for a synergistic view of linguistic disorder: Early phonological behavior in normal and language disordered children. *Journal of Speech and Hearing Disorders*, *45*, 357–377.

Semel E.M., Wiig, E.H., & Secord, W.A. (1987). *Clinical evaluation of language fundamentals–Revised.* NY: Harcourt Brace Jovanovich.

Shames, G.H., & Florance, C.L. (1980). *Stutter-free speech: A goal for therapy.* Columbus, OH: Merrill.

Shank, R.C., & Abelson, R.P. (1977). *Scripts, plans, goals, and understanding.* Hillsdale, NJ: Erlbaum.

Shapiro, D.A. (1985). Clinical supervision: A process in progress. *National Student Speech Language Hearing Association Journal, 13,* 89–108.

Shapiro, D.A. (1987). Myths in the method of supervision. *Hearsay—Journal of the Ohio Speech and Hearing Association,* Fall, 78–83.

Shapiro, D.A., & Anderson, J.L. (1988). An analysis of commitments made by student clinicians in speech-language pathology. *Journal of Speech and Hearing Disorders, 53,* 202–210.

Shapiro, D.A., & Moses, N. (1989). Creative problem-solving in public school supervision. *Language, Speech, and Hearing Services in Schools, 20,* 320–332.

Shapiro, H.R. (1992). Debatable issues underlying whole-language philosophy: A speech-language pathologist's perspective. *Language, Speech, and Hearing Services in Schools, 23,* 308–311.

Shatz, M. (1982). On mechanisms of language acquisition: Can features of the communicative environment account for development? In E. Wanner & L. Gleitman (Eds.), *Language acquisition: The state of the art* (pp. 86–103). Cambridge, MA: Cambridge University Press.

Shatz, M., & Ebling, K. (1991). Patterns of language learning-related behaviours: Evidence for self help in learning grammar. *Journal of Child Language, 18,* 315–338.

Shatz, M., & Gelman, R. (1973). The development of communication skills: Modifications in the speech of young children as a function of listeners. *Monographs of the Society on Research in Child Development, 38.*

Shaw, R.E., & Hazelett, W.M. Schemas in cognition. In V. McCabe & G. Balzano (Eds.), *Event cognition* (pp. 45–58). Hillsdale, NJ: Erlbaum.

Shine, R.E. (1980) Direct management of the beginning stutterer. *Seminars in Speech, Language and Hearing, 1,* 339–350.

Shipley, K.G., Maddox, M.A., & Driver, J.E. (1991). Children's development of irregular past tense verb forms. *Language, Speech and Hearing Services in Schools, 22,* 115–122.

Shriberg, L., & Kwiatkowski, J. (1982a). Phonological disorders 1: A diagnostic classification system. *Journal of Speech and Hearing Disorders, 47,* 226–241.

Shriberg, L., & Kwiatkowski, J. (1982b). Phonological disorders II: A conceptual framework for management. *Journal of Speech and Hearing Disorders, 47,* 242–256.

Shriberg, L., & Kwiatkowski, J. (1982c). Phonological disorders III: A procedure for assessing severity of involvement. *Journal of Speech and Hearing Disorders, 47,* 256–270.

Shriberg, L., & Kwiatkowski, J. (1990). Self-monitoring and generalization in preschool speech-delayed children. *Language, Speech, and Hearing Services in Schools, 21,* 157–170.

Sinclair, H. (1970). The transition from sensory-motor behavior to symbolic activity. *Interchange, 1,* 119–126.

Sinclair, H. (1987). Symbolic systems and interpersonal relations in infancy. In J. Montangero, A. Tryphon, & S. Dionnet (Eds.), *Symbolism and knowledge* (pp. 129–142). Geneva: Fondation Archives Jean Piaget.

Skinner, B.F. (1957). *Verbal behavior.* New York: Appleton-Century-Crofts.

Skinner, B.F. (1989). The origins of creative thought. *American Psychologist, 44,* 13–18.

Sloane, H.N., & McCauley, B.D. (Eds.). (1968). *Operant procedures in remedial speech and language training.* Boston: Houghton Mifflin.

Smith, L.B. (1984). Young children's understanding of attributes and dimensions: A comparison of conceptual and linguistic measures. *Child Development, 1984,* 363–380.

Smith, N.V. (1973). *The acquisition of phonology: A case study.* New York: Cambridge University Press.

Snow, C.E. (1977). Mothers' speech research: From input to interaction. In C. Snow & C. Ferguson (Eds.), *Talking to children* (pp. 31–50). Cambridge, MA: Cambridge University Press.

Sparrow, S.S., Balla, D.A., & Cicchetti, D.V. (1985). Vineland adaptive behavior scales. Circle Pines, MN: American Guidance Service.

Spector, C.C. (1990). Linguistic humor comprehension of normal and language-impaired adolescents. *Journal of Speech and Hearing Disorders, 55,* 533–541.

Spector, C.C. (1992). Remediating humor comprehension deficits in language- impaired students. *Language, Speech, and Hearing Services in the Schools, 23,* 20–27.

Stampe, D. (1969). The acquisition of phonetic representation. In R.T. Binnick, A. Davison, G. Green, & J.L. Morgan (Eds.), *Papers from the fifth regional meeting, Chicago Linguistic Society* (pp. 443–444).

Stampe, D. (1973). A dissertation on natural phonology. Unpublished doctoral dissertation, University of Chicago.

Stark, R. (1978). Features of infant sounds: The emergence of cooing. *Journal of Child Language, 5,* 379–390.

Stark, R. (1980). Stages of speech development in the first year of life. In G.H. Yeni-Komshian, J.F. Kavanagh, & C.A. Ferguson (Eds.), *Child phonology: Production* (Vol. 1, pp. 73–92). New York: Academic Press.

Stark, R., & Tallal, P. (1981). Selection of children with specific language deficit. *Journal of Speech and Hearing Disorders, 46,* 114–122.

Starkweather, C.W. (1980). A multiprocess behavioral approach to stuttering therapy. *Seminars in Speech, Language, and Hearing, 1,* 327–337.

Starkweather, C.W. (1984). On fluency. *Journal of the National Student Speech-Language-Hearing Association, 12,* 30–37.

Starkweather, C.W. (1987). *Fluency and stuttering.* Englewood Cliffs, NJ: Prentice-Hall.

Starkweather, C.W., & Gordon, P.A. (1983). Stuttering: The language connection. Short Course presented at the 1983 Annual Convention of the American Speech-Language-Hearing Association. Cincinnati, Ohio.

Starkweather, C.W., Gottwald, S., & Halfond, M.M. (1990). *Stuttering prevention: Clinical methods.* Englewood Cliffs, NJ: Prentice-Hall.

Stern, D. (1985). The interpersonal world of the infant. New York: Basic Books.

Stern, D., Jaffe, J., Beebe, B., & Bennett, S. (1975). Vocalizing in unison and in alternation: Two modes of communication within the mother-infant dyad. In D. Aronson & R. Rieber (Eds.), *Developmental psycholinguistic and communication disorders. Annals of the New York Academy of Sciences, 263,* 89–100.

Sternberg, R. (Ed.). (1984). *Mechanisms of cognitive development.* New York: Freeman.

St. Louis, K.O., & Ruscello, D.M. (1987). *Oral speech mechanism screening examination—revised (OSMSE-R).* Austin, TX: Pro Ed.

Stocker, B., & Parker, E. (1977). The relationship between auditory recall and dysfluency in young stutterers. *Journal of Fluency Disorders, 2,* 177–187.

Stoel-Gammon, C. (1985). Phonetic inventories, 15–24 months: A longitudinal study. *Journal of Speech and Hearing Research, 28,* 505–512.

Stoel-Gammon, C., & Cooper, J.A. (1984). Patterns of early lexical and phonologic development. *Journal of Child Language, 11,* 247–272.

Stoel-Gammon, C., & Dunn, C. (1985). *Normal and disordered phonology in children.* Baltimore: University Park Press.

Strauss, A.A., & Lehtinen, L.E. (1947). *Psychopathology and education of the brain injured child.* New York: Grune & Stratton.

Sugarman, S. (1978). A description of communicative development in the prelanguage child. In I. Markova (Ed.), *The social context of language.* New York: Wiley.

Sutton-Smith, B. (1979). *Play and learning.* New York: Gardner.

Tallal, P. (1975). Perceptual and linguistic factors in the language impairment of developmental dysphasics. *Cortex, 11,* 196–205.

Tallal, P. (1988). Developmental language disorders. In J.F. Kavanagh & T.J. Truss, Jr. (Eds.), *Learning Disabilities: Proceedings of the National Conference* (pp. 181–272). Parkton, MD: York Press.

Tallal, P., & Piercy, M. (1978). Deficits of auditory perception in children with developmental dysphasia. In M. Wyke (Ed.), *Developmental dysphasia* (pp. 63–84). London: Academic Press.

Taylor, O.L. (1986). *Treatment of communication disorders in culturally and linguistically diverse populations.* San Diego: College Hill Press.

Terrell, B.Y., & Hale, J.E. (1992). Serving a multicultural population: Different learning styles. *American Journal of Speech-Language Pathology: A Journal of Clinical Practice, 1,* 5–8.

Tomasello, M., Conti-Ramsden, G., & Ewert, B. (1990). Young children's conversations with their mothers and fathers: Differences in breakdown and repair. *Journal of Child Language, 17,* 115–130.

Tomasello, M., & Farrar, M.J. (1984). Cognitive bases of lexical development: Object permanence and relational words. *Journal of Child Language, 11,* 477–493.

Tomasello, M., & Farrar, M. (1986). Object permanence and relational words: A lexical training study. *Journal of Child Language, 13,* 495–505.

Tomes, L., & Shelton, R. L. (1989). Children's categorization of consonants by manner and place characteristics. *Journal of Speech and Hearing Research, 32,* 432–438.

Torgesen, J.K. (1982). The learning disabled child as an inactive learner. *Topics in Learning and Learning Disabilities, 2,* 45–52.

Tyack, D., & Gottsleben, R. (1974). *Language sampling, analysis and training: A handbook for teachers and clinicians.* Palo Alto, CA: Consulting Psychological Press.

Uzgiris, I., & Hunt, J. (1978). *Assessment in infancy.* Chicago: University of Illinois Press.

van Kleeck, A. (1984). Metalinguistic skills: Cutting across spoken and written language and problem-solving abilities. In G. Wallach & K. Butler (Eds.), *Language-learning disabilities in school-age children* (pp. 128–153). Baltimore: Williams and Wilkins.

van Kleeck, A. (1990). Emergent literacy: Learning about print before learning to read. *Topics in Language Disorders, 10,* 25–46.

van Kleeck, A., & Richardson, A. (1986). What's in an error? Wrong responses as language teaching opportunities. *NSSLHA Journal, 14,* 25–50.

van Riemsdijk, H., & Williams, E. (1986). *Introduction to the theory of grammar.* Cambridge, MA: Massachusetts Institute of Technology Press.

Van Riper, C. (1939). *Speech correction: Principles and methods.* Englewood Cliffs, NJ: Prentice-Hall.

Van Riper, C. (1954). *Speech correction: Principles and methods.* Englewood Cliffs, NJ: Prentice-Hall.

Van Riper, C. (1973). *The treatment of stuttering.* Englewood Cliffs, NJ: Prentice-Hall.

Van Riper, C. (1978). *Speech correction: Principles and methods* (6th Ed.). Englewood Cliffs, NJ: Prentice-Hall.

Van Riper, C., & Emerick, L. (1990). *Speech correction: Principles and methods* (8th Ed.). Englewood Cliffs, NJ: Prentice-Hall.

Vihman, M.M. (1976). From pre-speech to speech: On early phonology. *Papers and Reports on Child Language Development.* Palo Alto, CA: Stanford University.

Vihman, M.M. (1988). Early phonological development. In J.E. Bernthal, & N.W. Bankson, *Articulation and phonological disorders* (2nd ed., pp. 60–109). Englewood Cliffs, NJ: Prentice-Hall.

Vygotsky, L.S. (1962). *Thought and language.* Cambridge, MA: Massachusetts Institute of Technology Press.

Vygotsky, L.V. (1987). Thinking and speech. In R.W. Reiser & A.S. Carton (Eds.), *The collected works of L.S. Vygotsky.* New York: Plenum.

Wadle, S.L. (1991). Why speech-language pathologists should be in the classroom. *Language, Speech, and Hearing Services in Schools, 22,* 277.

Wall, M., & Myers, F. (1984). *Clinical management of childhood stuttering.* Baltimore: University Park Press.

Wansart, W.L. (1990). Learning to solve a problem: A microanalysis of the solution strategies of children with learning disabilities. *Journal of Learning Disabilities, 23,* 164–170.

Watzlawick, P., Beavin, J.H., & Jackson, D.D. (1967). *Pragmatics of human communication: A study of interactional patterns, pathologies, and paradoxes.* New York: Norton.

Wechsler, D. (1967). *Wechsler preschool and primary scale of intelligence (WPPSI).* New York: Psychological Corporation.

Wechsler, D. (1974). *Wechsler intelligence scale for children (WISC-R).* New York: Psychological Corporation.

Weiner, F. (1981). Treatment of phonological disability using the method of meaningful minimal contrast: Two case studies. *Journal of Speech and Hearing Disorders, 46,* 97–103.

Wepman, J.M. (1960). Auditory discrimination, speech, & reading. *Elementary School Journal, 60,* 325–333.

Wepman, J.M., Jones, L.V., Bock, R.D., & Van Pelt, D. (1960). Studies in aphasia: Background and theoretical formulations. *Journal of Speech and Hearing Disorders, 25,* 323–332.

Werker, J.F., & Pegg, J.E. Infant speech perception and phonological acquisition. In C.A. Ferguson, L. Menn, & C. Stoel-Gammon (Eds.), *Phonological development: Models, research, implications* (pp. 285–311). Timonium, MD: York Press.

Werner, H., & Kaplan, B. (1964). *Symbol formation.* New York: Wiley.

Wertsch, J.V. (1979). From social interaction to higher psychological processes: A clarification and application of Vygotsky's theory. *Human Development, 22,* 1–22.

Wertsch, J.V. (1984). The zone of proximal development: Some conceptual issues. In B. Rogoff & J.V. Wertsch (Eds.), *Children's learning in the zone of proximal development: New directions for child development* (pp. 7–18). San Francisco: Jossey-Bass.

West, R., Ansberry, M., & Carr, A. (1957). *The rehabilitation of speech.* New York: Harper & Row.

Westby, C. (1980). Assessment of cognitive and language abilities through play. *Language, Speech, and Hearing Services in Schools, 11,* 154–168.

Westby, C. (1988). Children's play: Reflections of social competence. *Seminars in Speech and Language, 9,* 1–14.

Wilson, D.K. (1987). *Voice problems of children* (3rd ed.). Baltimore: Williams & Wilkins.

Wingate, M.E. (1988). *The structure of stuttering: A psycholinguistic analysis.* New York: Springer-Verlag.

Winitz, H. (1969). *Articulatory acquisition and behavior.* Englewood Cliffs, NJ: Prentice-Hall.

Winitz, H. (1975). *From syllable to conversation.* Baltimore: University Park Press.

Wolfe, V., & Blocker, S. (1990). Consonant-vowel interaction in an unusual phonological system. *Journal of Speech and Hearing Disorders, 55,* 561–566.

Wozniak, R.H. (1972). Verbal regulation and motor behavior: Soviet research and non-Soviet replications. *Human Development, 15,* 13–57.

Yoder, P., & Kaiser, A. (1989). Alternative explanations for the relationship between maternal verbal interaction style and child language development. *Journal of Child Language, 16,* 141–160.

Appendix A

BOX A–1.   HIGHLIGHTS OF LAHEY'S CONTENT-FORM INTERACTIONS, PHASES 1 THROUGH 8 +

Phase	Selected Features of Development	Sample Utterances
1	Earliest content categories emerge, coded with single words: existence, nonexistence, recurrence, rejection, action, locative action	cat (existence), more (recurrence), eat (action)
2	Phase 1 content categories now coded with two words: • relational + substantive • two constituents	the book, no book go car, eat cookie
3	Two new content categories added, coded with 2 or 3 constituents: • locative state • state Action and locative action expand from 2 to 3 constituents Beginning of coordinated content categories: existence + attribution	baby crib I want cookie baby eat cookie, daddy go car that a big cookie
4	Two new content categories emerge: • notice/perception • temporal (some verbs inflected with -ing, -s, and irregular past) Additional coordinations, especially action + • attribution • recurrence • place Wh questions emerge with: • existence • locative state Beginning of complex content categories involving two verb relations, coding volition/intention	look at kitty I making cookie, that goes here, I did peepee make a big cookie make nother cookie make cookie there what's that? where's daddy? wanna go home, gonna eat cookie

(continued)

310

BOX A–1. *Continued*

5	Expansion of complex sentences to include additive	that's a cat and that's a dog
	Additional coordinations • existence + copula + who Q • action + intention and possession • state + attribution, + recurrence	that's a book who that I gonna eat my cookie want big doll want more cookie
6	Expansion of complex content categories: • temporal • causal	I go home and drink juice cup broke cause it fell
7	Continued expansion of complex content categories: • epistemic • adversative Further coordinations: • action + 'what,' 'how' Q • action + possibility (can) Increase in variety of connectives: • then, when (temporal) • so, and, because (causal)	I know what color that one is big but that one is little what you doing I can do it I go in room and then I come out you go home when I go to sleep get out cause I hafta go in let's get the peach so I can eat it
8	New complex content category: communication Further developments: • why Q • increase in variety of verbs and connectives notice—see if, see what, look what specification—that	tell mommy I want more why it broken look what I found the book that goes on the shelf
8 +	Narrative sentence sequences: additive, temporal, causal	There was a turtle walking down the street and he met a frog and they went to a pond....

Modified from Lahey's, 1988, Content-Form-Use Plan for Language Development Goals. For a more complete description of developmental changes, see Lahey (1988).

BOX A-2. A Plan for Language Development Goals: Use Interacting With Content Form*

USE

Function	Nonlinguistic		Linguistic
	Perceptual Support	Other	
		BSH:PHASES 1,2, AND 3	

1. Comment (most frequent including interactive & noninteractive, label, indicative etc.)
Regulate
2. Direct action
3. Call-focus attention
4. Protest/reject
5. Obtain object
6. Obtain response
7. Respond
8. Vocal play
9. Routines
(e.g., greet, transfer objects, etc.)
	10. Communicates about events and objects that are present (+ here + now)	11. Most utterances about
		  a. What child is about to do
		  b. What child is doing
		  c. What child wants others to do
		12. Awareness of listener May talk less to strangers
		13. Listener adaptation May repair, upon request, with phonetic recoding
			14. Most utterances follow (adjacent to) those of others; if contingent may be by
			  a. imitation (may be frequent)
			  b. Adding a related word (less frequent)
			  c. Contextually related (because both focus on the same topic) rather than linguistically related

		PHASES 4 AND 5	
As above plus 15. Obtain information (Many questions are asked that are not to obtain information but as routines or as request for conformation, etc.) 16. Greater variety of forms for all functions	17. Increasing number of utterances about immediate past and imminent future	18. Increasing number of utterances about what others are doing 19. Speaks more utterances/unit of time 20. Listener adaptation: Repair, upon request, with phonetic recoding and deletions	21. Number of nonadjacent utterances increases, but still adjacent are most frequent 22. More contingent utterances that add to prior utterance of another (with word or phase) plus some that repeat a part of prior utterance and add to it.

(continued)

BOX A-2. (continued)

Function	Context — Nonlinguistic: Perceptual Support	Context — Nonlinguistic: Other	Context — Linguistic
			23. Recoding of prior utterance, mainly pronominalization of object and change of agent (I/you)
PHASES 6, 7, AND 8			
24. Obtain information about what someone else has said	27. Increased distancing of utterances from referent (–here –now)	28. Deictic forms used (I/you, this/that, here/there, a/the)	30. The number of nonadjacent is now greater than the number of adjacent utterances
25. Increase in frequency of social functions		29. Listener adaptations: Politeness markers to strangers More explicit information Get attention before requests Repair, upon request, with phonetic recoding, deletions, and substitutions	31. Imitation is rare but other contingent utterances have increased and convey new information usually by repeat/recode/add
26. Inform or report			32. More utterances of a child are related to and add information to prior child utterance
			33. Some anaphoric ellipsis is used
			34. An increase in questions that are contingent on prior utterances

From Lahey, 1988. Used with permission.
*Numbers do not imply sequence but are used for reference.

Appendix B

Form B–1: Areas of Assessment for Intervention Planning

Name:_____ Age:_____ Primary Disorder:_____

Necessary Information	Source	Utility of Procedure
I. Language and speech A. Content-form		
B. Use		
C. Phonology 1. Phonetic		
2. Phonological		
D. Fluency		
E. Voice		
II. Maintaining factors A. Cognitive		

B. Sensorimotor
        1. Peripheral
            speech
            mechanism		

2. Body stability		
C. Psychosocial		

Form B–2: Summary of Baseline Data for Intervention Planning

Name:_____ Age:_____ Primary Disorder:_____

Area Assessed (include sources and results)
I.   Language and speech   A.   Content-form
B.   Use
C.   Phonology   1.   Phonetic
2.   Phonological
D.   Fluency
E.   Voice
II.   Maintaining factors   A.   Cognitive

B.   Sensorimotor
         1.   Peripheral
             speech
             mechanism

2.   Body stability
C.   Psychosocial

Form B–3: Management Plan

Long-Term Goals and Procedures

Client: _____   Clinician:_____

Supervisor: _____   Semester:_____

Long-Term Goals and Expected Duration:

Rationales with reference to:

Baseline data (how current linguistic performance motivates goals):

Maintaining factors (justification of long-term expectation):

Procedural Approach:

Maintaining factors addressed:

Guiding principles (from learning theories):

Reward system and rationale:

Form B-3: Short-Term Goals and Procedures

Client: _____

Short-Term Goals	Long-Term Goals Addressed	Prioritization Source
Procedural Contexts	Learning Principles	Maintaining Factors
Non-Linguistic Context (types of materials):		
Linguistic Context:		

Form B–3: Session Goals and Procedures

Client: _____ Clinician:_____

Supervisor: _____ Semester:_____

Date: _____

Short-Term Goal Addressed:

Session Goal: (child)_____will (observable behavior and context)

_____

(criterion frequency or percentage)_____

Session Procedure: Clinician will provide (materials):

Clinician will interact with the client by:

Derivation: Maintaining factor(s) addressed:

Principles from learning theory referenced:

Performance demands controlled:

Form B–4: IEP Conversion Form

Client: _____ Clinician:_____

Long-Term Goal(s):

Criterion goal(s):

1. (child)_____will (observable behavior)_____

(criterion frequency or percentage)._____

How measured: e.g., clinician observation, norm-referenced test)_____

Expected date of achievement_____

2. (child)_____will (observable behavior & context)_____

(criterion frequency or percentage)._____

How measured: (e.g., clinician observation, norm-referenced test)_____

Expected date of achievement_____

3. (child)_____will (observable behavior and context)_____

(criterion frequency or percentage)._____

How measured: (e.g., clinician observation, norm-referenced test)_____

Expected date of achievement_____

Appendix C
Developmental Sequences for Determination and Prioritization of Goals
at All Phases of Intervention Planning

Taxonomy	*Source*
Form-content interaction	Bloom & Lahey, 1978 Lahey, 1988 Nelson, 1993
Use	Lahey, 1988 Lund & Duchan, 1988 Nelson, 1993
Asking questions	Bloom, 1991 Brown, 1968
Answering questions	Parnell, Patterson, & Harding, 1984
Developmental morphemes	Brown, 1973
Figurative language	Nippold, 1985
Complex sentences and connectives	Bloom, 1991
Narrative development	Culatta; Page, & Ellis, 1983 Lahey, 1988
Humor comprehension	Spector, 1990, 1992
Irregular verbs	Shipley, Maddox, & Driver, 1991
Cognition	Forman & Hill, 1984 Gallagher & Reid, 1984 Piaget & Inhelder, 1969
Play	McCune-Nicolich, 1981 Nelson, 1993
Vocal tract structure and function	Kahane, 1983 Laitman & Crelin, 1976
Elimination of phonological processes	Grunwell, 1985 Stoel-Gammon & Dunn, 1985

Appendix D
Sources for Developing Session-Goal Sequences
(Based on Contextual and Physiological Performance Demands)

Disorder area	Source
Language	
Nonlinguistic context	Bloom & Lahey, 1978
	Forman & Hill, 1984
	Lahey, 1988
	Linder, 1990
	Lund & Duchan, 1988
	MacDonald & Carroll, 1992
	Nelson, 1993
Pragmatic context for content-form interactions	Lahey, 1988
	Lund & Duchan, 1988
Nonlinguistic & pragmatic context for narratives	Cullata, Horn, & Theodore, 1992
Phonologic influences	Klein & Spector, 1985
	Stoel-Gammon & Cooper, 1985
Conceptual complexity	
color and shape	Bornstein, 1984
color	Johnson, 1977
form, color, and size	Kagan, & Lemkin, 1961
Articulation and phonology	
Length of unit and position in word	Bernthal & Bankson, 1988
	Creaghead, Newman, & Secord, 1989
	Van Riper, 1978
	Winitz, 1969, 1975
Serial position	Klein, 1981b
	Klein & Spector, 1985
Stress level	Klein, 1981b
	Klein, 1984
	Klein & Spector, 1985
Phonetic context	Camarata & Gandour, 1984
	Hodson & Paden, 1991
	Kent, 1982
	Leonard, Devescove, & Ossela, 1987
	Wolfe & Blocker, 1990
Coarticulation (Assimilation)	Kent, 1982
	Macken, 1980
	Smith, 1973
	Grunwell, 1985

(*continued*)

Appendix D (*continued*)

Disorder area	Source
Language	
Phonological knowledge	Elbert & Gierut, 1986 Powell, 1991 Powell, Elbert, & Dinnsen, 1991
Perceptual support	
Stimulability	Creaghead, Newman & Secord, 1989 Powell, 1991 Powell, Elbert, & Dinnsen, 1991
Imitation	Bernthal & Bankson, 1988 Creaghead et al., 1989
Voice	
Awareness of impairment	Andrews, 1986 Wilson, 1987
Perceptual support	Andrews, 1986 Wilson, 1987
Physiological processes	Andrews, 1986
Phonetic context	Andrews, 1986 Wilson, 1987
Linguistic complexity	Andrews, 1986
Pragmatic context	Andrews, 1986
Fluency	
Psychosocial context	Conture, 1990 Starkweather, Gottwald, & Halfond, 1990 Wall & Myers, 1984
Phonetic context	Starkweather & Gordon, 1983 Wall & Myers, 1984
Linguistic complexity	Colburn & Mysak, 1982a, 1982b Starkweather, 1980 Ratner & Shi, 1987

Appendix E

Collaborative Management Plan

Child: _____ Term: _____

Specialist or Educator: _____

Present Developmental Level or Performance: _____

_____

_____

Long-Term Goals: _____

Short-Term Goals:	Session Goals and Procedures Applied by Allied Professionals	Criterion	MET
	Classroom or Adaptive Daily Living:		
	Educator:		
	Speech-Language Pathology:		
	Clinician:		
	Occupational or Physical Therapy		
Recommended Procedures:	Clinician:		
	At Home:		
	Parent:		

Name Index

Subject Index

Nonlinguistic context *(cont.)*
  phonology disorder, 165, 168
  voice disorder, 172, 175
  defined, 139–140
Nonstandardized assessment, 68–69
Nurses. *See* Allied professionals

O

Observable behavior, session goals and, 177
Occupational therapists. *See* Allied
  professionals
Operant learning theories, 32
  and other learning theories
   compared, 35–36
  principles derived from, 31
Orthographic symbol, perceptual
  support and, 193
Outcome prediction, 94

P

Parent. *See* Caregiver; Family(ies)
Pathology, speech-language, periods of
  influence of theories on, 43
Perception, speech-related, 19
Perceptual support
  articulation-phonology disorders and,
   192–193
  fluency disorder and, 197–198
  language disorders and, 186
  voice disorders and, 194–195
Performance
  best, specification of, long-term goals
   and, 96–97
  clinician's, developmental patterns in.
   See Staff development issues
  linguistic. *See* Linguistic performance
  variability of, performance demands
   and, 185
Performance demands
  causal reasoning and, 268–269
  generalization and, 185–186
  influence on session goals and
   procedures, 184–186
   developmental language disability
    and, 186–189, 204–206
   fluency disorders and, 196–198,
    214–218
   phonology disorder and, 190–193,
    227–233
   voice disorders and, 194–196,
    242–243
  and performance variability, 185
  session-goal sequence development
   sources, 321–322

Peripheral deafness, differential
  diagnosis of, 46
Peripheral speech mechanism, 14–16
Perspective taking, in supervision,
  277–282
  anchored instruction and, 281
  child's point of view, 265–266, 270
  procedures for facilitating, 279
  Shapiro and Moses recommendations,
   279–281
  viewing from different theoretic
   perspectives, 266, 277–279
Phonation training, 195
Phonetic context, voice treatment and, 195
Phonetic environment, 191–192
Phonological knowledge, 192
Phonology
  articulation and, 190–193
  impact on dysfluency, 198
  impact on language learning, 189
  sources for session-goal sequences,
   321–322
Phonology disorder
  delineated procedural context and,
   158, 160, 163, 165–167, 168
  deriving long-term goals and
   procedural approaches for,
   115–121
  evaluation of, 81–82, 83–88
  long-term goal statements, 116
   derivation of, 116–119
  long-term procedural approach, 116
   derivation of, 119–121
  management plan for, 120, 122, 125,
   128
  performance demands and, 190–193
  session planning in, 226
   effect of performance demands on,
    190–193
   goal-approach strategy in, 226
   goal construction in, factors
    influencing, 226–227
   sample goals and procedures,
    234–239
   short-term goals for, 158
   derivation of, 160–163, 164
   sources for session-goal sequences,
    321–322
Physical therapists. *See* Allied professionals
Physiological process, of voice
  production, 195
PLAI. *See* Preschool Language
  Assessment Instrument (PLAI)